THE
PSYCHIATRY
OF

RESOLVING SCHIZOPHRENIA PSYCHOANALYTICALLY

How visualizing the therapeutic
process can assist success

Dr Gillian Steggles

First published in 2019 by
Free Association Books

Copyright © 2019 Dr Gillian Steggles

The author's rights are fully asserted. The rights of
Dr Gillian Steggles to be identified as the author of
this work has been asserted by her in accordance with the
Copyright, Designs and Patents Act 1988

A CIP Catalogue of this book is available from
the British Library

ISBN: 978-1-91138-331-4

All rights reserved; no part of this publication may be reproduced, stored in a retrieval system, or transmitted, in any form or by any means, electronic, mechanical, photocopying, recording or otherwise, without the prior written permission of the publisher. Nor be circulated in any form of binding or cover other than that in which it is published and a similar condition including this condition being imposed on the subsequent purchaser.

Typeset by
Typo•glyphix
www.typoglyphix.co.uk

Cover design by
Candescent

Printed in the UK

DEDICATION

This book is dedicated to the late Dr Elvin Semrad, and to those like him, who taught their students at the Massachusetts Mental Health Centre in Boston and in other therapeutic centres across the world how to sit with their schizophrenic patients while these courageous individuals are brave enough to address the terrible experiences they have previously lived through, earlier in their lives, in their quest for mental health.

In this way, the kindness and wisdom of the late Dr Leslie Sohn, together with his gentle humour, are remembered in the calm confidence with which he enlightened his own schizoaffective patients from the Maudsley Hospital in London. He represents all that is best in Psychiatric Psychoanalysis. The late Dr Murray Jackson tended his patients who were suffering the ravages of schizophrenic illness with deep insight; as more patients with schizophrenic illness are treated, more will be learned about their frailties and needs, so that successful approaches and techniques will be built upon.

The book honours the excellent supportive psychotherapy units in the McLean Hospital in Belmont, Massachusetts and in the Maudsley Hospital in London, where these extremely frail patients are psychodynamically nurtured at needful times while in treatment.

But this book was primarily written to enlighten, in an encouraging way, British Psychiatrists into the kinds of revelations that only psychoanalytic thinking can provide into the mental processes underlying psychosis. In this way, more Psychiatrists will identify those schizophrenic patients who could benefit from psychoanalytic treatment. Some Psychiatrists could indeed themselves train in Psychoanalysis at the Institute of Psychoanalysis in London so as to become able to alleviate the extreme psychological distress of schizophrenic illness. The enlightenment of this endeavour has been the intention of the following pages, and its dedication is to those pursuing it.

CONTENTS

Foreword   vii
PROFESSOR R D HINSHELWOOD

Preface   xv
DR GILLIAN STEGGLES

Glossary of terms   xxiv

CHAPTER 1   Introduction   1
DR MIOMIR MILOVANOVIC

PART I
Illness: Schizophrenia and Schizoaffective Disorder   11
DR GILLIAN STEGGLES

CHAPTER 2   The Symptomatic Distress of Schizophrenic Illness   13

CHAPTER 3   The Cost to Society of Schizophrenia   20

CHAPTER 4   Organic Aspects of Schizophrenic Illness and its Treatment   27

CHAPTER 5   The Need for Effective Remedial Therapy for Schizophrenia   33

CHAPTER 6   Psychiatric Help for Patients with "Reactive" Schizophrenia   39

PART II
The PPCC Model   45
DR GILLIAN STEGGLES

CHAPTER 7   The Development of the PPCC Model   47

CONTENTS

CHAPTER 8	The Structure of the PPCC Model	57
CHAPTER 9	The Adaptability of the PPCC Model	67
CHAPTER 10	The Overall Structural PPCC Sequence of the Recovering Schizophrenic or Schizoaffective Mind	79

PART III
Successful Psychoanalytic Psychotherapy for Schizophrenia 87
DR GILLIAN STEGGLES

CHAPTER 11	The Psychoanalytic Concepts of the PPCC Theory	89
CHAPTER 12	Aspects of Psychoanalytic Psychotherapy that are Helpful for Schizophrenic and Schizoaffective Patients	102
CHAPTER 13	Some Psychoanalytic Psychotherapists of Schizophrenic Patients	118
CHAPTER 14	The Seven Therapeutic Stages of Successful Psychoanalytic Psychotherapy for Schizophrenia (identified by Dr Michael Robbins MD)	132

PART IV
Case Study 1: Included herein by kind permission of
Dr Michael Robbins MD and of The Guilford Press 141

CHAPTER 15	Case Study 1: "Emily: An Unusually Successful Treatment": The work of Dr Michael Robbins MD	143
CHAPTER 16	Visualization of Case Study 1 (Dr Robbins) using the PPCC Model: Dr Steggles	171
CHAPTER 17	Commentary on Dr Robbins' Case Study 1 and its Visualization: Dr Steggles	179

PART V
Case Study 2: Included herein by kind permission of
Dr Michael Robbins MD and of The Guilford Press 185

CHAPTER 18	Case Study 2: "The Successful Psychoanalytic Therapy of a Schizophrenic Woman": The work of Dr Michael Robbins MD	187

CONTENTS

CHAPTER 19   Visualization of Case Study 2 (Dr Robbins) using the PPCC Model: Dr Steggles   222

CHAPTER 20   Commentary on Dr Robbins' Case Study 2 and its Visualization: Dr Steggles   229

PART VI
A Proposed National Health Schedule for Schizophrenia   235
DR GILLIAN STEGGLES

CHAPTER 21   Principal Available Treatments for Schizophrenia and Schizoaffective Disorder   237

CHAPTER 22   Patient Safety during the Psychoanalytic Psychotherapeutic Treatment of Schizophrenic and Schizoaffective Patients   246

CHAPTER 23   Funding, on a Par with Physical Treatments: Conceptual Blocks   254

PART VII
Psychiatry and Related Philosophical Concepts of Healing   261
DR GILLIAN STEGGLES

CHAPTER 24   Medical Ethics: The Ethics of Transformative Mental Health Treatments   263

CHAPTER 25   The Philosophy and Values of the NHS in Relation to Psychiatric Patients   269

CHAPTER 26   The Human Mind's Structural and Constitutional Beauty   282

CHAPTER 27   Motivation: The Patient Experience and the Human Spirit in All its Guises   292

References   298
Table of Figures   306
Acknowledgements   308
Index   310

FOREWORD

This is a book that every psychiatrist should know. It is a powerful attempt to convince us of the fact that the person in a schizophrenic episode is as much a human being as anyone else. It is just that their human experiences are invariably of the most painful and terrifying kind. Psychoanalysis and psychoanalytic psychotherapy methods have been employed over many decades with some of the most tortured people. It has never become a standard treatment – for reasons that are of interest in themselves. Here however is an account of a methodical process that can be replicated from one therapist to another, or from one patient to another.

Even if some psychiatrists may dismiss this work, they should, out of obligation to their patients, be clear with themselves why they do not agree. It is all too easy to disagree and turn away on the basis of hearsay and popular reputation. But with this book to inform us, we cannot justify turning-the-back without a fully informed knowledge of why we do so.

In fact there are two mountainous issues to be overcome. One is the easier one – to master the kinds of practice this book, and others like it, prescribe for the more receptive of schizophrenia sufferers. The other, the more difficult, is to tackle the interdisciplinary barriers that exist between more medically oriented approaches and more psychological ones. The US anthropologist, Tania Luhrmann, conducted a fieldwork study of a psychiatric service, and came to the unsurprising conclusion:

> *In the one domain, there is the scientist, the fearless investigator of truth. In the other there is the psychoanalyst, the wise wizard of insight. These two ideals embody different moral sensibilities, different fundamental commitments, different bottom lines.*
> (Luhrmann 2000, p. 158)

FOREWORD

This colourful description draws the line between the two sets of sensibilities and commitments which have been well established over long periods. In fact more than a hundred years ago, Freud could write bitterly:

> *You will grant that there is nothing in the nature of psychiatric work which could be opposed to psycho-analytic research. What is opposed to psycho-analysis is not psychiatry but psychiatrists.*
> (Freud 1917, p. 254)

I would not be as cruelly condemning because I think there are reasons why people develop such fundamentally different 'bottom lines' and get into their incomprehensible opposition with each other. I have discussed this at length elsewhere (Hinshelwood 2004), and that is not my purpose here.

If the hurdle separating the different disciplines is to be overcome, one strategy is to meet the antagonisms where they exist – with information. That is the great virtue of the book; it informs us.

Some schizophrenic patients have made remarkable recoveries. And almost certainly they would not have done had there not been an intensive psychoanalytic psychotherapy intervention. We really need to cultivate a curiosity to prick the interest, even the conscience, of psychiatrists who tend to dismiss a listening approach.

What is of interest in the approach of this book is just that – it is a listening approach. It is led by the patient and her attempts to conceptualise her own mind and what is happening to it. It is surely very easy to take the position that mad people don't know what they are talking about and therefore the doctor knows best. But this book starts in the opposite direction. The patient knows something if only it can be grasped – in this case, in a visual way. In terms of standard medicine this is turning the practice upside down. Those who are to be professionally treated by knowledgeable and experienced mental health workers are being given the opportunity to contribute in their own way, however odd and convoluted that might be. The job of the professional is then to try to smooth out the convolutions. This is not so distant from an ordinary human approach. It is a characteristic of the human species *par excellence* to try to listen to another person's point of view. Of course human beings go the other way too, and stifle others than themselves. But the most human of actions is to listen, and something in the evolutionary tree has found it to have an adaptational value for the survival of the fittest that we can attend to what someone else is attending to.

My own career long ago was via the therapeutic community. That was a movement, and still is, which decided to take the standard roles of traditional age-old psychiatry and to soften the hard boundary between those who treat and those who are treated. Such a softening, whilst keeping sufficient boundaries of care, has now a long history and is an inspiring achievement. It was not the overthrow of psychiatry as some had wished, and some had feared. It is simply an adjustment to the rigidity of the roles of carer and cared-for. My greatest learning from the therapeutic community was that a patient in a psychotic state, however severe the state, still retains a sensible side to himself, albeit a temporarily hidden sensible side. I was interested a long time later to read Freud saying the same things late in his life:

[O]ne learns from patients after their recovery [after psychosis] that at the time in some corner of their mind (as they put it) there was a normal person hidden, who, like a detached spectator, watched the hubbub of illness go past him.

(Freud 1940, p. 202)

We used the mantra, 'support the person's healthy side, not the ill one'. It all seemed to depend on which side of the patient one concentrated on, the healthy or the ill. The professional service could, it seems, bring out one side or the other. Or at least to a degree it could bring out one side or the other.

So, the issue then is whether we dismiss all hallucinations and delusions as insane nonsense to be disregarded, or whether there is a grain of healthy sense embedded there to be cultivated in whatever way might be possible. It is the brilliance of this book to show that Gillian Steggles' patient had a sense which could be cultivated through the use of visual analogies.

The appeal to psychiatrists to attend to the grain of health in another person which might be induced to grow and flower, cannot, I believe, fall on deaf ears. My own career moved on to nearly two decades of work in a traditional mental hospital, one of those in the process of closing down. However this one was closing slowly, and hung on for a while after most others. I had therefore a long acquaintance with the traditional attitudes to the 'mad', and indeed the traditional attitudes to each other's disciplines.

I had the good fortune to work there as a psychoanalyst, with the responsibility for helping medical students and qualified doctors (as well as many other staff) to think a little about their patient's point of view, and to enjoy, even, the opportunity to listen as opposed to the tiring onus of always knowing best. Needless to say, I was therefore a bit of a focus of conflict in that respect. I could pose the question to colleagues of all disciplines: choose between the professionally correct demand to know and do, or the human task of listening and responding.

It was, I came to be sure, not only my conflict. I was very sure that, as I followed some people through from being medical students to becoming trainee psychiatrists and eventually qualified consultants, I could see a characteristic progression. The younger the person – the medical student – the more fascination there was with the experience of the 'mad', whilst the older and more trained the person became, the more their serious responsibility weighed down heavily and demanded professional correctness. It seemed a sad progression as humane interest gave way to professional propriety. Nevertheless, I do not believe the underlying fascination ever disappeared. Somewhere there survives in all of us – whether we work in psychiatry or not – a human interest in those suffering from the most painful of horrors which drive people mad. This book asks us to turn on our heels and at least glance back at that side of ourselves – that fellow-feeling side of ourselves – which tries to stand as close as possible with someone who suffers, and to listen in to that suffering.

In the course of my work with these colleagues in the mental hospital, I tried to listen in to the stress of the work, and what it meant about the patients in their care. I made arrangements for them to explore for themselves various aspects of the work, and the experiences of the people they were working with. The aim was to allow their interest in those experiences and their care for those who suffered them, to endure, and not to fade away under the various pressures of the institution, of their sense of burdening responsibility and of their own career progress.

There was some thirst amongst many of the staff (not just the medics) for a psychodynamic alternative to the largely routine treatment methods of the general psychiatrist, and I remember one day a realisation came to me. I realised then that I was seen by some of the staff in a very particular, and perhaps unique, way. I was an enlightening alternative, an alternative to standard psychiatry. These staff included a few nurses, none of the qualified psychiatrists, but a lot of the trainee psychiatrists, and many of the other professionals, like art and music therapists. I responded to this and set up regular case discussion seminars. I also needed to avoid being seen as an *agent provocateur*, someone seeking to undermine the establishment of the institutions. Not surprisingly, in a psychiatric service there was a sensitive paranoia around amongst the authorities. The hospital had after all been a custodian of disorder for well over a century.

I also had a role teaching medical students, many of whom appeared fascinated by the tales of the unconscious which I told them. They came from the university for six-week placements to the hospital, and no doubt had hardly grown up beyond their adolescence. So they were often looking not just for teaching but for some ideas which might orient them to their own personal needs. The trainee psychiatrists were not necessarily much beyond that level of maturity, though they were aligned in a definite career direction. Their training required them to have a minimal acquaintance with psychotherapy. Although their interest gradually changed as they passed through their training period, many did respond and seriously considered some form of further psychotherapy or psychoanalytic training. I understood that psychotherapy did not come up much in their examinations, and so their attention was increasingly absorbed in diagnostic puzzles, and pharmacological treatments. Nevertheless, I took a lot of interest in them as the future leaders of the profession. So, I spent some time thinking about how to develop their interest.

In fact, as I have said, it was not so much that they needed to develop an interest, but the opposite. It appeared to me, as I compared medical students, trainee psychiatrists and my trained colleagues, that what happened in the course of this professional development was that there was a gradual movement away from taking an interest in the individual person of each patient. There was more than just this career pull, because the ethos of the whole hospital was to house long-standing cases, who had lost most of their capacities to be ordinary persons, and were stubbornly resistant to the empathic identification that newcomers and neophytes tried to make. Therefore my efforts were not to take an interest in the sad humanity incarcerated in the hospital, but to work in the opposite direction and encourage staff, especially the young ones, to retain the fascination that they had started with. I wanted to stop as much as possible the blunting of empathy and humanity that occurs in the course of a psychiatric career. So, as well as concentration on the formal teaching, I started work discussion and reflective kinds of groups, and indeed many of the other non-medical staff took an interest too.

Another mode of training had an 'experiential' form. There were two options. First of all, I ran a study group for trainee psychiatrists. It was *not* group therapy, but the kind of study group that has been pioneered by the Tavistock Institute – to study oneself in the context of a group for purposes of understanding what groups do to people's behaviour and experience. It was not intended to be curative in any way – rather to be exploratory of groups and how ordinary people find themselves in roles without negotiation, and seemingly intent on tasks that had no apparent meaning in the group. It was a method for individuals to discover how people come together in ways that are not always conscious; and how cultures develop and myths become socially constructed.

I found, surprisingly, that a considerable proportion of the psychiatric trainees took part in these experiential groups. The study groups were weekly, lasting six months, and were reconstituted every six months. Sometimes keen people stayed for several of these six-month periods.

I was explicit that I wanted them to explore the group, as a group entity. I had learned this from the Group Relations conferences at Leicester, run by the Tavistock Institute. When people tried to make personal revelations about themselves, I took the view that they were trying to tell the group about the experience they brought from the wider group, the hospital. They emanated from shared impressions. I helped them to consider whether the group was able to listen, or if the group was being handicapped in various ways. My observations were that the group struggled with certain kinds of problems, which were:

- conflict over being too like a patient
- the need to retreat from danger, as if the group was safe, and must be kept separate from the work
- the insecurity of being a doctor, and the 'superiority' of the study group as a group of doctors, over other groups.

These were purely my own impressions, and I do not claim this as a reliable piece of research. The point was to help the study group members try to work at locating what *their* experiences were, how these experiences developed as group phenomena, and where they came from.

The second experiential thing I did was to offer the trainees the opportunity to make a formal observation of a ward. The aim was to help them keep a focus on their own reactions. I based this idea on the baby observation course in my own psychoanalytic training at the British Institute of Psychoanalysis. Instead of observing a baby, these trainees observed a ward. The purpose was to develop the ability to observe a social context – the mother with her baby and sometimes in the midst of a family, and this transferred to become an observation of the place of a professional mental health worker in the social context of a psychiatric service. It was intended as a method of developing one's own capacity for observing emotionally, and at the same time observing oneself in the context of an emotional setting. This is a double kind of observation – I take it as the essence of psychoanalytic observing – both observing one's relational context, and one's own experiencing of it.

FOREWORD

This method evolved into a form of 'observing organisations' of various kinds (Hinshelwood and Skogstad 2000). Observers, without their stethoscopes, white coats, and the emblems of official medical authority, simply went and sat in one place for one hour every week for three months. The aim was that trainees might retain their human sensitivity to others without the expectation of role-performance in the working situation. This was solidified by a weekly seminar in which three or four trainees would meet with me to discuss in a formal way their observations (which I asked to be written up each week). I was astonished at the interest in doing this. At the same time, I might say, there was a considerable enthusiasm in the staff of wards who observers asked permission to observe. It was as if those wards felt starved of interest from outside and felt forgotten most of the time. So, they welcomed someone coming to see what happened.

These kinds of activities drew my attention, as well as that of colleagues, to the institutional processes within psychiatry. I decided that this could be important in psychiatric training. People in institutions behave quite compliantly according to what is required by the culture of the organisation they are in. Such a recognition goes back to the French social psychologist, Gustave Le Bon in the 19th Century, who described people as different when in a group compared with when we are separate individuals on our own (Le Bon 1895). When we get together, we represent group ideas and group beliefs as if they were our own. Of course they *are* our own, but only while we are in that group! I take it that it is the psychiatrist's job to be in a situation (with his patient) but also to be aware of how he is being influenced by that situation. Eventually, I wrote up some of this interest in the organisational dynamics of institutions which have the particular job of working with 'insanity', in my book *Suffering Insanity* (2004). I had noticed how, under the stresses of a career in psychiatry with the horrors that patients bring to their carers, there is an understandable tendency to retreat to an emotional distance. It gives some relief for staff, but it leaves the patient as it were stranded, as if an inanimate object.

This tendency to relate to an inanimate object in the patient – that is, the illness he becomes – then becomes institutionalised as a scientific attitude. Of course there is nothing wrong with science. I am convinced that it has brought, in the form of medication, an enormous relief to very many people. However, there may be something about the way it is used – i.e. if it is used to keep an emotional distance, a focus on remote aetiology (as Freud said), to protect us from feeling the suffering of other persons. Then, it is *used* as a kind of psychological defence, and not just as a means towards some important knowledge, or the controlled use of some effective pharmacological product.

What I have to ask the reader to do now is to expand his/her perception. I ask them to face towards the specific challenge of understanding what an individual patient means and experiences when he is hampered by the psychotic disturbance to his ability to conceptualise, verbalise, and communicate. This book's *raison d'etre* is to persuade the reader that there are serious avenues of advance that can be made with even the most disturbed patients in giving a shape and concepts to what seem like inexpressible experiences. With the right coaxing, some of the most severe patients can allow their most horrific feelings to be channelled into shapes that have some new-found coherence for them. They in their most intimate being can be grasped in new ways, seen from different angles, and given coherent diagrammatic form. Please read on to consider the dedicated kind of focusing that could bring many of our most disturbed patients back home, as it were.

Bob Hinshelwood
Fellow of the British Psychoanalytical Society
Fellow of the Royal College of Psychiatrists
March 2018

References

Freud, S (1917). Psycho-analysis and psychiatry. In The Standard Edition of the Complete Psychological Works of Sigmund Freud, Vol. XVI. 241–256. London: Hogarth.

Freud, S (1940). An outline of psycho-analysis. In S.E. Vol. XXIII. 139–208. London: Hogarth.

Hinshelwood, R (2004). Suffering Insanity. London: Routledge.

Hinshelwood, R and Skogstad, W (2000). Observing organisations. London: Routledge.

Le Bon, Gustave (1895). Psychologie des foules. Paris: Alcan. English translation (1995) as The Crowd. Brunswick (US) and London (UK): Transaction Publishers.

Luhrmann, T (2000). Of two minds. New York: Alfred Knopf.

PREFACE

DR GILLIAN STEGGLES

The subject of schizophrenia tends to arouse people's deepest-seated fears of mental illness. And this is especially so when it relates to a loved one or to personal experience. So it becomes particularly important that services organising efficient, effective and capable care for individuals suffering from psychosis are available to them and their families.

This book offers a scientific, explanatory, visual model of the mind affected by schizophrenia or schizoaffective disorder, the general pathway it follows when it receives remedial treatment with psychoanalytic psychotherapy, and a way of visually conceptualising its resolution when treated by this method. The therapeutic stages of successful recovery in this way, identified by Dr Michael Robbins MD, are outlined. Not all patients suffering from schizophrenia or schizoaffective disorder are suited to this treatment method, which makes very heavy demands in several different ways on the patient. Sometimes finding a carer, the help of a community psychiatric nurse or psychiatric social worker, family therapy, and social skills therapy can, together, be more effective than the expensive, solitary, stressful life of a psychoanalytic psychotherapy patient. And this treatment method does not always result in success.

Dr Michael Robbins MD, in addition to practising, very successfully, psychoanalytic psychotherapy with his paranoid schizophrenic patients from which he identified his seven therapeutic stages of successful recovery, has also developed his own wide-ranging and engaging approach to the unconscious mind generally. This approach is developed in detail in his many writings, but perhaps nowhere more clearly than in his book "The Primordial Mind in Health and Illness: A Cross-Cultural Perspective" (Robbins, 2011). Here he studies a wide range of models of the mind in terms of his own progressive thinking during his professional development. Starting with "Experiences of Schizophrenia", which he published in 1993, Dr Robbins' ideas have increasingly explored in depth the nature of the unconscious mind, most recently examining the engagement between psychoanalysis and psychosis in relation to attachment and separation. This author (GS) admires Dr Robbins' grasp of the characteristics of the unconscious mind and his ability to contain it clinically within the therapy he administers to his patients.

Dr Miomir Milovanovic outlines his insightful regard for psychiatry's biological, psychological, and social approaches in his Introduction. This author (GS) adheres to biological psychiatry, especially if the demonstrable psychological/psychoanalytical truths manifest in so much psychoanalytical psychotherapeutic literature are *as rigorously* adhered to as are biological paradigms, in furtherance of the "psycho" element of biopsychosocial psychiatry. Much has been written about this psychological component in connection with psychosis, eg. Evans, 2016; Lucas, 2009; and Martindale and Summers, 2013a and 2013b; as being one of the most important dimensions of all in a psychiatry that endeavours to alleviate some of the most extreme mental distress encountered in its patients.

The costs referred to in the text are those of the 2012 Schizophrenia Commission's calculations. In 2019, at £100 per day, the cost of five times per week analytic treatment per patient for a year would amount to £23,000 per year (including the analyst's holidays of six weeks). But even for a period of four to eight years, this would be well worth spending in relation to the £1.8 million (even at 2012 figures) that society spends on the lifetime care of a largely untreated schizophrenic patient. Treating newly-diagnosed patients who are suitable for psychoanalytic psychotherapy in due course, after a period of stabilisation, provides them with the opportunity for greatly improved mental health; and this in itself, as well as being an essentially necessary humanitarian consideration, is very likely to save society the large sums involved in the maintenance support required for chronic illness.

The Psychodynamic Pentapointed Cognitive Construct (PPCC) model illustrates graphically the major phases of how a schizophrenic patient's mind changes, during its psychoanalytic psychotherapeutic journey, from being uncomfortably restricted in its initial circumstance where the illness has developed, to its smoothly functioning as an independent and autonomous entirety. Some of this journey can be experienced with other forms of help than psychoanalytic psychotherapy, but the whole process that permits ultimate autonomous individuation requires the gruelling extent of exposure and self-scrutiny that only psychoanalytic psychotherapy provides. The PPCC model's graphic illustrations enable these remedial processes to be visualized, making the psychological processes easier to understand.

Practical considerations are described, particularly the absolute requirement for patient safety at all times. Patient safety is more important than the sum of all other considerations grouped together. Physical safety and preservation goes hand in hand with maintenance of a healthily progressing mental state that is sustained by psychological therapy. These issues are discussed in terms of ward management and the strong relationships and links that patients develop with ward staff, which affect this safety and persist long after discharge from hospital.

The experience of psychoanalytic psychotherapy is outlined, along with personal attributes required of the patient. Perhaps most needed of all is a dogged determination in the patient to see their therapy worked through, starting with an insightful motivation and followed up with tolerance and patience to see themselves through their worst of times. Dr Michael Robbins' accounts of his own cases bear witness to the struggles his patients have had to work through, by way of examples.

This book aims to illustrate the very real possibility for future flourishing that working through difficulties like these makes possible for patients who persevere. The scale of these projects, embarking on and completing in each case an expensive, major personal enterprise, is what puts healthcare authorities off supportive attitudes towards them. These authorities rationalise away from endorsing them, even though the ultimate costs of not doing so regularly outstrip the overall inclusively required financial outlay, great as this is. The long term is simply disregarded in face of the initial shocks of necessary expense and necessary investment of time: the long time-frame for psychological treatments is quite different from that of shorter mainstream physical treatments. The key to its validation is the healthy motivation and ambition lying deep within many young schizophrenic patients' being, where they powerfully want, with their whole self, to be well and happy. Prior demonstration in their past history of significant achievement in some form augurs well for the patient. Health services should capitalise on such innate streaks of essential human wellbeing in these psychologically ill patients, just as in all their other patients in every branch of physical medicine who are trying to respond to all treatments. What is needed is a perceptual shift towards investment in the future, in psychological medicine and physical medicine equally, as in so many other unrelated contexts.

Some aspects of the psychoanalytic psychotherapist's tasks are described which have emerged from clinicians' experiences of working with psychotic patients. A grounding in psychiatry is necessary for delivering psychoanalytic psychotherapy to schizophrenic patients because of the obligatory ability to recognise early any inclination in the patient towards unrealistic or psychotic thinking in his or her sessions. Moreover, the ability to know how to respond to a psychotic patient in the consulting room is essential, and this best develops through psychiatric work on hospital wards. Psychotic thinking in a patient demands specific techniques of understanding and clinical handling and, while this book is not a manual for guidance in doing this work, it contains experience-based aspects of successful management of the schizophrenic or schizoaffective patient, derived from experienced clinicians and particularly from Dr Michael Robbins, as well as anecdotes from patients. One of the most enduring elements of psychoanalytic treatments which can sustain a patient for many years after cessation of therapy sessions is the memory of a kind, understanding, attentive fellow human being, who has not judged the patient but has instead communicated strength and has held an evenly suspended positive regard towards the patient based upon possibilities that the patient can believe to be true about themselves. The transference, the essential relationship between the patient and the analyst, holds the most substantial key as to how, or not, the patient will ultimately thrive. In order to achieve this experience for the patient while effectively delivering the therapy, the therapist must be absolutely secure in recognising and handling the psychotic elements in their patient, in addition to maintaining an emotionally sustaining engagement with them.

When treating severe mental illness such as schizophrenia and schizoaffective disorder it is sometimes important to take into account the patient's own explanatory narrative insight concerning their own life story in addition to their understanding a little of the medical insight that psychiatrists depend upon to do their work. Their own explanatory narrative insight is often the best way a patient with severe illness can make sense of the confusion they now suffer from. Meaning is paramount to their fresh acquisition of aspects of mental health for themselves. The psychiatrist identifies all the features necessary for medical insight, and enlightens their patient in this as far as the patient wishes towards their psychiatric treatment and management. But if the psychiatrist is also able to work with the patient to understand their experiences in the patient's own terms, according to his or her own explanatory narrative insight, then the patient's insight into their own condition may be considerably improved (Bouvet et al, 2018), with implications both for their peace of mind and more effective psychiatric management. The PPCC Theory was developed from a schizoaffective patient's explanatory narrative insight, and was found by this author (GS) to be equally applicable in detail to the therapy of two paranoid schizophrenic patients by Dr Michael Robbins throughout their treatment process. It is clear, in the case of this schizoaffective patient certainly, that the patient's own explanatory narrative was greatly influential in her eventual attainment of mental health.

Dr Robbins' work with schizophrenic patients is written up by him in many papers and in his seminal work "Experiences of Schizophrenia". Some of his case studies are written up in his book, while others are recounted separately, eg. "The successful psychoanalytic therapy of a schizophrenic woman". His accounts are clear and concise and the treatments may be readily understood from his perspective. The PPCC offers lucidity from the position of the patient. This approach, that of trying to understand the psychoanalytic psychotherapy of schizophrenia as the patient experiences the treatment as much as from the therapist's intention to provide understanding to the patient, is adhered to throughout the following pages. The difficulties experienced by the patient in necessarily moving through mental changes, sometimes from one very painful state of mind to another, form the reality underlying the graphic geometric PPCC model's phases. Dr Robbins' written-up case studies, including those quoted in Parts IV and V herein, present these terribly painful changes in narrative context as they occur during his patients' progress. The PPCC model provides in graphic form the core facts relating to these changes through the emerging transformations of the patient's mind between one state of comprehension in treatment and the next. Dr Robbins has identified the stages of the therapy he has practised with his patients in his "seven stages of psychoanalytic psychotherapy". These stages have been aligned with the PPCC model's phases of recovery, giving a lucid account from both the therapist's and the patient's perspectives of the entire process of the psychological alleviation of schizophrenia when seen through to its resolution, in an autonomous and independent individual.

Dr Robbins' portfolio of cases illustrates what it is possible to achieve through the skilled psychoanalytic psychotherapy of suitable cases of schizophrenia. In order for every suitable patient to receive this treatment and emerge subsequently into mental health it would require an adaptable National Health Schedule for Schizophrenia, which allocates to each schizophrenia patient the form or forms of therapy for which they are best suited, including psychoanalytic psychotherapy. In this way, patients who could benefit from psychoanalytic psychotherapy would not be overlooked but would receive their remedial treatment. Such a treatment schedule's greatest obstacles so far as NHS managers and politicians are concerned would be its financial considerations, particularly for the psychoanalytic psychotherapy-treated patients; and the scarcity of psychiatrically trained psychoanalysts for delivery of the therapy to these patients. Currently, sums of £190,000 per patient are being discussed in relation to some six-month drug course treatments for cancer. Physical treatments are readily conceptualised and identified with, visibly and tangibly, while psychological treatments are usually complex to grasp conceptually, impossible to grasp physically, and invisible. The difficulty of grasping the staple ideas involved in psychological treatments renders them unconsciously distasteful to politicians and others involved in funding them, for fear that what is not understood cannot demonstrably be proven justifiable; what the potential funders are unable to discuss becomes feared as an unknown quantity. It is a form of unintended prejudice in people who would surely be shocked if they were aware of it. There is also the factor of lack of effective treatments for many mental illnesses, where no amount of money spent on them would be likely to bring about appreciable clinical benefit to the patients. Psychoanalytic psychotherapy has been proven effective for some determined schizophrenic patients by one clinician, Dr Michael Robbins, in the USA, and it remains for those in the UK who are in a position to do so, to replicate his findings in Britain.

The proportion of schizophrenic or schizoaffective patients who could benefit from psychoanalytic psychotherapy is unknown, but it is unlikely to be greater than 5-7%. Nonetheless, it is known that this therapy can assist some schizophrenic patients in living their lives even when complete resolution is not achieved. And the concept of improving the lot of patients despite their carrying a substantial burden of illness permeates the whole of NHS policy. So when long-term savings in the expenses of accommodation, clinician time, and welfare payments are reviewed in line with transformative treatments in other medical specialties, and combined with the positive benefits to the patients and their families, a condensed, intensive psychological treatment, albeit paid with a major sum initially, seems a good investment. Dr Michael Robbins, an experienced and psychiatrically trained psychoanalyst specialising in the treatment of paranoid schizophrenic patients, achieved "a positive result" in half of his patients. Training psychiatrists in psychoanalysis needs good morale and support for the trainees if they are to succeed. Following in the footsteps of Bion, Segal, Rosenfeld, Lucas, Sohn, and Murray Jackson could appeal as an enticing career for those already engaged in medical prescribing for mental illness together with the straightforward addressing of the patient's problems at a practical level. When the current, apparent problems are addressed in psychotherapy, the patient's fundamental abilities to cope better in future situations may not necessarily be enhanced if her underlying debility has not been alleviated. A really good case can be made for integrating judicious prescribing with skilled psychoanalytic consultations; that intervening psychologically at a profound level can shape a patient's fragmented mind into the patient's own, self-reliant source of beneficence and harmony, strengthening their autonomy and independence which is the goal of a successful psychoanalytic psychotherapy treatment.

Psychiatry is deeply rooted in medical ethics, and psychoanalysis is also practised by clinicians with the highest ethical standards, particularly so because their work relates to the patients' very minds, and thus close contact with their souls may be made. The psychiatrist and the psychoanalyst alike utilise the whole of themselves in their work, which can extend in their cases to the depths of their own souls, or "psyches". Clinicians clearly need to take the greatest care of themselves while working so that they do not succumb in any untoward way to adverse effects of engagement with their patients, including especially long-term strains. All their decisions take as a primary concern the patient's best interests. They balance beneficence with any possibility or inevitability of maleficence that might be incurred from adopting a particular stance, and they always try to sustain their patients' autonomy so far as this exists within the patient by refraining from being prescriptive or didactic. They try to deliver justice as an overall goal for their patients when a patient cannot obtain this for themselves.

Philosophy sometimes has to be turned to during very difficult spells in a patient's therapy. On occasion, the patient can become very disturbed in a wide variety of ways, leaving the analyst dismayed and concerned. He or she must use all their repertoire of clinical skills to contain the patient, and when they have reached their conclusions each day they need to address the wider picture within which their practice rests, including perhaps from a philosophical, pragmatic perspective. This can help them retain their own mind intact, strengthening it with fantasy, imagination, rest, and reassurance through their personal contacts and relationships. Their own psychoanalysis and clinical supervision of their work help them to address and balance their workload so that it does not overwhelm them. Joint presentations and academic sessions can greatly refresh their state of mind and sense of self. Spiritual peace may be reached anew after sufficient rest and recuperation deep within the analyst's own personal world, away from the clinical scene.

Sheer interest in his work may sustain the psychoanalyst for long tracts of time spent working clinically. His humanitarian interest in his patients

PREFACE

may occupy the larger part of his time away from the actual clinical business of interpreting his patients' expressed troubles in his consulting room. The very many and various applications of psychoanalytic theory throughout the worlds of art, literature, and culture generally, may also provide him with readily sustainable interest, as may an interest in philosophical ideas. The PPCC model, for example, demonstrates the Golden Ratio, otherwise known as the Golden Rectangle, the Golden Triangle or the Golden Spiral. This is an extraordinarily beautiful philosophical phenomenon of the world, with examples to be seen and appreciated everywhere on earth. Thus the philosophical considerations of this Golden Ratio have their own beauty and truth, and stimulate an interest in the wider world. The PPCC model connects science, psychiatry, psychoanalysis, philosophy, mathematics, health, and the beauties of human culture; but although theological, sacred, and divine properties have been attributed to the Golden Ratio, these are not considered to be properties of the PPCC model, and are not discussed in this book.

Sound science, with its evidence, underpins in this book a description of one of the most complex and baffling of all mental illnesses, against a backdrop of what has been found, in fact, to obtain after thirty years' study by the author of this book, and after at least forty-six years' clinical work with schizophrenic patients in the case of her clinician colleague, Dr Michael Robbins. The facts are assembled diligently and methodically, and the ensuing conclusions reached logically. We each have encountered and tried to contribute to the field in its current state of knowledge, admitting and accepting all the many avenues which have simply not, as yet, been embarked upon from an exploratory or explanatory viewpoint. It could also be argued, however, that if schizophrenia is a great mountain, we have dug a tunnel of understanding through it which has emerged out into daylight at the far end which is manifestly the same as the daylight where we started. The author, Dr Steggles', patient had a memory of being perfectly happy at the age of six, before her molestation aged eight which immediately precipitated nine episodes of behaviour disturbance and parental relationship difficulties and distorted her life for the next thirty years. The written-up account of this research patient's remedial psychoanalytic psychotherapy, presented here as the PPCC model, which allowed her to recover her mental faculties, albeit with a few circumscribed deficits, and develop her personal perspective, forms this early tunnel successfully dug through the mountain of schizophrenia. Similar experiences were provided to his patients by Dr Robbins, thus constructing other, connecting tunnels. We need further tunnels to be dug through the schizophrenia mountain to daylight, and to connect with the tunnels already dug. Bright, intelligent, heartbreakingly distressed schizophrenic patients are crying out for talking therapy to resolve and save their lives. Brave and determined psychiatrists are the people, after training in psychoanalysis, who could share this understood daylight of psychoanalytic psychotherapy with these patients, buried as they are in the depths of schizophrenia, in the night of their distress. Simply, what the patients require is their own understanding of the meaning to them of their life's experiences.

This book tries to present visually the overall sum of the changes these schizophrenic minds undergo during remedial psychoanalytic psychotherapy. It hopes thereby to illustrate the overall nature of their changing internal capacities and strengths as they interact with their psychoanalyst during their recovery from their schizophrenia to become independent individuals. Summarising this process emphasises its completeness and reality, demonstrating it as a clinical phenomenon. Clinicians with the skill of Dr Michael Robbins and all the others summarised in Chapter 13 are those gifted to bring the opportunity of mental health to schizophrenic patients who are prepared to work for their health and achieve it.

GLOSSARY

Abreaction: discharge verbally of painful previously unconscious memories.
Abstract transitional object: a transitional object (see below) which is abstract but which nonetheless provides comfort to the patient.
Analyst: a psychoanalyst.
Analysand: a person receiving a psychoanalysis.
Catharsis: an intense verbal outpouring of psychological content which has built up over time.
Cathexis: an emotional investment in an entity.
Countertransference: the feelings a psychoanalyst may experience for their patient.
Defence mechanism: a measure that the mind's ego (see below) adopts to protect itself when it feels under threat from aspects of other people. There are many examples, such as splitting, projection, projective identification, repression, intellectualisation, and displacement (see below).
Depressive position: a state of mind where another person is regarded as a whole, with both good and bad attributes, and where the patient feels guilty and wishes to make reparations to the other for any hurt they may have caused to them.
Differentiation: becoming a unique, characterised individual different from others.
Displacement: a defence mechanism (see above) where a feeling is transferred from where it arises to another person or situation.
Ego: the individual, personal self.
Evacuating: emptying the self of a feeling.
Feeling states: states of experiencing specific feelings.
Fixation: an arrest of some aspects of development at a time of traumatic experience, which may sometimes be located and alleviated by psychoanalytic psychotherapy.
Golden Ratio: a ratio relating to a divided line where the ratio of the smaller length to the larger of the two resulting lengths is the same as the ratio of the larger length to the whole length.
Individuation: becoming an integrated and unique individual.
Intellectualisation: a defence mechanism (see above) where a situation or idea that the patient has difficulty in accepting or tolerating is converted into elaborate thought.

GLOSSARY

Internal good object: a good person who the patient has taken into themselves metaphorically, or internalised, so that the good person has a very real identity within the patient and can influence them in the person's absence.

Internalisation: taking in, by adoption, into the patient's self of an entity such as a feeling, an idea or another person's identity as an internal object: similar to introjection (see below).

Internal object: a person who the patient has internalised, or metaphorically taken into themselves, and who exists psychologically within the patient and can influence them during the person's absence from the patient.

Introjection: an external entity being psychologically taken inside the self: similar to internalisation (see above).

"Links": Wilfred Bion's "Links" of Love, Hate and Knowledge are bonds, with other people, that he saw schizophrenic patients destroying as part of their illness. These bonds are formed by healthy people with others, and sustain them in their normal, everyday relationships with others during life. Love, Hate and Knowledge summarise as broad categories the characteristics of these bonds.

Narcissism: a person is narcissistic who relates everything to his own self and denies the separateness and integrity of another person as a defence (see above) against envy (thick-skinned narcissism) and dependence (thin-skinned narcissism).

Object: a person other than the patient to whom the patient relates.

Object-cathexis: an emotional investment in an object (another person).

Object relations: a differentiated, consistent and relatively realistic representation of the self and other people in interaction.

Paranoia: a highly anxious feeling in a patient that others around him are threatening him and are about to attack him.

Paranoid: a state of mind, or a patient experiencing it, where the patient is anxious about being attacked; and which may initiate an unjustified attack on a feared person in deluded self-defence.

Paranoid-schizoid position: a state of mind where the patient regards another person as all good or all bad, as extremes of perceptual experience which bear little relation to each other. The patient's mind has become split (see below) into different parts as a defence mechanism (see above) which prevents the patient from functioning as a capable, strong individual. In this state of mind the patient commonly suffers from considerable paranoid (see above) anxiety.

"Pathosymbiosis": a primitive and pathological symbiotic relationship conceived of by Dr Michael Robbins MD between the analyst and the patient near the start of therapy which is a transference (see below) relationship consisting of the patient's passive and disabled state enacted and repeated from its earlier manifestation in her family of origin. It exacerbates her constitutional vulnerability and is a feature of her schizophrenic illness.

PPCC model: the shapes describing a schizoaffective patient's mind as it recovers into mental health, as illustrated by the PPCC Theory.

GLOSSARY

PPCC pentagram: one of the series of larger and smaller PPCC constructs according to the Golden Ratio.

PPCC Theory: the changes a schizoaffective patient's mind undergoes as it recovers into health through psychoanalytic psychotherapy may be illustrated accurately, and conceptually visualized, as geometric shapes.

The PPCC/The PPCC construct: the pentapointed PPCC shape.

Projection: a defence mechanism (see above) that involves several different ways of the patient unconsciously sending their own feelings outwards to other people.

Projective identification: a defence mechanism (see above) common in schizophrenic patients where bad feelings in the patient are unconsciously evacuated (see above) out of themselves and into another person. This may lead to the patient disowning the feelings and the other person experiencing the feelings rather than the patient. Thus the patient may attribute part of their self to another person.

"Protopathosymbiosis": the passive, global, indiscriminate adaptation of the untreated schizophrenic patient towards others, which manifests as extreme passivity somewhat resembling "parasitism", and is a term conceived of by Dr Michael Robbins MD.

Regression: a return by an individual's unconscious mind to an earlier stage of psychological life.

Representational world: Joseph Sandler's and Bernard Rosenblatt's conception of a patient's ongoing conceptualisation, since childhood, of meaningful aspects of their successive external environments.

Repression: a defence mechanism (see above) in which a painful or traumatic memory is buried deep into the unconscious psyche, where it remains unobserved by the patient, who is unaware that it exists. If a passing connection, eg. a spoken word or a perception, connects with a repressed memory, it may burst back into consciousness, taking the patient unawares. This process may take the form of a precipitated psychotic episode.

Splitting: a defence mechanism (see above) where the patient's mind becomes separated into different parts which may be contradictory towards each other, eg. both good and bad perceptions of another person.

Therapeutic alliance: Elizabeth Zetzel's concept of the working relationship between the psychoanalyst and the patient.

Therapeutic dyad: the two participants in therapy, the psychoanalyst and the patient.

Therapeutic hour: the fifty minutes in the day during which the patient consults the psychoanalyst and they work together to resolve the patient's problems.

Thing-cathexis: emotional investment in an inanimate entity.

Thing-presentation: an inanimate entity considered as the abstract constitution of the information being received.

Transference: the personal feelings that the patient generally has for other people may be transferred on to the psychoanalyst. The transference may be positive (agreeable) or negative (antagonistic).

GLOSSARY

Transitional object: Donald Winnicott's conception of a child's soft toy or comfort blanket which helps the child to separate from its mother around the time of weaning, by being both "me" (the child) and "not-me" (the mother). The transitional object is completely within the control of the child, so the child can monitor its own feelings as it wishes, and gain a sense of its own independence from its mother.

Word-cathexis: emotional investment in a word.

Word-presentation: a word considered as the abstract constitution of the information being received.

CHAPTER 1

INTRODUCTION

Almost full circle: Is it time to improve further the basic paradigm in Psychiatry?

DR MIOMIR MILOVANOVIC

Dr Steggles' book "The Psychiatry of Resolving Schizophrenia Psychoanalytically: How visualizing the therapeutic process can assist success" will be a bit surprising and certainly a demanding and inspiring read for many psychiatrists, clinicians working within the field of mental health, psychotherapists, patients, and the general public. It aims to improve the psychological science component of psychiatry's biopsychosocial model into being the best it can be. And all of these groups should read it.

Reasons for this include the present situation in psychiatry and the whole field of mental health. Improving psychiatry's approach to the psychological aspects of mental illnesses is an idea rich in potential. Psychiatry is, however, dominated by so called medical or biological approaches to understanding and helping patients with mental disorders.

Perhaps one of the best illustrations of this is Kaplan and Sadock's Comprehensive Textbook of Psychiatry, a well-known and one of the most prestigious psychiatric textbooks in the world. Its last, tenth edition was published on its fiftieth anniversary last year. The very first sixteen pages (immediately after the book cover and before the title page) contain a Colour Atlas of Psychiatry with numerous coloured images, mostly of the brain taken using different imaging techniques and technologies that are available today. After the Title Page, Contents, and lengthy Contributors' List, the first 450 of its pages are devoted to neuroscience, then there are 200 pages devoted to neuropsychiatry and behavioural neurology, and then about 100 pages of psychological sciences (including chapters on sensation, perception, learning, biology of memory etc). Only at the end of these 950 pages of general introduction are there eighty pages (or 8.5%) devoted to psychoanalysis and its different schools.

The section "Schizophrenia and Other Psychotic Disorders" starts with a page and a half long "Introduction and Overview" written by Carol Tamminga (page 1405). It is very interestingly written, particularly if we read it with attention to minute detail.

She starts by saying:

"Schizophrenia is arguably one of the most puzzling yet disabling of **brain diseases**, with its severe and persistent psychotic manifestations accompanied by variable cognitive dysfunction and profound psychosocial impairment."

She continues, "**Substantial progress in understanding and treating schizophrenia will depend** on discovering the neural mechanisms of the elements of the condition, one of those being the mechanism for psychosis. This understanding is necessary for developing drug targets, novel therapeutics, and for biologically based disease definitions. **It is hard to conceive of the exact neuro mechanisms** whose dysfunction could interfere so extensively with such broad cognitive functions as does psychosis… In this section the curious reader will find the facts of psychosis presentation and the sum of manifestations and biomarkers that any model **needs to take into account** in the formulation of a disease model… Therefore, it might be optimistically predicted that it will eventually be possible to describe the genes, cellular and molecular mechanisms, and rational treatments for psychosis manifestations over the next several decades." (Tamminga C, 2017) (Emphasis in bold added by MM).

Dr Tamminga's tone is very confident, optimistic and self-assured, without any doubts, uncertainties, or awareness that we are facing the unknown and unimaginably complex reality of the human being, his/her brain, and equally complex states and conditions when they function in ways that bring suffering to self and/or others.

Her confidence is based on a sense of certainty that she is very clear what schizophrenia is and that we now have very reliable and powerful tools that will provide us with an explanation of what schizophrenia is and how it develops. If we read the text carefully we can see that this confidence is not about something that is already known but of something that is based on knowledge that we will acquire in several decades' time in the future.

Of course, in this eagerness we often forget that the brain in structure and function is an incomparably more complex organ than any other organ in the body or indeed any other phenomenon in the universe. If we look into the history of "modern psychiatry" we can see that these dreams are not new. They have already been dreamt by the founding fathers of modern psychiatry, such as Flechsig, Alzheimer, and others, all of whom were either

INTRODUCTION

professors of psychiatry or professors of psychiatry and neurology although when we think of them we remember them as neuroanatomists, neuropathologists, neurohistologists etc. With the same passion and the same beliefs as their heirs today they were chasing to obtain cadavers (and their brains) or struggling to obtain permission to dissect/slice and investigate histologically brains of particular patients they knew very well and followed over a long time, thus using the best technologies available to them at that time in their search for the causes of mental illness. They didn't achieve the goals they were working towards but they did produce extremely valuable neuro-scientific research on which present day research is founded. Tamminga has written "Substantial progress... will depend on discovering the neural mechanisms..." when Dr Robbins has already produced substantial progress, demonstrated in this volume, without mention of the neural mechanisms behind it. Enhancing the "psycho" element of biopsychosocial psychiatry is a paradigm of enormous potential.

Within neuro research the Dopamine Hypothesis of Schizophrenia (DHS) has an important place:

"The articulation of a modern biological hypothesis for schizophrenia began with dopamine. The pivotal observation that drugs that diminish dopamine-mediated neurotransmission in the brain reduce psychotic symptoms was made only in the mid-20th century. The first antipsychotic drug (chlorpromazine) was discovered serendipitously **but with a strong clinical rationale and astute observation (?)**. The experimental result that implicated the action of the chlorpromazine connected to dopamine receptor blockade was a hypothesis that fuelled decades of drug discovery and was the basis for a related etiological hypothesis that dopamine was indeed the core pathophysiology of schizophrenia. The speculative extension of this **well-supported treatment hypothesis (?)** has been harder to prove and to establish as the basis for schizophrenia pathophysiology, although ideas are still being tested. Although data have consistently supported the dopamine mechanism of antipsychotic drug action, support for the dopamine hypothesis of pathophysiology has been inconsistent." (Tamminga C, 2017) (Emphasis in bold and question marks added by MM)

The DHS has been one of the main connections between neuro research and at least some potentially understandable aspects of the pathophysiology of schizophrenia. It has kept alive the hope of a breakthrough in neuro research into the genesis of schizophrenia for decades. Although extremely reductionistic (the unimaginable complexity of both brain and schizophrenia was reduced to one neurotransmitter only), on the whole, and after years of dedicated research, it is not supported by good evidence. Kenneth Kendler, one of the leading researchers into psychiatric disorders and genetics, provides an elegant discussion of the DHS and the wider context that it has established (Kendler, 2015). Antipsychotic medications did not live up to their initial huge expectations - to be a cure for schizophrenia and psychotic disorders and to provide a model for their understanding: antipsychotics are helpful in reducing some symptoms in some patients with psychosis, but they did not help further the DHS. They are well known to cause a number of side effects, some of which can be quite serious (tardive dyskinesia, heart problems, and possible enlargement of brain ventricles, for example).

I want to point out the importance of noticing:

(i) how neuro researchers in psychiatry in pursuing this Holy Grail seem to have forgotten that:
- our patients, as all of us, have minds and an internal world as well as brains; mind and brain are not two, but one, single entity. But because of our very primitive level of knowledge of the brain, we can only think about, approach and research them as two, and not one.
- it seems that every new step in advancement in research (whether in terms of technical advancement or new research ideas or design) that brings a hope of leading to major breakthrough in understanding reality has usually brought us to a more complex and diverse view of reality.

(ii) harmful effects of the medical model:
1. Alienation of the person from important aspects of self, and of the person from others, by sometimes labelling thoughts, feelings, and behaviours as meaningless consequences of brain abnormality.
2. Stigmatising the mentally ill with social judgements of abnormality, and enabling misuse sometimes in some countries of labels for political purposes.
3. Using medication sometimes to suppress and anesthetise parts of the person rather than understanding them.

(iii) points made by Dr Michael Robbins:
- To date no physical finding has been discovered that distinguishes schizophrenic persons from "normal" ones. The same is true of most mental illnesses. (The Brain and Behavior Research Foundation, funded by NIMH, summarises the current status of research findings.)

- While there is a higher incidence of schizophrenia among biologically related persons, no specific causal gene or cluster of genes has been discovered that is present in all instances or that distinguishes schizophrenic persons from others.

(iv) some axioms of the psychosocial model of the mind:

1. Mind and personality, normal or abnormal, has a neurobiological substrate. There is a reciprocal relationship between brain and environment. According to the principle of neural plasticity, environmental factors affect brain structure and function.
2. In instances where there is no specific physical cause for a personality condition that society labels abnormal, psychosocial factors may be the most important determinants.
3. Interactions with family members have greatest impact on personality formation during infancy and childhood because of the state of utter physical and psychological dependence of the infant on the primary caregiver(s), and because of the immaturity of the brain.
4. A particular genetic predisposition may lead to what society judges as ability or disability, depending on environmental circumstances.
5. All psychosocial therapies are not created equal. To do the work I describe requires extensive supervised clinical training and a knowledge of theory of how the mind works. (Robbins, 1993).

Another very important approach within psychiatric research that has been neglected, but has been gaining influence in recent decades, particularly in the UK, has been research of different environmental factors that increase the risk of schizophrenia. There is good evidence that environmental factors such as childhood adversity, frequent moves in adolescence, being a migrant or belonging to an ethnic minority group, adverse life events, living in a city, cannabis use, etc., increase the risk of somebody developing schizophrenia or another psychotic disorder. Researchers from this group, although recognising the importance of neuro research and dysregulation of the dopaminergic system in the brain, have been less convinced that schizophrenia is a brain disease and are more open to the idea that social and psychological factors play a major causal role. This in turn has led to recognition that, in the treatment of patients with schizophrenia and psychosis, social and psychological factors are very important.

This line of research has an important connection with the aims and demands of patients' and carers' groups and initiatives which strenuously seek a different approach to the understanding and care of patients with schizophrenia and psychosis: recognition that patients and their families should be treated with respect and care, taken seriously and listened to, their views regarding care and treatment respected, their experiences accepted as important, that they be supported in making sense of their experiences in a way they find helpful, through on-going relationships and dialogue; and that they be given the opportunity to choose amongst a number of different therapeutic approaches and supports. Help should be provided as early as possible, at their home, and by the same clinicians over the treatment period.

So in recently developed models of schizophrenia (the Neurodevelopmental Hypothesis of Schizophrenia, the Sociodevelopmental-cognitive Model, and the Developmental Risk Factor Model) different research lines are brought together into an increasingly integrated and interactive system where genetic vulnerabilities interact with adverse environmental, social, and psychological factors, which in turn affect the brain and in particular the dopaminergic system, as well as salient cognitive and emotional systems resulting in psychosis and schizophrenia.

In this integrated model psychoanalysts can easily recognise the general psychoanalytic model, and in particular psychoanalytic models of psychosis, that have been discussed and used over the years, starting with Freud, Abraham, Sullivan, Searles, Rosenfeld, Bion, Segal, and recently Michael Robbins, as well as work led by Yrjo Alanen in Finland which resulted in developing the Need Adapted Approach/Open Dialogue Approach. Psychoanalysts have recognised that some people are more vulnerable than others to developing different mental disorders. Some speak about genetic vulnerability. Psychoanalysis has made major contributions in studying very closely the development of human beings from their birth, within extremely complex networks of early (emotional) relationships. The baby is born within a family where he/she is an active member, while being at the same time very sensitive to being affected by complex emotional relationships. Psychoanalysis (and psychoanalytically informed approaches to research) has been studying how different relationships affect a young child, eventually resulting in the development of particular behavioural, relational, and emotional patterns, many of which we label as particular mental disorders.

The problem here is that the wider research community is not sufficiently well acquainted with the psychoanalytic approach nor with psychoanalytic research developed and amassed over past decades. I want to point out here that a number of neuroscientists have found psychoanalytic models very helpful and have successfully applied them in research. This has been

INTRODUCTION

a part of the discipline of Neuropsychoanalysis that has been developing recently, founded by Mark Solms and colleagues.

Dr Steggles' book addresses this gap. The book starts with general information about schizophrenia (symptomatic distress, cost to society, organic aspects, and physical treatments). Although in these chapters Dr Steggles covers basics, what I found very impressive is that she writes about all of these issues from the perspective of the patient in a lively, persuasive and powerful way. She presents a number of points about different aspects, processes, interactions and experiences that describe psychosis/schizophrenia as experienced, perceived, and lived by a patient. Some of these points are present throughout the book, although in a number of different ways and not necessarily highlighted as such.

There are a number of books written by patients who have had first-hand experience of psychosis/schizophrenia, but in her book Dr Steggles presents something much wider and more rounded than just presenting someone's experiences (valuable as they are). It is more about her thinking through the whole field of mental health/social care/social and political aspects as relevant to psychosis/schizophrenia from the points of view of patients' lived experience in all their complexity.

The main part of her book is about the Psychodynamic Pentapointed Cognitive Construct (PPCC) model. Complementary to the impressive psychoanalytic work of Dr Michael Robbins, Dr Steggles developed her PPCC model by observing a patient with schizoaffective disorder who was treated by another psychoanalyst, and then applied it to two of Dr Robbins' patients (Case Studies 1 and 2). Over the years, she discussed with her patient the details of her experiences and thoughts, and followed her progress as her health improved.

Dr Robbins is a psychoanalyst who has devoted his professional career to the intensive psychotherapeutic treatment of severely disturbed psychotic patients. He presents his work in an important book, "Experiences of Schizophrenia: An Integration of the Personal, Scientific, and Therapeutic", that he published in 1993. Combining results from different fields of research with his own extensive clinical work and theoretical thinking, he has compellingly demonstrated the importance of thinking pluralistically about the treatment of schizophrenia, integrating a psychoanalytic model of understanding and treatment with neurobiological, social, and psychological perspectives while openly discussing his failures and credibly presenting his successes.

Dr Steggles compares the Stages of Psychological Therapy of Schizophrenia that Dr Robbins has delineated from his clinical work with her detailed case study of a patient's recovery from schizoaffective disorder. These two data sources are juxtaposed and examined. Dr Robbins' therapeutic stages are found to parallel exactly Dr Steggles' findings from her case study, which she summarises as her PPCC model of her schizoaffective patient's experience. The PPCC is a graphical representation of clinical work that enables understanding of complex and frequently baffling (to patient as well as to analyst) therapeutic processes, and importantly it provides the possibility of reflecting on these processes later.

Dr Steggles, and also Dr Robbins and other clinicians who have devoted substantial time, energy, thought, and passion to working with severely unwell patients, leave us with very important and difficult questions: what should be our aims and goals in treating and helping patients with any, and in particular any severe, mental disorder, of which schizophrenia is perhaps one of the most severe? These disorders are extremely crippling in many, and particularly in the most intimate, spheres of life: they interfere with the capacity to engage positively and rewardingly in intimate relationships, to follow the person's talents, and to feel fulfilled and able to make important contributions to society and to other people, as some of Dr Robbins' patients and Dr Steggles' patient demonstrated themselves able to do. As both authors highlight very clearly, not all patients with schizophrenia will be able to use the most promising help, such as intensive psychoanalysis or the Open Dialogue Approach and achieve very high goals. And again, as we see from their work, this cannot be predicted precisely at the beginning, during psychodynamic assessment. But for that reason it is crucial that patients who present with a capacity to engage in an intensive and very demanding endeavour are given an opportunity to have treatment. This is a particularly important issue at the present time when the whole fabric of the welfare state, and, amongst other institutions, the NHS, is under merciless attack resulting in severe cuts in resources and, with important consequences, in providing often barely basic support, care, and treatment for people who need these most.

Dr Miomir Milovanovic MRCPsych, MInst.Psychoanal.
Consultant Psychiatrist in Psychotherapy
Psychoanalyst, Member of the British Psychoanalytical Society

References

Bebbington, P (2015). Unravelling psychosis: Psychological epidemiology, mechanism, and meaning. Shanghai Arch. Psychiatry. 2015 Jun 25; 27(3): 70-81.

Kendler, K (2015). The dopamine hypothesis of schizophrenia: an updated perspective. In Kendler, K; Parnas, J, Eds. Philosophical Issues in Psychiatry IV, 283-294. Oxford University Press.

Murray, R; Sideli, L; La Cascia, C; La Barbera, D (2015). Bridging the gap between research into biological and psychosocial models of psychosis. Shanghai Arch. Psychiatry. 2015 Jun 25; 27(3): 139–143.

Robbins, M (1993). Experiences of Schizophrenia: An Integration of the Personal, Scientific and Therapeutic. New York: The Guilford Press.

Tamminga, C (2017). Introduction and Overview. In Sadock, B; Sadock, V; Ruiz, P; Eds: Kaplan and Sadock's Comprehensive Textbook of Psychiatry, 10th Edition, 1405-6. Wolters Kluwer.

PART I
ILLNESS
Schizophrenia and Schizoaffective Disorder

·····················

DR GILLIAN STEGGLES

CHAPTER 2

THE SYMPTOMATIC DISTRESS OF SCHIZOPHRENIC ILLNESS

The degree of suffering that is experienced by schizophrenic and schizoaffective patients is unimaginable to those who do not suffer from it. Every waking moment in life for a schizophrenic patient is compromised by their underlying confusion and incapacity to understand so much of what the world consists of, including, in particular, other people.

Lack of insight

This potentially blanket disconnection by the illness from every artery of life support available to these patients can make them despair, and all the more so as insight increases. Approximately 5.6% of schizophrenic patients commit suicide, and deliberate self-harm or suicide attempt is common (25-45%) in cases of schizophrenia and other psychotic disorders (Wasserman and Wasserman, 2009, pp.282-283).

In cases of severe negative symptoms it is unclear what the level of awareness is, but consciousness for these patients cannot be pleasant. As the level of consciousness increases, the level of awareness of suffering is so much greater. Commonly at the time of first presentation insight is scant; except for a sure knowledge that something is very wrong for the patient. Understanding is almost absent; just an awareness of stress, incredulity, great anxiety and often terror, piteousness in face of monstrous injustice in the world, sometimes rage and, somewhere, the patient's own personality with perhaps some fleeting memories of a happier, earlier time. Awareness often extends to an acceptance of needing help, but by no means in all cases. Sometimes a flat refusal of help is symptomatic of deep hurt from a previous incident, or of the patient's general fearfulness. There is a long, steep road for the patient to climb patiently towards reflection, understanding, growth and independence. All of these processes require mental effort by the patient with ward staff's help, and especially with their psychoanalytic psychotherapist if they are fortunate enough to receive this treatment.

Lack of security

The world is a frightening place for the schizophrenic patient. Because they can make so little sense of it, their own place in it is not understood at all. Reliable havens become restricted to, perhaps, a drop-in centre or cafe, and many live on the streets despite provision of hostel places; the subdued, restricting effect of a fixed abode interferes with the patient's mind's usual nonsensical but free-roaming habits. A fixed abode forces them to start addressing their life-issues, and usually this is far too painful for them to start attempting it.

Those patients who are trying hard to cooperate with analytic treatment are likely to need sheltered accommodation until the analyst judges that they have truly mastered the therapeutic process, have learnt to use their minds constructively, to tolerate pain, and with some insight can work towards their own self-help. During this time they will need all their available mental resources to concentrate on the therapy, particularly if they are scarcely managing their intensely painful and difficult psychological problems, because distraction by accommodation issues may inhibit full clinical concentration.

Fear and paranoia

Fear can easily develop into paranoia if the stresses of the environment prove too intense to contain manageably. Widespread, indeed universal and constant, fear can lead to misattribution of the causes of these fears and then to attacks on other individuals, with disastrous consequences for all concerned. Treatment is usually by medication, commonly fortnightly injections, with as much social support as can be organised to help the patient. Compliance with tablets or fortnightly injections is commonly difficult to sustain, especially in peripatetic patients, when supervision becomes difficult to monitor.

Acute compared with chronic illness

Difficulties in maintaining management of a patient's chronic ill-health generally develop in patients when debility has permeated the whole of their mental functioning, and fresh access to their personality, which could have proved helpful, is now unlikely to be reached. The best opportunities for success in remedial treatment are available to early-onset, acute psychoses where the greater part of the patient's personality is still accessible, relatively coherent, and optimistic. These patients are often comparatively young, in their late teens or early adult life, in their early twenties. Their minds are beginning to open up to the wider world from the relative restrictedness in some way of their earlier life. But, for these individuals, this problem in their early life has caused interference with their healthy adjustment to living where they were trying to develop. Part of them has not succeeded in this. It has been held back, caught up or trapped in a niche which ultimately is now preventing normal responses to new environments. Their representational world is distorted and cannot help them relate to new environments in the external world around them. There may also be deeper fault lines, for example in unconscious memories, preventing healthy mental activity.

Psychotic delusions

Patients suffering from schizophrenic illness spend the time when they are psychotic apparently in another world, barely acknowledging other people or their immediate environment. Delusions seem to form an alternative world which is widely believed to be less intimidating than the real one. The delusional world may have a tenuous relation to a core psychological difficulty the patient has experienced. As also mentioned in Chapter 6, Marcus Evans (2016, p.107) recounts the case of a young woman who felt she "had a large man sitting on top of [her] head". In fact, her father had been bullying her to get married; she experienced the stress of this as an oppressive and strange weight bearing down on her head. Relating to this fanciful person who did not harm her but only exerted some influence on her was much less irksome to her than in fact her aggressive father appeared to be.

Hallucinations

Hallucinations suffered by schizophrenic patients are usually auditory and can cause great distress if they are commands in the second person. These commands are all too often instructions to injure or maim the self, and sometimes to end life itself. A second person command can, also, paranoaically order the death of an acquaintance or a stranger. Whispering third person voices can be equally distressing, sometimes leading to paranoid thoughts and delusional ideas or schemes which, again, may have a harmful intent. Patients often have to struggle to ignore or resist auditory hallucinations.

Schizoaffective disorder compared with schizophrenia

Schizoaffective disorder is different from the illness of schizophrenia with secondary depression, and should be distinguished from it because the prognoses of the two illnesses differ. Schizoaffective disorder, consisting of mixed symptoms of schizophrenia, depression, and sometimes also mania, is a treatable disorder which usually consists of episodes of these illnesses in early adult life which then cease with treatment. Schizophrenia affects nearly all of the patient's mind and does not, itself, involve specific affective states. It can be treated, as demonstrated herein, but is even more serious an illness, and its treatment takes longer, than schizoaffective disorder. The patient may be racked with distress and pain during treatment, the price of having to address often terrible truths about their life thus far, before being able to ameliorate these. Depression can be a secondary, reactive response to the pain, distress, and the shock of having to live with schizophrenia. Its onset follows suffering from psychosis after a clear interval of time, not starting at the same time. In schizoaffective disorder the emotional life of the patient is caught up in the confusion of psychosis, accompanying it very shortly afterwards or just preceding it or emerging at the same time. Sometimes mania is superimposed upon the psychotic confusion, or may cause it. Some clinical experience bestows expertise to the clinician in distinguishing between schizophrenia and schizoaffective disorder, and frequently diagnostic clarity can only be established after the passage of time with careful observation.

Psychotic depression

The experience of intense, psychotic depression is truly terrible to live through. The world seems completely black and bleak, with no light anywhere and no relief available. The patient feels numbed, surrounded by cold facts of stark, hard, harsh walls and entrapped as in a living tomb with no way out. No human contact offers any succour, merely appearing irritating. Movement is sometimes difficult or painful, or both, so sitting quite still permits the least disturbance physically. There seems no end in sight for the patient affected in this way. Even carers have difficulty making meaningful contact at the illness' worst. Death by suicide commonly appears to be a welcome option.

Mania

Mania can be equally dangerous in a worldly sense. If the patient becomes megalomanic, euphoric, and grandiose, they may turn to wildly improbable ideas and fantasies as a defence against their depressive experiences. In this state they may make business deals and financial investments that dangerously risk their own savings and property and that of their dependents. Whole families can fall apart if the breadwinner's health subsides into chaos without restraint. This is clearly a preventable tragedy, but general practitioners and hospital staff need to be aware of its possibility in vulnerable individuals known to them. There may be a prodromal period during which the patient could be identified clinically and duly protected, sometimes by admission under a Section of the Mental Health Act. The patient should be protected from the experience of blowing a fortune irretrievably as far as ever possible; the spouse should be made aware of their partner's diagnosis and warned to take immediate steps if the picture of the patient's health changes.

Self-care

The patient with schizoaffective disorder can themselves be primed during their intervals of normality with regards to what to watch out for in their own health. This illness reverts to neutral, interim normality between psychotic episodes, with no lasting personality change or damage. Psychotic episodes of schizophrenia, by contrast, are longer and tend to be irreversibly debilitating, with a steady downward course towards chronicity. Schizoaffective episodes have a greater emotional content and lead to a better prognosis than in the case of episodes of acute schizophrenia. The normal intervals in schizoaffective disorder provide opportunities for the patient to reflect and consolidate their health and learn about their own attitudes, beliefs, tendencies, good and bad habits, and to work out ways of strengthening themselves with resilience techniques. The schizoaffective patient is fortunate in having recourse to these spells of normal lucidity during which personal strengthening can be built up. Friends, relatives, clinicians, and fellow sufferers can all help if the patient remains accessible to their offers of support. Schizophrenia sufferers do not have such helpful lucid intervals in the same way. They remain in a state of fluctuating accessibility and commonly, without help, sink lower and lower in their self-care towards destitution.

Communication difficulties

Schizophrenic and schizoaffective patients experience marked communication difficulties, especially while in the throes of a psychosis. As noted in Chapter 8, a number of authoritative psychoanalysts, Wilfred Bion (1967, pp.43-64), Richard Lucas (2009, p.6), Murray Jackson (2001, p.334) and Leslie Sohn (1999, p.15), were of the view that psychotic patients have a non-psychotic part to their minds. Using this non-psychotic part, it is possible for the patient to inter-relate at a practical level with staff and communicate their needs while on the ward. While psychotic, however, the patient tends to be in a world of their own, remote and very difficult to reach in any practical way. Psychosis can completely distort a patient's language, giving rise to word salads, neologisms, clang associations, and a wide range of incomprehensible expressions. The patient tends to try to communicate in their own idiosyncratic way; Richard Lucas described this as "the psychotic wavelength" (Lucas, 2009), and Marcus Evans has also elucidated the importance of trying to help the patient feel understood even within this bizarre mode of communication (Evans, 2016).

At this time the patient's facial expression may be distracted and their behaviour erratic. The experience of psychosis, while the patient is unable to make logical sense, is very frightening for them. The patient needs to hold on tight to their best relationships and hope that this distressing phase passes quickly. If they become too familiar over time with psychosis they can feel less distraught and thus less keen to gain good health itself; but in doing so their mental health begins to slide downwards; tolerating psychosis becomes habitual, and the drive for fighting it less acutely felt. Tolerance is necessary in order to cope with psychotic episodes, but efforts should be made by staff not to let the edge of the patient's resistance to psychosis become blunted from over-exposure to it. Efforts to maintain the patient's personality throughout their early illness should be strenuous. Staff's efforts to communicate with the patient "on the psychotic wavelength" until they can be reached non-psychotically will help this endeavour.

Isolation

The young schizophrenic or schizoaffective patient tends to be isolated in preoccupation with their thoughts whatever company surrounds them. It seems that preoccupation with painful issues and experiences prevents exchange of whatever aspects of life the patient might have in common with others. Living through the unpleasant experiences and trying to tolerate the worst symptoms leads to introversion that is hard to overcome. The patient's internal world becomes crowded with issues they try to avoid, and this takes up their spare energy, leaving little left over for interpersonal exchanges.

Schizophrenic patients often are mild and gentle people when they have lived a long time with their illness that has now become chronic. They become tolerant and benign towards others when they have become tolerant and benign towards their own symptoms. Their suffering can move the heart of an observer, and also their willingness to reach out towards friendships, when they have been helped into a social equilibrium in a therapeutic community. They sometimes have a mild sense of humour and cooperatively respond to social conventions when their needs are met.

This long term characteristic cooperation and interaction occurs when the chronic illness has been fully stabilised. These patients are often able to draw comfort from their long-term relationships with staff and other patients. Acute illness in young people, by contrast, has a very isolating effect and this remains so for many years. Its painfulness is the main reason why depression can set in and entirely prevent social involvement. This situation can lead to suicidal ideation or enactment.

Lack of sanctuary

One of the most painful aspects of schizophrenia is its unrelenting blocking of access to peace of mind. Schizoaffective patients can at least utilise their intervals of normality between psychotic episodes, which can be very helpful. Schizophrenic patients have little respite of this kind. They can benefit from a determination and drive to ameliorate the painful nature of the developmental niche they have occupied within their family of birth or childhood. They may not have a clear objective of what they want to emerge into, only a determination to leave where they have been stuck for so long. They have received some stimulus which allures them into a concept of "something better", and psychoanalytic psychotherapy, which may permit realistic access to these imagined possibilities, is given to those who appear most determined and most insightful. Many obstacles of attitude, lack of strength, confusions, unhappiness, and often anxiety may have to be overcome; but for the determined, joy may await at the end of the therapeutic road. Eventually, a university course, a marriage, coming off medication or other achievement may be undertaken and enjoyed. Once a route in to the illness has been achieved by the analyst and the patient, and a good relationship established, hard work together is the way that peace of mind can indeed be reached, a wonderful reward for the patient, and gratifying for the analyst.

CHAPTER 3
THE COST TO SOCIETY OF SCHIZOPHRENIA

The Schizophrenia Commission Report of 2012 (Andrews et al, 2012) provides a measure of the cost to society of schizophrenia according to 2010/11 prices per person with schizophrenia. It finds that the total societal cost of schizophrenia in England during the year 2010/11 is £11.8 billion; the cost to the public sector is £7.2 billion. Societal costs include those relating to excessive unemployment, premature mortality, and unpaid care; public sector costs include income tax and indirect tax (eg. VAT) forgone, and social security payments. Health and social care costs and institutional costs are common to both societal and public sector costs. The average annual cost to society is £60,000, and to the public sector is £36,000 per person with schizophrenia. In direct comparison, the cost of treating a schizophrenic patient with five sessions per week for a year of psychoanalytic psychotherapy, including six weeks' holiday, at £60 per session, would be £13,800 in addition to the usual, anticipated as diminishing, hospital accommodation costs. If with initiative, confidence, and professional expertise a patient's schizophrenia could be alleviated, the savings would be immense.

The costs of caring for schizophrenic patients include direct costs, that is inpatient hospital costs and support from community mental health teams, and unpaid care from family and friends. This unpaid care amounts to very real costs for society but has no impact on public spending. There are huge costs for society that translate into indirect costs for the public sector via loss of tax revenue. The loss of potential output is due to higher unemployment rates and premature mortality.

There are eight key cost drivers associated with schizophrenia: inpatient time, disrupted or loss of employment, disrupted education, homelessness, physical health problems, substance misuse, contact with the criminal justice system, and impact on the family. The estimated number of people with schizophrenia in England was recently uprated by NICE and found to be 197,000. The inpatient time of these patients accounted for 38% of all health, social care, and institutional costs associated with the condition, and for 21% of all public sector costs. The cost of a night in a mental health inpatient bed is £321 (Curtis, 2011). The median length of admission is thirty-eight days, so the estimated cost of an admission is £12,198 per admission. Formal admissions, under a Section of the Mental Health Act, are longer than the thirty-eight day average.

The employment rate for all adults aged sixteen to sixty-five years in England is 71%. For schizophrenic patients the employment rate is 5-15%; at an averaged 18% rate for both direct (income tax) and indirect (VAT) tax, £715 million of tax revenue is lost through schizophrenic patients' unemployment, ie. £5,500 per service user per annum, in addition to payments of social security benefits. Schizophrenic patients' education is also usually disrupted to some extent by their condition. Only 27.4% of schizophrenic patients return to an undergraduate degree following onset of their illness.

33% of schizophrenic patients have been homeless at some stage. 13% have actually been roofless at some time during their illness. This lack of care and support leads to considerable physical health problems for them. The age-adjusted all-cause mortality rate for people with schizophrenia is 2.58 times higher than for the general population (Saha et al. 2007). Clinical records show that among a sample of 1.7 million people, 61% of people with schizophrenia smoked compared with 33% of people without schizophrenia. 33% of schizophrenic people were obese whereas only 21% of people without schizophrenia were obese (Hippisley-Cox and Pringle, 2005). Some medications, for example especially olanzapine, can precipitate obesity in its users. Substance misuse is common in schizophrenia sufferers and may have serious consequences. Alcohol misuse occurs at a rate of 26% in those with schizophrenia compared with 11.9% of those in the general population. All other substance abuse affects 17.8% of schizophrenic people compared with 7.0% in the general population. These physically self-damaging habits of schizophrenic patients add to the costs to their own lives of their mental illness.

Contact with the criminal justice system affects a proportion of sufferers. However, Fazel and colleagues found that the elevated risk of someone with schizophrenia committing a violent crime can be almost entirely accounted for by the high levels of substance abuse in this group (Fazel et al, 2009a). It was found that this co-morbidity leads to a risk of committing a violent crime that is increased from that in the general population by a factor of 4.4 (95% CI: 3.9 – 5.0). By comparison, individuals who had schizophrenia but did not abuse substances had an elevated risk of just 1.2 greater (95% CI: 1.1 – 1.4). A recent systematic review (Fazel et al, 2009b) confirmed these findings. Violent crime causes economic and social costs totalling £44.6 billion per year in England and Wales (a Home Office estimate in 2005). 8% of the prison population has psychosis, and 2% of prisoners have schizophrenia. These figures compare with 0.2 - 0.5% having psychosis or schizophrenia in the general household population (Singleton et al, 2000; Saha et al, 2005; Mangalore and Knapp, 2007). The contemporary annual cost of a prison place is £40,000 (Ministry of Justice, 2011), but this expenditure is remarkably ineffective at preventing reoffending.

The financial cost to the family of a schizophrenic member is very considerable. 4.8% of carers had terminated their employment to provide care and support for their dependent relative (Mangalore and Knapp, 2007). 15.5% took a mean of 12.5 days off work per year specifically because of being a carer. This was a mean annual economic loss to them of £517 at 2011/12 prices. A mean of 5.6 hours of support per day is given to schizophrenic patients, which is equivalent to £34,000 per person with schizophrenia being cared for by a family member per year. 31% of schizophrenic patients are living in private households, which could be evaluated as an aggregate cost to society of as much as £1.24 billion per year.

The economic output of schizophrenia sufferers is greatly decreased because the illness adversely affects their capacity for cognition and understanding, and undermines their autonomy. Their ability to engage with other staff at a place of employment is likely to be affected by their introversion, which may cause them to become isolated, and they may consequently need tailored training in social skills to relate comfortably to their work colleagues. Practical skills can be taught by their employer, thus utilising their learning ability, and they may become able to accept responsibility and take initiative for projects.

Quite apart from financial considerations in relation to how the schizophrenic individual copes with the world, the cost to themselves of their illness is terrible to contemplate. They endure a much lesser degree of competency in their level of engaging with the world than if they were well. This affects their self-regard, self-compassion, and self-esteem. They must accept every last detail and effect of their lesser functioning. It can be a miserable realisation for them, and yet to survive they must remain on good terms with the world. If they are treated promptly at the time of their first episode then most of their personality can be rescued and preserved. This bodes well for their future. Their determination to help themselves must be enlisted, and the cost to themselves in terms of lost opportunities, achievements, and skills tolerated with as good grace as they can summon up. If they find their outlook too much to manage, especially at the time of onset of their symptoms, they may feel depressed and may actually develop a full-blown secondary depression. At this time particularly they are in great need of psychological resuscitation by the clinical staff tending them. It may appear to them that every hour that passes is intolerable, so how on earth are they going to survive the rest of their life?

Their organising skills are likely to be poor, which otherwise they could employ to help themselves re-engage with what their life situation offers them as it stands at the moment. The acute onset stage of illness precludes every consideration other than the patient reconciling themselves to their present moments and learning to tolerate the experiences they are living through. These may be very harsh and frightening. The cost to their peace of mind is swingeing, and this will continue for the foreseeable future. Loved ones are needed like never before, with encouragement towards patience, trusting communication with those around them, and any spiritual benefits available such as music, artwork, and the hospital chapel. Occupational therapy in the hospital can be of tremendous assistance in picking up the patient's self-belief.

Hope is commonly a costly casualty when a person develops schizophrenia. The patient may feel sure that they will never again experience their own independence in an adjusted experience of life. This may be a devastating blow. Their inclination is to curl up in a ball and shut the world out. But they cannot escape the contents of their mind, so they require help to address its terrible pain. Life becomes confined to the ward and practical issues like the next meal or whether or not they will have a visitor that day. As the weeks go by, the patient's perspective expands to include any green spaces around the hospital where they could walk and get some exercise, and to where they will live when they leave hospital. There is also the question of work, and the Social Services department may be able to help with work experience in relation to the patient's preparedness to apply themselves, given the opportunity to get their life back with whatever means is open to them. Loss of mental ability or personal capacity for some kinds of work will lie heavily with the patient. Disappointment must not, however, be allowed to prevent them from doing what they are capable of doing once their mind grows back together, collecting all the good remnants that have survived the onslaught of the illness. Psychoanalytic psychotherapy for the lucky ones, CBT for some, family therapy for all who need it, social skills therapy, anticipatory pleasure skills training to help motivation, avatar therapy for those who are hearing disturbing voices, and local supportive ventures for rehabilitation can all be helpful when appropriately applied; therapies of many kinds can help the patient counter the losses they have sustained from their illness in an optimistic but measured way, and can help them develop accordingly from the good nature that is left in them and that can be utilised to move forward into new areas of life.

The patient themself is responsible for nurturing their own determination and quality of mind. They can feel crestfallen at what has happened to them. It is a big blow to their self-belief and self-esteem to find themselves spending long periods of time in a mental hospital. The costs to the self of mental illness, and especially one as severe as schizophrenia, are almost so severe as to necessitate the patient regrowing their mind from scratch (see Chapter 5 describing patient recovery) in therapy. Before therapy, the patient feels that while they can remember details of their past life they are not capable of understanding themselves or, particularly in relation to responses and reactions to other people, why actually they have repeatedly collapsed at work or experienced their serious symptoms, or what they can do about this. They are completely dependent on their therapists to guide them; all they can do is be obedient to the ward staff, and listen to everything that is going on from which they can learn. This costs time, and effort, and goodwill. But it is the best endeavour that the patient could possibly find available to them, because it is understanding that the patient lacks in sufficient quantity and that leads to the massive misunderstanding that is schizophrenia. No matter how this arose, perhaps tacit assumptions where they grew up that prevented normal growth, or particularly distressing experiences, the patient learns to use their mind. When a mind first breaks down it has completely stopped functioning for the first time. The forces acting upon it throughout the past have aggregated sufficiently to cause functional block. This is indicated on the triangular model of the PPCC construct in schizophrenia (see Chapter 8 and Figure 10b). This is the ultimate cost to the patient of schizophrenia: the cost of non-functioning of their mind. Perhaps it is a biological mechanism for preventing excessive pain; instead, the mind detaches from reality and engages in fantasy or psychosis to protect itself from the harshness of reality. It has been said that the survival value of schizophrenia is to protect enemy soldiers who are committing atrocities from being aware of what they are doing. Not every patient is behaving like that. But schizophrenia could be nature's way of protecting a mind from unbearable unpleasantness. It is a high price to pay for having to try to develop among unbearable unpleasantness.

The human cost of schizophrenic illness to the family is also, often, considerable. The family of a schizophrenic person usually suffers deeply, like the patient themselves. There is often a sense of guilt and responsibility. But sometimes the word "illness" is used ubiquitously in the family to explain why the patient's problems are nothing to do with anyone else. This can be maintained even when a serious event such as a molestation in the family that is known about is swept under the carpet and never referred to by the unacknowledging parent or the perpetrator. The past is gone. Other siblings should not be bothered by unpleasant knowledge. This knowledge is a high cost paid by the patient so that family life can continue undisturbed. Staff in mental hospital wards are familiar with issues like these, and are trained in how to nurse patients who have fallen victim to such occurrences.

Families of schizophrenic patients are often equally disturbed and distressed in other ways, additionally. They may simply not know how to relate to their afflicted family member. They may try very hard to accommodate their own feelings so that these do not impinge on the already complex situation around the patient; or emotion may be liberally expressed among the family members. Unaffected siblings may experience difficulty enjoying their own health when the patient is clearly so troubled. They may worry about themselves, wondering whether they, too, will develop schizophrenia, the terrible illness that they observe their brother or sister having to endure. Unhappy memories from a time before the condition was diagnosed may give them guilt feelings about a preferable kinder approach that could have been demonstrated to the one who is now sick. These young family members, inexperienced in life, may develop a troubled self-image, rightly or wrongly, due to worrying about their ill brother or sister. Their own self-esteem, self-confidence, and achievements may be set aside while they try to adjust to the illness in the family, wondering how much of it is due to their own behaviour and attitudes. They may experience prejudice from other people, the neighbours or school classmates, or they may live through stranger abuse, victimisation or bullying by people they hardly know in the street. Their own stamina and self-efficacy may suffer from their situation and the unfortunate turn their lives have taken. The parents tend to respond to the new knowledge that their son or daughter is seriously ill either with denial, being unable to assimilate the news, or with great concern and a fear of not being able to do enough to adjust the family to coping effectively and to assist the patient adequately. Over time the situation becomes steadier. But the family's usual level of functioning can be drastically affected by the diagnosis, even though the parents may have suspected something was wrong for some time, possibly a number of years. The diagnosis may then come as no surprise, but the arrangements that subsequently have to be made nonetheless amount to a huge cost to the family's life together. The burden of caring for the suffering family member commonly amounts to a heavy toll emotionally, physically, and in terms of making appropriate arrangements on a daily basis to accommodate the patient's needs. Other siblings' needs may temporarily not be met due to the focus on the young person suddenly taken ill.

In England, in approximately 2002, the cost of premature mortality, much of which was due to suicide, was £562 million (Wasserman and Wasserman, 2009, p. 360). In Scotland at approximately this time, the average cost of each completed suicide was £1.29 million (Platt et al, 2006). These financial figures relate to the suicides of fit, otherwise healthy adults, and of course schizophrenic patients are not often the main breadwinner in a family. But the death of a loved schizophrenic member of the family can still be a dreadful loss, and a heavy emotional cost for the rest of the family to bear as a consequence of schizophrenic illness. Unaffected siblings may suffer from guilt feelings relating to previous incidents when the undefended patient came off worst. The effects of schizophrenia can extend beyond the patient's concerns as a family member to their close family members' entire lives outside the home, and all at a very heavy cost to each individual.

CHAPTER 4

ORGANIC ASPECTS OF SCHIZOPHRENIC ILLNESS AND ITS TREATMENT

Schizophrenia is primarily a psychological condition, but it also frequently has physical concomitants. There is a need therefore to observe physical changes and care equally for these physical aspects in order to preserve patients' lives.

Schizophrenic patients may have minor physical abnormalities such as hypertelorism, an enlarged gap between the first and second toes, which are not, however, detrimental to their lives. These changes suggest intrauterine hindrances to normal development, which could perhaps extend to contemporaneous differences in intrauterine brain development. Other changes such as tremor unrelated to medication may be affected by genetic or environmental factors.

Abnormal foetal growth and development such as low birth weight, congenital malformations and reduced head circumference appear to be more common in schizophrenic patients who become ill at an early age, but with no relationship to any family history of schizophrenia or gender specificity (Verdoux et al, 1997). Perinatal hypoxia is implicated in some studies (Cannon et al, 2002), the hippocampus being particularly vulnerable to hypoxia and thus adversely affected during stressful births of this kind. Hypoxic damage to the hippocampus causes enhanced dopaminergic sensitivity in the nucleus accumbens, part of the mesolimbic system, which is also affected by hypoxic damage to the medial prefrontal cortex (Williamson, 2006). Schizophrenic patients manifest a similar mesolimbic dopaminergic hyper responsivity, which becomes the rationale for anti-D2 receptor medications for the treatment of schizophrenia. Winter births are unusually common among schizophrenic patients, but the explanation for this remains unknown.

Intrauterine development is adversely affected by maternal starvation (Williamson, 2006, p.36). Schizophrenia's incidence is increased under these conditions. Evidence for this is to be found in careful medical notes taken by the Dutch authorities when, during World War II, the Nazis deliberately starved the Dutch occupants of several cities they besieged. Two investigations of the data obtained (Susser and Lin, 1992; Susser et al, 1996) revealed an increase in the incidence of schizophrenia associated with these patients' maternal malnutrition.

Genetic factors are very strongly influential in the incidence of schizophrenia. Family members may manifest related conditions such as schizotypal personality disorder and schizoaffective disorder as well as schizophrenia itself. Heritability is in the range 60%-90% (Kendler et al, 1993), (Cardno and Gottesman, 2000), (Ingraham and Kety, 2000), and the risk is increased ten times in a first-degree relative to 10% (from 1% in the general population), and to 50% in identical twins.

The EEG contains very low-voltage changes within the first 400 milliseconds following a stimulus. It is possible to record an Event-Related Potential (ERP) associated with the stimulus. ERPs at the positions P50 and P300 on EEGs are affected in schizophrenic patients. Early components vary with the physical properties of the stimulus, whereas late components (particularly P300) reflect cognitive processes associated with the stimulus. The P50 is measured by presenting two auditory stimuli 500ms apart. Of these, schizophrenic patients when tested fail to suppress the second tone, unlike non-schizophrenic subjects. In schizophrenia, too, the amplitude of the P300 ERP is reduced, although P300 abnormalities are also found in other conditions such as dementia, alcoholism, and major depression (Friedman and Squires-Wheeler, 1994). Overall, ERP studies suggest that schizophrenic patients have difficulty distinguishing relevant stimuli worthy of attention from irrelevant stimuli (Williamson, 2006, pp. 62, 125).

Studies involving pre-pulse inhibition suggest that in schizophrenia there is a widespread failure to suppress the startle response. If a weak pre-pulse precedes a startling stimulus, the response to the startling stimulus is reduced in normal subjects, but not in schizophrenia. This phenomenon has similarities to schizophrenic patients' failure to suppress the second of two auditory stimuli presented closely together (as above). Both of these characteristics may be related to defective sensorimotor gating at the subcortical level (Freedman et al, 1987).

Antipsychotic medications characteristically have significant side-effects that adversely affect the patients taking them (Rang et al, 2012, p. 560). Extrapyramidal symptoms (EPS) are the most characteristic side-effects of antipsychotic medications. They arise due to dopamine D2 receptor blockade in the nigrostriatal pathway, which arises as a side-effect when D2 receptors in the psychosis-mediating mesolimbic pathway are deliberately blocked with the antipsychotic medication. Extrapyramidal side-effects consist of acute dystonias, which are involuntary movements such as akathisia (restlessness), tardive dyskinesia (lip smacking and movements of the trunk and limbs), symptoms of Parkinson's disease such as tremors at rest, hypokinesia eg. difficulty initiating walking, with a shuffling, festinant gait and then difficulty stopping, cogwheel muscular rigidity, and some cognitive impairment. The extrapyramidal side-effects tend to decrease within a few weeks of starting the medication, but anticholinergic drugs are commonly required to counteract them at the start of antipsychotic drug therapy.

Unwanted endocrine side-effects of antipsychotic medications include breast swelling and lactation from increased prolactin levels, sometimes occurring in men as well as in women. Drowsiness and sedation can occur, especially early in the drug treatment of psychosis, but tend to decrease gradually. A change in antipsychotic medication may resolve these issues.

Increases in weight and in the incidence of cardiovascular disease and diabetes are very undesirable side-effects of antipsychotic medications, but regularly develop from the time of commencement of treatment with atypical antipsychotics as much as with the older typical antipsychotic medications. Agranulocytosis is a serious side effect most commonly associated with clozapine, which then should be immediately withdrawn. Neuroleptic malignant syndrome rarely occurs but is a potentially dangerous idiosyncratic reaction that needs prompt treatment with bromocriptine or apomorphine.

The possibility of metabolic physical side effects of antipsychotic medications, such as weight gain and the possibility or reality of diabetes and cardiovascular disease, needs careful vigilance or, if present, monitoring by the general practitioner. The life span of schizophrenic patients is fifteen to twenty years less than their non-schizophrenic contemporaries, so all due care must be provided to them wherever possible. Continuity of care can be difficult to provide if they are peripatetic, but in this instance full assessments should be done at every opportunity when they do present themselves for a check-up. They require intensive management and support at community level to prevent escalation requiring hospital treatment.

Lithium carbonate can be very effective in stabilising the mood of schizoaffective patients while they are undergoing psychoanalytic psychotherapy. Christopher Baethge's review (Baethge, 2007) of the long-term psychopharmacological treatment of schizoaffective disorder is still one of the most authoritative sources of information available on this subject. The long-term psychopharmacological treatment of schizoaffective disorder recommended by Baethge consists of lithium carbonate and carbamazepine for patients experiencing mainly affective episodes, and antipsychotics, especially olanzapine, although this tends to cause weight gain, for patients mainly experiencing schizophrenic episodes (Marneros and Akiskal, 2007). Alternatively, to combine antipsychotic management with affective symptom control, risperidone may prove a useful choice in combination with lithium carbonate, together with an anticholinergic such as procyclidine if required.

Once medication that stabilises the patient's symptoms has been established, the psychoanalytic treatment may proceed and allow the patient's past and present mind itself to be what both the patient and the analyst try to fathom. Extremes of self-reinforcing mood, whether depression or elation, are not helpful if they incapacitate the patient; these mental states may be contrasted clinically with contextual anger or disappointment which needs to be analysed. Psychiatric training is necessary to make accurate ongoing clinical psychoanalytic decisions in these situations with a potentially psychotic patient. A skilled psychiatrically trained psychoanalyst is in a position to link the patient's moods to what is currently under consideration in the consulting room, and to discuss his or her views regarding medication with the patient's ward consultant who has his own perspective of the patient's progress, as referred to by Dr Michael Robbins in Case Study 2 (see Part V herein). As Dr Robbins holds, when the role of medication is understood, it can be both necessary in allowing the analysis to continue, and extremely useful in facilitating optimal use of the psychoanalytic sessions by the patient. Not infrequently the patient requires both a psychoanalysis, that can be visualized, and also lifelong medication, in order for them to gain sufficient insight and self-knowledge to continue their life independently; and in a National Health Schedule for Schizophrenia the aim would be to make these two arms of treatment available to all those patients who could benefit from them, with this opportunity in view.

Schizophrenic patients consume alcohol and drugs and smoke much more than non-schizophrenic people (see Chapter 3). Their smoking levels are double, their alcoholism levels and substance abuse levels are more than double, and their obesity levels increased by 50%, compared with the mentally fit average. It is believed, as referred to above, that defective gating at the subcortical level prevents schizophrenic patients from being able to suppress the second of two tones 500 ms apart. This defect can be genetically transmitted in association with a variant of the a7 nicotinic acetylcholine receptor subunit gene (Leonard et al, 2002). Nicotine itself reverses the defect, and this calming effect may explain why so many schizophrenic patients are so addicted to cigarette smoking (Williamson, 2006, p. 62).

Schizophrenic patients have low self-esteem in general, little hope, little to look forward to, and very little to depend upon to meet their needs. Their self-discipline, motivation, and anticipatory pleasure skills tend to be at rock bottom when they reach a chronic state of illness, so they have very little incentive to keep to any programme of self-improvement. It is hard for them to see any benefit for themselves in adhering to a self-management programme even if this is drawn up with their input. Improvements in diet, cigarette and alcohol moderation, and exercising activities do not appeal to their sense of survival. Because of their introversion they establish links with others with difficulty, and with equal difficulty are barely able to sustain them. So isolation from others, including from help with their health at clinics they are encouraged to attend by welcoming staff, is the nature of their survival pattern.

These are the main physical issues faced by patients suffering from chronic schizophrenia. The objective in treating schizophrenia is to reach young people as soon as they manifest psychotic symptoms, catch and retain as much of their personality as possible, bring the patient to a state of acceptance, and begin psychoanalytic psychotherapy early, long before breakdown of their physical health becomes a possibility. Rescue of their mind enables them to think their own way to physical self-preservation through a good diet, exercise, and avoidance of excessive alcohol, nicotine or other dangerous substances. Much has been learned about the damage schizophrenia characteristically does to its sufferers, so clinicians' intention needs to be to help the patient find their mind without delay and find a life where they can use it to preserve themselves from undue physical or mental schizophrenic decline.

These physical and psychological characteristics of schizophrenic patients are mainly those of the chronic illness; if patients are not helped adequately at the time of onset of illness they tend to slide into this chronic state if they don't tragically end their own lives. It is clear that early intervention is essential to prevent these debilitating secondary effects of schizophrenic illness; resuscitation from the acute throes needs to be followed by a period of stability, and then engagement of the patient's mind in active, productive, motivating therapy to stimulate and strengthen their own initiative regarding the one life they have, to make the most of it. Younger patients are often only too pleased to have this opportunity. Others may be too cowed by their illness to overcome self-doubt and flourish in this way. But every patient should be given their chance, ideally in a National Health Schedule for Schizophrenia, to think optimally using psychoanalytic psychotherapy, or other stimulating and enlightening talking therapy.

What is believed to be the organic basis for the underpinning of schizophrenia's psychological effects, ie. dopaminergic hyperactivity in the nucleus accumbens and hypo activity in the prefrontal cortex, due to NMDA receptor hypofunction, thus needs to be considered in the context of all these features; and then, all attention given to understanding how they are experienced.

CHAPTER 5

THE NEED FOR EFFECTIVE REMEDIAL THERAPY FOR SCHIZOPHRENIA

The humanitarian consideration that every human in need should be helped hardly requires introduction or expansion. In the UK we are particularly fortunate that, as far as our health goes, every human in need has a statutory right to be helped, with a view towards them helping themselves as far as possible.

Yet schizophrenic patients are a group of humans who collectively have remained sorely in need, and this seems so in spite of decades of efforts to direct aid and assistance specifically towards them. It appears that we have not known how best we can help them, given that large numbers of this population stolidly remain on our streets, inhabiting hostels only reluctantly, drifting and scavenging when robust help with accommodation, nourishment, and support could be accessed. They seem to like their independence more than comfort and security.

The minds of the drifters have long ago been lost to the wayside. But acutely psychotically ill young adults still retain their personalities. Work by Early Intervention Services has shown beyond doubt (described by The Schizophrenia Commission, 2012) that, if these young adults can be engaged fully by skilled clinicians, they often prove able to talk their way through the early psychosis, perhaps with the help of some medication, into identifying helpful measures that can be adopted by themselves and caring family and friends. Retaining the goodwill and trust of such patients is a skill. The patients are nearly always very frightened about what is happening to them. They crave security and comfort at this stage. It is clear that in a general way the work of Early Intervention Services must be followed by continuous intensive care and treatment for a further period if its good results are to have long-term effectiveness in the patients' lives. Those patients who strike out on their own independently create great concern and require careful management because if they become over-assertive they can prove a danger to themselves and to others. These are cases where sedation is clearly required and which cause considerable management difficulties.

Schizophrenia affects many aspects of the personality of the patient. Her determination and initiative suffer. Her self-efficacy and self-compassion disappear. Her sense of optimism, hope for the future, sociability, anticipatory pleasure skills regarding tangible and intangible rewards, her creativity, her ability to commit herself to any person or cause, and her courage all fall by the wayside. Her sense of shared ethics and compassion for others, her sense of common humanity and of self-worth, of love for her fellow man and woman, and her appreciation of others are lost. Her sense of enjoyment of life for its own sake, all hobbies and interests and aesthetic sense are completely overcome by her dismay at her own overwhelming need and despair.

Schizophrenic illness breaks down self-efficacy into two main groups: one group experiences being overly dependent on others, and the other refuses to be dependent on anyone else in any way. Finding a middle way becomes possible only after considerable interaction with staff on a hospital ward or at a mental health centre, when the individual's needs have been examined and discussed with her, and a plan acceptable to her drawn up. Every schizophrenic patient is a unique person with his or her own personality and characteristics as well as having a diagnosis common to many, and clinicians are aware that every patient's particular combination of symptoms also marks him or her out as having unique diagnostic characteristics. The response of every individual to his or her particular combination of problems also varies from that of other individuals; a very wide range of problems, responses, and symptoms all occur among those patients considered to fit a diagnosis of "schizophrenia", so sensitivity about how the patient regards aspects of her particular situation is always needed when making any assumptions or reaching for any conclusions about treatment for her.

Their profound neediness and the extreme difficulty of understanding them makes schizophrenia sufferers difficult for the public at large to relate to them. Turning away, ridicule, fascination, pain, kind gestures or major attempts to reach out towards them all feature much more prevalently among the public's responses than does indifference. That it is so common, with around 1% of the population suffering from it, makes the reality of the suffering it causes, and its sufferers as people, impossible to ignore. Undoubtedly, every mentally well person will at some time have worried about his or her mental health and then been extremely relieved to find that in a general way they are actually quite mentally fit. Mostly this experience has the effect of generosity towards those afflicted, leading to the provision of wider assistance becoming available for those suffering.

So with the rejection of offered help, the undoubted loss of mental function which becomes permanent and chronic if not treated early, the considerable difficulties of helping and treating early illness, the intense neediness of schizophrenia sufferers, and the extreme difficulty of understanding them, what is to be done about resolving the impact this illness has on patients, their families and friends, the public, and the many different kinds of costs and losses it causes to society?

The best plan to alleviate all these aspects of difficulty that schizophrenia causes would be to "Catch them before they fall", the title of a book by Christopher Bollas (Bollas, 2013), so that each case of schizophrenic illness would become resolved into a treatment path that could direct and help the patient positively in a gradual upward, forward direction. In this supervised kind of plan each patient would be prevented from coming to a catastrophic "stop!" in her life, but would be helped forwards at her own pace towards her best adjustment to what has befallen her. Her goodwill could be fostered at an early stage, familiarity together with realism and optimism about the illness conclusively accepted, and steady encouragement offered in outpatients once the initial acute phase has been successfully endured.

This leaves the long-standing, chronic cases to be helped as much as the patients will allow. Services exist which remove people from the streets and place them temporarily in accommodation, but the homeless have to respond to help themselves if they are going to live fulfilling lives in any sense. Those who do respond occasionally thrive subsequent to the unfortunate ordeal that made them homeless. But mentally ill people such as those suffering from schizophrenia cannot constructively help themselves to any very competent extent, and although they are expected to respond to help offered, returning to the streets apparently enables what part of their mind does function to sustain themselves at this level. This part cannot bear to be trampled by other people's rules and regulations and requirements. And so a revolving door policy does generally operate with this population, where they return temporarily for succour when they feel completely and desperately needy, only to leave again to face their destitution when they have revived somewhat. Perhaps the best that can be done for them is to make sure they know where and how to receive the help they need, when they feel they need it.

Society's provisions for schizophrenic and other mentally ill patients who are unable to significantly help themselves due to their illness are grouped according to the patients' styles of self-management. Hostels offering temporary accommodation and staffed by wardens, social workers, and charity workers and other staff provide some provisional safety and security, and keep a proportion of schizophrenic patients off the streets for some duration. It is often the police who initially collect rough sleepers and take them to hostels, and though some are kindly mannered, sometimes police need to be much kinder to the rough sleepers who may be suffering from schizophrenia or another mental illness. Police cells and prisons are the wrong places for the mentally ill, who are taken there sometimes because they are suspected of committing an offence, but often because there is nowhere else for them to be taken in the first instance. There is not a simple answer for their plight. These mentally ill vagrants need accommodating, reviewing and treating; and then encouraging, and given a forward-looking plan they agree with, for rehabilitating them once any sentence, reprimand or caution has been implemented, if appropriate; otherwise, their illness will prevent completely the effectiveness of any formal rebuke, and their illness is likely to degenerate. Probation officers and wardens need to be creative in engaging with the patients, and give them a second opportunity at life, supporting them in their new roles. And as it is, care in hospitals is already orientated towards doing all that can be done for chronically ill schizophrenia sufferers, involving community placements and as much supervision as the patients need to meet their own levels of self-care.

It is unfortunately the case that young adults whose first episode of psychosis has been resolved in a positive way by a clinical Early Intervention Service sometimes then find themselves struggling to progress forwards in a positive way. They are orientated mostly in terms of reality, but their cognitive functions will have suffered from their illness, they have fallen out of their original stream of life, and are now having difficulty in orientating themselves again, positively, back into their life-flow. They may have fallen out of education or employment, and lost touch with their friends and main peer group. What is to be done?

Only by finding answers to the questions thus far unformed in their minds can this group of schizophrenic patients resolve the issues lying underneath and behind their schizophrenia syndrome. They don't know where to begin in helping themselves. They do need help to begin being able to use their minds again; and this help can be provided by psychoanalytic psychotherapy. Analytic treatment suggests to them the questions they need to ask themselves, so that by providing their own answers they can resolve their own, schizophrenic conundrums so unkindly presented to them by their early experiences. Early developmental experiences have not been understood, and so, with an Analyst's help, the meaning of these experiences to the patient can be gently explored with her, for her own consideration and evaluation. Thus the patient's sense of how she used to feel in comparison to how she feels now is mutually developed, and she is thereby helped to gain a sense of herself, for clarification and ongoing growth.

When the patient finds her own meaning within her past experiences she begins to find a self-identity. With psychoanalytic psychotherapy this self-identity can even develop into becoming intact, and the patient therefore becomes so much more robustly able to function as an individual.

If all young adults with a recent first psychotic episode now resolved into stability were assessed, and then those deemed most suitable were given this opportunity of psychoanalytic psychotherapy, a cohort of recovered schizophrenic patients might be returned to the economy. Careful patient selection is key to the success of this element of the National Health Schedule for Schizophrenia. All the young adults with a schizophrenic illness could be considered for psychoanalytic psychotherapy, and those who proved to have sufficient potential would be offered it. Those who had not demonstrated application, high intelligence, patience, a good nature, or a willingness to work hard, and a determination to help themselves would be offered other, more suitable, treatments within the National Health Schedule for Schizophrenia. But those who were prepared to work hard for their health should be given this opportunity as being equivalent medically to cardiac patients for whom only a heart transplant or coronary bypass operation will save their life. Young adult first-episode psychosis patients have minds that are at death's door. Their minds will fail, like a car's engine, unless given the succour of paced, nurturing mental exercise such as is provided in an active psychoanalytic psychotherapy treatment. They need to be helped to "use their minds", work out for themselves why their minds became so weak: what was it about their past that they really couldn't stand? What did they hate the most? What change would they like to see in their life? What is stopping them from making this change?

Their analyst's perspicacity would enable him or her to broach these issues with the patient in such a way as to initiate self-scrutiny and critical thinking. Starting to think constructively can be a painful business for a schizophrenic patient, for to do so opens up the terrible realities of her life and experiences into her conscious awareness, something she has been blocking out for the anaesthetic properties of doing so. But gentle persistence and support, as illustrated in Case Studies 1 and 2, Parts IV and

V herein, can be understood as the means whereby the analyst can indeed support the patient while she works at her tasks. It takes time, finance, and all the personal attributes enumerated above. But the potential rewards are tremendous, and with the high prevalence of schizophrenia (1% of the population) even the small proportion of young adult patients deemed suitable for psychoanalytic psychotherapy amount to very many people for whom effective treatment would make a fundamental difference. A greater enthusiasm is needed to treat all schizophrenic patients effectively with the most suitable treatments for them each as an individual, and to train psychiatrists in psychoanalysis so that this intensely skilled therapy becomes more widely available for these very needful patients. There is no reason why this talking therapy should not take its place as a standard treatment for this group of patients within today's standard psychiatric care. Medication would be prescribed and used as needed, but the emphasis would be on enabling the patients to learn to use their minds in understanding themselves, finding their own meaning for themselves in their lives, and fostering a positive outlook on the world around them. Good morale in the treatment settings and skilled treatment will enable these patients to make the best of themselves even after such a shock as being diagnosed with schizophrenia.

CHAPTER 6

PSYCHIATRIC HELP FOR PATIENTS WITH "REACTIVE" SCHIZOPHRENIA

Schizophrenia is thus a severely distressing, long-term, commonly incapacitating condition. Traditionally, since the 1960s, phenothiazines and then atypical neuroleptics have provided the mainstay of psychiatric treatment. These drugs help to banish psychotic symptoms and thus convince doctors that the patient's illness has remitted, that they feel better, they can think more clearly, and that psychiatric medicine has worked. For decades, this process has served the NHS well. A revolving door policy has been applied for those who relapse intermittently.

Susan Hingley writes about "a small subgroup of sufferers fulfilling DSM-III-R criteria for schizophrenia who can respond to intensive, often long-term, psychodynamically-oriented psychotherapy… These may well be individuals who have a high loading on environmental and/or traumatogenic origins to their vulnerability, and rather less genetic predisposition" (Hingley, 2006). Here Hingley is distinguishing between "reactive" schizophrenic illness, where she says the patient is reacting to external influences, and "process" schizophrenic illness, where the patient experiences endogenous development of confusion primarily due to constitutional factors. Psychiatry consultants are well placed to discern this difference in their newly-presenting patients, which may relate to the intensity or otherwise of affective symptoms and also the relative proportions of positive and negative symptoms (a greater presence of affective and positive symptoms generally augurs well for progress in psychotherapy). Those patients who have indeed suffered early abuse but are otherwise essentially psychologically intact will be grateful lifelong to a psychiatrist who gives them the chance to reverse these effects of their early terrible adversity.

It is well-known that environmental adversity in childhood can severely affect mental health in adulthood. In a study of adult outpatient schizophrenia sufferers 35% had suffered emotional abuse as children, 42% physical neglect, and 73% emotional neglect (Holowka et al, 2003). Among 139 female outpatients, 78% of those diagnosed "schizophrenic" had suffered child sexual abuse (Friedman et al, 2002). These environmental influences prevented normal development due to the children's reactions to them as they tried to grow up. Few psychiatrists doubt the importance of a patient's early experiences in the aetiology of their illness, or in shaping the nature of their symptoms.

An adult patient's difficulty may actually be revealed by examining the exact nature of their symptoms. For example, if a child has been sexually molested in their bed in the silence and darkness of the night, their mind may not be able to process this horror; it may emerge later, no longer repressed but rather released into conscious awareness by current adult experiences of a related emotional nature, such as active student life. An adult illness might present, in such a case, as a sleep paralysis hallucinatory experience of a black psychopath outside their window (representing in psychoanalytic terms the spectacles behind which this perceived horror of a mind was operating in the dark), once again terrifyingly trying to control them as they lie in their bed in the darkness. The molester may thus eventually be hallucinated as a fantastical terror, following a trigger experience; just prior to breakdown, another real person who also wore similar spectacles and who the patient, in their extreme anxiety, becomes afraid of, may simply look like the father and be behaving in a hostile manner to the mother in a similar way to how the hated father behaved towards her, which had led to divorce on grounds of mental cruelty. The anger and fear aroused by the father becomes transferred by projection on to the mother's unpleasant work colleague who had caused the mother difficulties at work, in case he, too, should assault the patient. This becomes a trigger symptom of the developing illness that is based upon fear and dislike of the person who terrifyingly mistreated the patient as a child, to such an extent as to cause the patient's mind and brain to dysfunction. Thus this symptom of transferred projection may unconsciously, in the patient's great anxiety which was blocking fresh, appealing student feelings, be illustrating to the patient the possibility of further danger to themselves, sufficient to cause breakdown from this psychic conflict.

In their 2013 paper "The Psychodynamics of Psychosis" (Martindale and Summers, 2013a), Brian Martindale and Alison Summers illustrate some common alternative responses other than hallucinations that the human mind may adopt in order to address the severe psychic pain of unpleasant realities. Their examples include several instances of delusional thinking, rather than hallucination as in the above example. In some of their cases, delusional symptoms reflect the patient's painful reality, but in a muted form rather than in a repetition of the original horror as in a hallucination. More than twenty examples are offered in Martindale's and Summers' paper, showing how patients' minds may find an alternative "new reality" that is easier to tolerate than the original painful truth. Hallucination, by contrast, may simply be a new expression of the original fear. But as "patches" that the psychotic mind uses to cover areas of intense psychic pain, delusions and delusional systems soften parts of the patient's experience which otherwise would dominate their mind destructively; the patient can live with this lesser pain more tolerably. As also mentioned in Chapter 2 herein, Marcus Evans, in his book "Making Room for Madness in Mental Health" (Evans, 2016), cites the case of a young woman who was admitted to a psychiatric ward complaining of "a large man sitting on top of [her] head". In fact, her father had been bullying her to get married, and she apparently found this fanciful person less irksome than her aggressive father in the way he was behaving towards her. Enlightening her about this plausible substitution in her preoccupations helped to calm her. It may be that hallucinations starkly re-present trauma in another graphic form whereas delusional thinking is the mind's way of producing a more tolerable version of unpleasant or traumatic realities.

These examples illustrate how the patient may be better understood, and their subsequent welfare greatly improved through clarification of the focus of their illness, by applying psychodynamic principles when the patient first presents with their psychotic symptoms. The patient has become ill when their mind can no longer address the adverse realities challenging them. As Martindale and Summers point out, both internal and external realities may contribute to the patient's collapse when these become too intensely challenging, unpleasant or painful, causing the appearance of hallucinations or delusions. This fresh appearance of new psychological phenomena is a good point of entry for interpretive care, which may then be able to access aspects of the deeply disturbing experiences underlying the patient's struggles.

Patients suffer terribly when they become psychiatric patients. They crave clear thinking and understanding. Kindness, too, is always needed absolutely on the psychiatric ward. It is kindness to try to understand what the patient means by his or her pronouncements that "a large man is sitting on top of my head" or "a black psychopath was terrifyingly trying to control me in my bed from outside my bedroom window". Without psychoanalytic understanding of symbolism or psychodynamics, such patients may spend many years in psychiatric care and in corrosive family relationships before the root cause of their disturbance becomes apparent. Richard Lucas wrote his book "The Psychotic Wavelength" to foster understanding of how patients may be addressed effectively while they are psychotic, to help them develop trust with their caring staff before calmness and relative sanity can be reached.

Outreach services these days are much better than previously at alleviating the effects of the first psychotic breakdown of newly ill young patients. By listening to the patients and talking kindly, constructively, and helpfully with them, the young person may then feel understood and able to express what is really troubling them: "My father is upsetting me" may then be addressed practically, and family therapy initiated. If clearly detrimental factors such as this are overlooked, the time for possible amelioration may elapse and positive resolution be delayed until it becomes no longer a possibility, perhaps preparing the way for repeated relapses of acute "reactive" illness, if not chronic schizophrenia itself.

Psychiatrists are in a key position to make the best use possible of available understanding for their schizophrenic and schizoaffective patients. Martindale and Summers emphasise that their psychodynamic illustrations should be used "to complement and enrich other frameworks rather than compete with them". Patients are tremendously grateful for understanding proffered by both ward staff, along with their kindness, and by a therapist such as a psychoanalyst who is skilled in enabling his or her patients to develop self-awareness, insight, autonomy, and then independence. This outcome is what psychiatrists wish for their patients, and is what Dr Michael Robbins' work (see Parts IV and V herein) and the PPCC model have shown is possible even for patients suffering from schizophrenic illness.

In a further paper in 2013 (Martindale and Summers, 2013b), Martindale and Summers illustrate "Using psychodynamic principles in formulation in everyday practice". This approach to developing formulations is again emphasised as being "complementary to other frameworks for understanding psychosis", and they conclude by summarising that "as stated in the NICE guidance (2009), psychodynamic principles can be used to generate hypotheses that may be helpful in better understanding people with psychosis and in guiding their general clinical care". These ideas may already be providing constructive opportunities for psychiatrists seeking fresh ways of alleviating distress in their schizophrenic patients.

Eric Kandel, in his 1999 paper "Biology and the Future of Psychoanalysis: A New Intellectual Framework for Psychiatry Revisited" (Kandel, 1999), stated that "psychoanalysis still represents the most coherent and intellectually satisfying view of the mind". Martindale and Summers have elucidated how psychoanalytic thinking may inform and support traditional psychiatric practice, possibly proving already to be to the substantive benefit of current patients. The PPCC model outlined herein, especially in Part II and also in Parts III, IV and V, provides a scientific basis, through its origin in scientifically derived data, for understanding the changes in a schizoaffectively disordered mind during remedial psychoanalytic psychotherapy.

These testaments to the value of psychoanalytic concepts should, I argue, be interpreted and directed towards deeply needful schizophrenic and schizoaffective patients. The contents of this book summarise the accuracy of the PPCC model; its value in reflecting the sequence of therapeutically-derived psychological changes in a healing schizophrenic or schizoaffective mind; its confirmation not only of the reality of psychological resolution of schizophrenic illness but of how this is brought about; its versatility in its descriptive potential; its core foundation confirmed as that of a valid theory by the criteria set out in The Shorter Oxford Textbook of Psychiatry (Gelder, Harrison and Cowen, 2006, p.89); and the PPCC model also points to the coinciding of Sigmund Freud's, Wilfred Bion's and Jerry Fodor's dynamic theoretical models of interacting factors both inside and outside the mind, producing outcomes which are described elsewhere (Steggles, 2012). Eric Kandel's, Michael Robbins', Brian Martindale's, Alison Summers', Susan Hingley's, and Marcus Evans' work, my own work, and the wealth of contributory findings supported by those seminal figures included in Chapter 13 and many others, all point to the value of psychoanalytic thinking.

Both the application of psychoanalytic ideas to routine psychiatric practice, as helpfully expounded by Brian Martindale and Alison Summers, and psychoanalytic psychotherapy as an individual therapeutic process, as elaborated by Michael Robbins and myself, open up the minds of all concerned to the origins, nature, and effects of psychological factors which by upsetting the "reactive" schizophrenic or schizoaffective patient have led to the development of their mental affliction and suffering from it. Through collaboration and teamwork, the core difficulty that is compromising a patient may be identified sooner rather than later, and resolved. Psychoanalytic ideas may make both routine psychiatric practice and long-term psychotherapy more effective. They reach to the origin of psychological difficulties back in the roots of the mind; CBT offers only short-term effectiveness for seriously debilitating mental illness. Circumstantial methods of coping with symptoms, which CBT provides, usually do result in helpful changes in the patient's life. But sooner or later the long-term difficulties arise again unless the patient has been enabled to trace their difficulties in their own understanding to their source. Once identified, this can be ameliorated, and the patient's illness of schizophrenia or schizoaffective disorder resolved. £1.8 million is the financial saving involved for the public purse per treated schizophrenic patient's lifetime, less the £58,000 cost of therapy for a psychoanalytic treatment of eight years plus the overheads common to both treated and untreated patients such as GP care, medication, and the community support required. Psychoanalytic understanding is the key to this greatly reduced clinical supervision required by the patient.

The weight of responsibility for the mental health of the population could be eased for those carrying it if they adopted the "most coherent view" of their patients' minds, and allowed their own experience to become to them "most intellectually satisfying", through a psychoanalytic approach as recommended by Eric Kandel, now that psychoanalytic thinking is becoming integrated with neuroscience through the new specialty of neuropsychoanalysis; and allowed their patients to become profoundly grateful to them for promoting their long-sought and autonomous self-understanding. Application of psychoanalytic thinking to psychological symptoms in psychiatric disorders even as severe as schizophrenia allows clarity to be bestowed upon thoroughly confused and distressed minds. Psychiatrists' work, if they respond to Kandel's inspiration, could really make a huge difference to those patients trapped by circumstantial adversity, even if the signs and symptoms of this have become nearly submerged within the classical symptoms of schizophrenic illness, ie. schizophrenia or schizoaffective disorder. A spark of initiative, determination, true insight, or a history of premorbid application and effort in a patient with schizophrenic illness should be enough to alert their psychiatrist that their human spirit is still alive and well, despite being buried beneath layers of symptomatology; and surely, like a heart transplant patient, they equally deserve their opportunity of rescue and rehabilitation.

PART II
THE PPCC MODEL

....

DR GILLIAN STEGGLES

CHAPTER 7
THE DEVELOPMENT OF THE PPCC MODEL

Schizophrenia and schizoaffective disorder are confusing and frightening conditions to experience. Trust in personal relationships provides the substantive basis for a patient's psychological development and progress forwards, out of her predicament. Psychoanalytic psychotherapy effectively helps an analysand, or patient, in this way. Through emotional and personal engagement with another human being, her psychoanalytic psychotherapist, the analysand learns about herself in a manner previously unknown to her; and she gains elemental knowledge and experience of herself as an individual human being.

The patient learns in psychoanalytic psychotherapy at a deep, unconscious level how she can exist with parts of her mind, parts of herself, that previously had caused so much disturbance that she was very distressed and far from being able to live independently. Within a relationship of trust and learning, her psychoanalyst's insights, articulated through interpretations, are now able to facilitate understanding and resolution of conflicts, incorrect assumptions, and unhelpful beliefs, and permit stabilisation, growth and integration and, ultimately, independence. This is the unfolding process hoped for when a patient embarks on a psychoanalytic treatment.

The PPCC model of the progress of a schizoaffective mind into mental health during a psychoanalytic psychotherapy treatment was developed from a single case study. A different approach, that of studying the effects of psychoanalytic psychotherapy on a population of schizophrenic patients to identify a common pathway as far as possible, was adopted by Bent Rosenbaum and others in Denmark (Rosenbaum et al, 2005). His team studied 562 patients in a prospective, longitudinal, multicentre investigation of their first episode of psychosis. The study revealed that after two years of treatment those patients receiving psychoanalytic psychotherapy showed greater improvement than those not receiving it. Deep psychodynamic understanding of the general nature of the treatment process was reached, and is described by Rosenbaum as the Initial Phase, the Middle Phase, and the Termination Phase of the therapy (Rosenbaum, 2009). Autonomy was encouraged in the Termination Phase, but consistent details of the experiences worked through by the patients during the three psychological phases while the patients achieved their improved health were not derived in the study. The PPCC model provides detail, and its details correspond with the details of Dr Robbins' two cited case studies, as visualized in Chapters 16 and 19.

The source of the PPCC construct

The Psychodynamic Pentapointed Cognitive Construct (PPCC) model was developed from observation of a schizoaffectively disordered patient who underwent this therapeutic process. She made a small study of her own mind when she had become so interested in her psychoanalytic psychotherapy treatment and felt so happy with her new knowledge gained from her analyst that she wanted to investigate what effect it was having on her mind. She wanted to write a novel about what she was so invigoratingly discovering about her thinking, which she realised lay on the cusp between the effect her illness was having on her, and what she was discovering afresh in her analyst's consulting room. She had been in her treatment for four and a half months, attending her analyst for fifty minutes, five days a week.

She was thinking about the chapter headings for her novel, and decided to use a Buddhist meditation technique that she knew of, to still her mind to utter, quiet passivity and stillness, and then to note carefully what entered it by way of thoughts. She did this, with a pencil and paper beside her, and wrote down each idea as it popped into her mind. In total, twenty-nine ideas individually entered her mind at approximately one-second intervals, grouped into five groups with four naturally-occurring breaks. Each of these ideas formed a chapter heading for her book. When she looked at them she was pleased with the range of ideas they covered, and she wanted to celebrate them as all being relevant to herself, and therefore as making sense to her in a valuable way. So she arranged the five groups on a pentapointed pattern with the group headed "Problems" at the top (see Figure 1). She drew out this shape and felt extremely satisfied at being able to look at its assembled ideas, being the content of her mind during her study.

The original interest of the PPCC construct

This author (GS) was, at this time, a Research Senior House Officer in Psychiatry and had made contact with this interesting patient as a subject

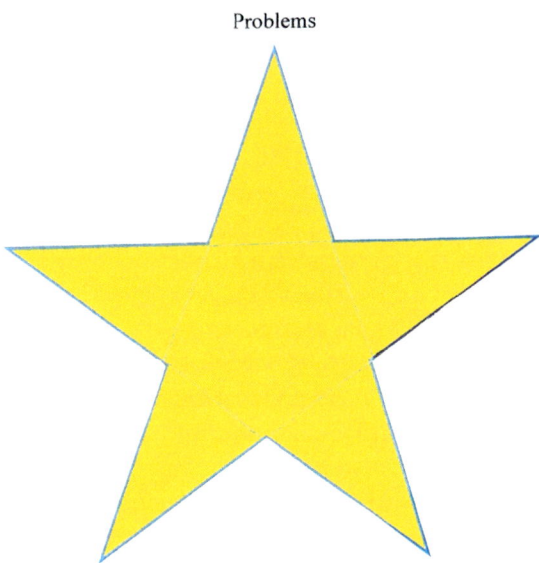

Figure 1 A schizoaffective patient's original representational world
© BMJ 2017

for a research project for the Westminster Board of Psychiatrists. As a Research SHO, the author asked the patient if she could look at what she had produced, and found it of great fascination, particularly when the patient told her she could talk with her about herself and about her progress in her therapy. Of course the author thanked her, and so began a thirty-year research relationship during which this author observed how the patient changed in her therapy and gradually overcame her psychological difficulties. As changes occurred in the patient's mind, so the author developed the PPCC model through its geometric phases towards its final form. The patient was quite interested in the author's work, including her initial surprise at the author's enthusiasm for her pentapointed diagram and her naming of the five variables. She was polite and patient when the author talked with her at length over subsequent years to follow her progress, and so the PPCC model developed. The author-researcher built up the PPCC model around the patient's progress, and recognised psychoanalytical phenomena that she demonstrated as her illness receded.

The evolution of the PPCC model

The PPCC model's actual structure and structural changes both describe and represent changes in the mind of a schizoaffective patient (see Figure

2a). For example, the therapeutic dyad, or working therapeutic couple, is described in terms of two individuals communicating with each other, directional arrows depicting the communication of each participant with the other; the patient was very close to her analyst, and in time "Analyst" replaced "Problems" at the top of the diagram when he became internalised, or introjected, by her. The other four variables are parts of the analysand's mind. In this way he became part of her Representational World, in a very influential position with respect to her mind. This decision, thus graphically described, illustrates his attaining access to her mind in due course so that he could heal it, and also represents his responsibility for helping her with her problems. Thus the analyst was included or internalised in the patient's world, both in psychoanalytic terms of the patient's mind and in the structure of the PPCC model. And in the same way, External Reality is described and represented around the therapeutic dyad; and the patient's Internal Space is represented in the centre of the model. Thus the PPCC model describes and represents aspects of the patient's mind in an observable, visual form.

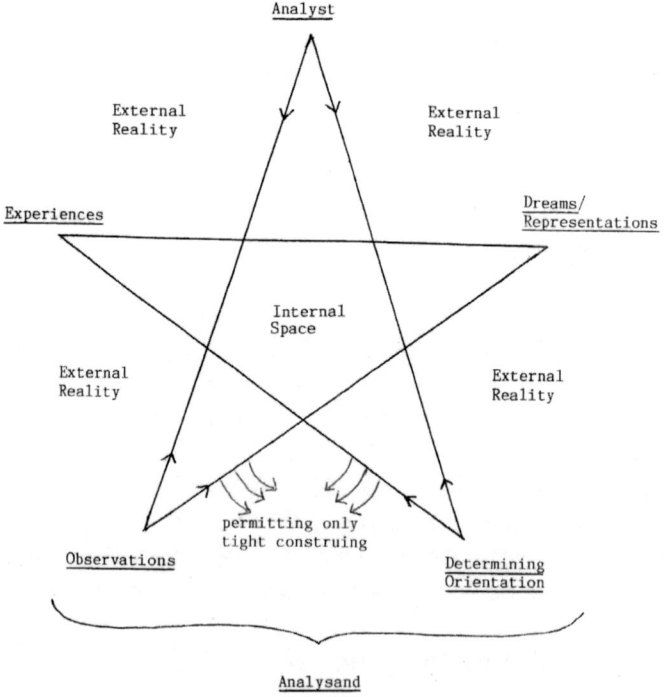

Figure 2a The PPCC model in the paranoid-schizoid position
© BMJ 2017

The patient's representational world was identified by her small study of her mind, emerging from her preconscious into her conscious mind. This representational world is a collection of significant aspects of an individual's environments as they live their life, starting from when they are a small child. Joseph Sandler, who became the Freud Memorial Professor of Psychoanalysis at University College London, and Bernard Rosenblatt, in 1962 devised this concept to illustrate how a young child regards the world around them, and how their impressions of it change over time (Sandler and Rosenblatt, 1962). The representational world changes and develops with time, and new experiences revise the child's feelings for people in their environment, different places and its memories of them. These changes affect the representational world, which is constantly updated in this way. The patient had elicited from her preconscious mind, closely connected with her unconscious mind, what she recalled of the world as she had lived in it, her most meaningful impressions of it. Structurally, in the PPCC model, the representational world occupies the border between External Reality and the patient's Internal Space, which represents its psychological function as an adjustable, internal guide to External Reality in the mind of a child becoming adjusted to finding its way in consecutive, sometimes difficult or confusing, environments.

The constituents of the PPCC model

The author observed the nature of the five groups of chapter headings, the characteristics that distinguished the different groups from each other, and gave the groups names. The four groups other than the Analyst variable appeared to her to consist of "Experiences"; "Dreams" or "Representations"; "Observations"; and "Facts or Fantasies" (later to become the "Determining Orientation" variable). These four analysand variables coincide precisely with the four variables that the Shorter Oxford Textbook of Psychiatry describes as providing the data derived from psychoanalytic treatments upon which psychoanalytic theories mainly depend (Gelder et al, 2006, p. 89). Childhood experiences, identified by the Textbook, are represented by Experiences; dreams by Dreams/Representations; thoughts by spoken thoughts or Observations; and fantasies by Determining Orientation which includes unrestrained Fantasies for psychotic mania, stark unrelenting Facts for psychotic aspects of depression, and Schizophrenic Global Perspectives (limited, extremely unpleasant outlook options for the schizophrenic patient) for schizophrenia. The fourth variable, Determining Orientation, thus describes the three functional psychoses which constitute schizoaffective disorder, ie. mania, depression, and schizophrenia, whichever psychosis is being suffered by the patient at any time when they are not in their neutral, non-psychotic state between episodes (which is represented by the pentapointed PPCC structure).

So the five points of the PPCC construct are five in number because of the derived content of the patient's mind when she examined it. The nature of the variables at the PPCC's five points form the different categories of the patient's representational world. "Problems", taken over by the Analyst variable, represent the patient's problems in her life and in the world. "Experiences" represent the patient's past experiences up to and including the present time, and "Dreams/Representations" represent the patient's dreams up to and including the present time, and her representations of people and places and events. "Observations" are her sane thoughts, and "Determining Orientation" is the variable related to what psychosis her mind is manifesting or tending towards. The PPCC's graphic nature is due to the patient's eidetic imagery and the creative appeal for her of visualising her mind while she began to study in more detail what she had obtained for herself. Her curiosity extended to taking an interest in the author's work with her, even though she did not understand its psychoanalytic or medical content.

Thus the five variables of the PPCC constitute symbolically the main elements of the schizoaffective patient's mind that together formed her representational world. She utilised and adapted this to successive experiences in different environments like an unconscious personal construct (Kelly, 1955), and to successive experiences that she encountered within the therapeutic alliance (Zetzel, 1970) in her analyst's consulting room. Constructing a patient's representational world in this manner can also be a way of preparing the analyst's mind for that patient's psychoanalysis with himself or herself, by establishing an overview of the patient's experiences received from their early environments.

Relations of the PPCC to psychoanalytic concepts
(see also Chapter 11)

The early development of the PPCC as an extension of the model beyond the paranoid-schizoid (Figure 2a) position to the depressive position reflected Melanie Klein's early psychoanalytic work. Melanie Klein identified these two states of psychological being as they occur in healthy people. The paranoid-schizoid position (Klein, 1946) describes a separation of the good and the bad sides of a person in an individual's perception of them; the depressive position (Klein, 1935) describes a mature willingness to accept both of these at one and the same time. The depressive position, which is only very distantly related to the illness of depression, consists of a concerned desire to love and care for another person who manifests good and bad attributes. In the paranoid-schizoid position, the good and bad aspects are only observed separately and often with a brittle, paranoid anxiety, which must be overcome to arrive at the depressive position. The depressive position of the PPCC (see Figure 3), represented by a marquise structure which graphically allows freer, looser construing and more relaxed and imaginative mental movement within the therapeutic dyad, illustrates fusion of the sane Observations variable with the psychotic Determining Orientation variable. This leaves the patient with much more flexibility in her approach and responses to the analyst. The two positions alternate quite frequently as recurring aspects of normality. Via the pentapointed paranoid-schizoid position, the depressive position connects with the Closure of the Vertex, where the five variables of the PPCC's representational world fold backwards together and enclose all of the patient's past as an experienced and comprehended life (see Figure 4).

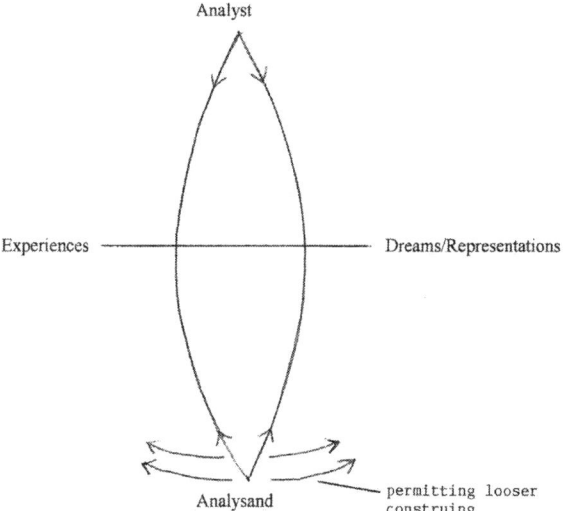

Figure 3 The PPCC model in the depressive position
© BMJ 2017

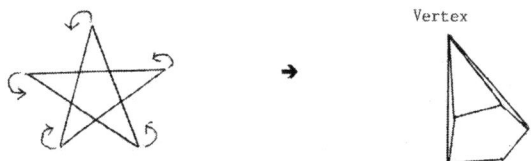

Figure 4 Closure of the PPCC's vertex
© BMJ 2017

The dynamic movements within the stages of the PPCC model

In all its forms during the early stages of remedial therapy, the PPCC model represents the dynamics of communication exchanges between the analyst and the patient through its linear connections between them, with arrows indicating the initial directions of conversational flow. Later forms illustrate increasing solidity of the patient's mind as it becomes more stable, and here the simple lines of communication do not persist: rather, the increasingly substantial nature of the patient's mind relates as a whole to the internalised analyst, and the patient's solid, stronger identity becomes apparent.

The appearance of solidity in the PPCC model is functional, another example of how the PPCC's structure describes and represents the changes in the patient's mind. Initially, at closure of the vertex when the five variables fold back to form a five-sided pyramid, what is enclosed is the totality of the patient's memories, now orientated in Time, Place and Person. The patient has become able to relate to all earlier memories that had previously been disturbing to the point of producing psychotic episodes in conjunction with current pathogenic stimuli. Once the pathological "sting" has been taken out of these past disturbing memories they are no longer psychotically stimulating to the patient. The patient can remember the occasions and has thought about them in terms of alternative possible responses to them that might have led to less traumatic sequelae. Thus the solid five-sided pyramid represents the containment of previously pathogenic experiences, now harmlessly modified. Similarly, the solid sphere that represents the endpoint of the recovery process represents the patient's personality "with all its corners rubbed off" (see Figure 5). In general, it functions smoothly in whatever circumstances the patient finds herself.

The PPCC model's final, spherical form of the recovered schizophrenic mind could contain Freud's latest diagram of the healthy conscious and unconscious mind (see Figure 6). Perhaps Freud's model could be thought of as having a self-righting mechanism keeping it upright within its spherical PPCC model as this rolls on smoothly while the patient now moves comfortably among other people.

Useful projections of the PPCC model

The PPCC can be developed into a comparison between the three functional psychoses, depression, mania and schizophrenia, that sometimes form episodes in a schizoaffective patient (see Chapters 8 and 9 and Figures 8, 9 and 10). It is also used to construct a dynamic comparison between

THE DEVELOPMENT OF THE PPCC MODEL

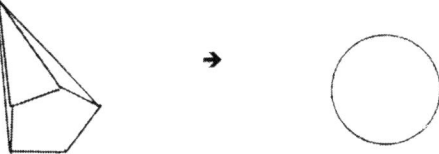

Figure 5 The endpoint of the recovery process: the patient's mind maturing "with all its corners rubbed off"
© BMJ 2017

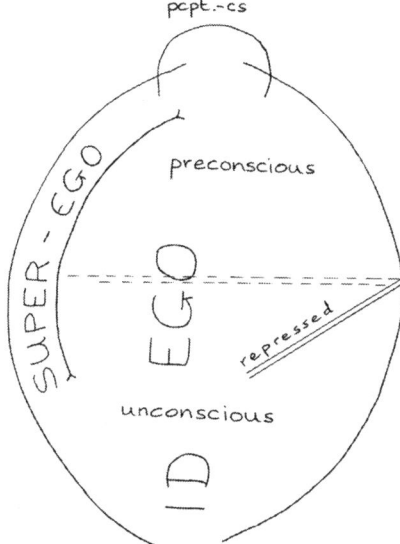

Figure 6 Freud's latest model of a healthy mind
(Ref. The Standard Edition of the Complete Psychological Works of Sigmund Freud, Volume XXII, Ed. James Strachey, Vintage, 2001, p.78)

Bion's, Freud's and Jerry Fodor's theories of mental processes; in each case, an element internal to the mind engages with an element in the external environment to produce a mental function (see Chapter 9 and Figures 12 and 13).

Overview of the PPCC model

The PPCC model started its existence, as described, in the form of representations of the world around the original schizoaffective patient studied. These parts of the environmental world, once internalised, became part of the structure of the patient's working mind, the part accessible to her analyst which he could observe and relate to as he tried to understand her relationships with the world, and how she herself functioned. The overall sequence of the PPCC model's changes over time is shown in Figure 7. Its structural properties and its symbolic changes help understanding and visualisation of the patient's mind in its ever-improving individuation as it heals from schizophrenia or schizoaffective disorder through the effects of psychoanalytic psychotherapy. The patient's mind grows in tiny steps on a daily basis during psychoanalytic sessions. Gradually, over time, these incremental changes accumulate and interrelate with all the patient's experiences and memories and responses, laying down new psychological fabric upon which the patient can build her perspective and modify traumatised conclusions that she has reached concerning past times. The amount of work required for the patient to move from one mode of the PPCC model to the next can take years to accomplish. The PPCC Theory summarises these steps with the implicit assumption that the clinical psychoanalytic psychotherapeutic work is done on a daily basis observing orthodox parameters and maintaining classical requirements such as patient safety and respect for therapist and patient likewise. The overarching geometric designs of the PPCC illustrate transformations in the patient that have been conclusively reached after all this work has been achieved, and when the patient's mind has eventually evolved into its new awareness.

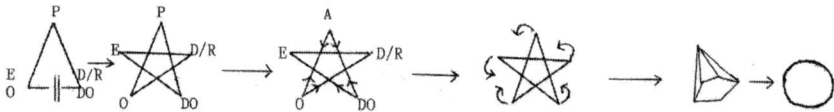

Figure 7 The overall PPCC sequence of recovery from schizophrenia
© BMJ 2017

CHAPTER 8

THE STRUCTURE OF THE PPCC MODEL

The PPCC is a dynamic, active model that describes the changes occurring in the mind of a schizoaffective or schizophrenic patient during psychoanalytic psychotherapy. The model is understandable by considering each of the forms that represent the patient's mind at its different phases of recovery, and also by considering what might be involved as one form matures into the next form. The PPCC model is a highly visual way of understanding the psychological transformations of therapy. This persistence in using geometric shapes to develop the model was deliberate, following on from observing the graphic enterprise of the schizoaffective patient originally studied (Figure 1). Visible, tangible and readily understandable treatments such as remedies for many physical medical conditions, for example electronic prostheses, technically elaborate implants and mobility chairs, may be comfortably related to and used in debate and argument about financing treatment. The treatment of psychological illnesses that are invisible, intangible, and very difficult to conceptualise, tends to elude people's grasp and comprehension. They thus may be highly reluctant to refer to them in debate relating to necessary finance or resource provision owing to their apparent obscurity and the consequent fears of making incorrect or false statements about them.

Fear about mental illness is widespread, partly because it is so difficult to comprehend, partly because it is such a serious form of illness, and partly because of an easily understandable horror and compassion for those in the throes of an acute episode. The clear, lucid shapes of the PPCC model convey absolute concepts such as inclusion/rejection (the analyst in the patient's representational world), solidity/containment (the patient being able to accept understandingly all her past experiences in an adjusted and realistic way), and the process of evolution itself from one state into another. Anyone may observe the PPCC's geometric changes for themselves and understand these simple concepts. In so doing, they will be helping themselves to recognise the terrible difficulties that schizophrenic patients have experienced throughout their lives until they reach treatment (this is the sorrow of a patient having a deeply unpleasant representational world around herself in which she has found it impossible to develop); and the rigours of this treatment's radical, difficult transformations of the patients in the endeavour of self-understanding. The clear elucidation of the sequence of changes in remedial schizophrenia treatment provided by the PPCC model may enable reference to the therapeutic process during financial discussions to be made much more confidently during healthcare planning meetings, for example when discussing resource allocation.

The original role of the PPCC

The PPCC's structure followed on from the examination of her own mind made by the schizoaffective patient the author studied for thirty years. Her ideas flowed into her mind, once she had stilled it, in five groups. She constructed the pentapointed shape to accommodate her study's findings because she had eidetic imagery, and because this shape appealed to her aesthetic sense in the context of her being very needful of being able to hold on to her mind's integrity, at least as she knew it to be. She was frightened of being ill with a schizoaffective disorder, she clung on to any hope available to her, and she was prepared to work very hard to preserve herself, hopefully to emerge at some future point into the person she felt herself to be, but currently unsuccessfully. Her pentapointed diagram was a part of herself that she could look at, scrutinise, and reflect upon. It gave her some sense at least of being a person made of a fabric open to inspection, and not just by her analyst. She could look at herself with a view to progress, not simply a constant image in a mirror. The original PPCC construct, the patient's pentapointed diagram, was a bright, attractive focus for her, yellow by choice, and, rather than merely a constant image, a constant companion (see Figure 1). She could think in depth about the issues that it raised for her, stimulated by the twenty-nine individual ideas that it comprised. She could feel happy in this, her temporarily settled state.

The PPCC construct's role in the patient's life developed into that of an abstract Transitional Object. She became attached to her diagram, since it consisted of the contents of her mind and in this way comprised part of herself. She painted it yellow, and it cheered her up at times when she felt disconsolate or anxious. It represented her analyst being present with her in her mind in his absence from her physically, and formed part of her own identity when she felt disintegrated or lost. Thus it even filled the role of an abstract "transitional object" for her. Donald Winnicott developed the idea of a transitional object, which is a soft toy or blanket which a young child becomes emotionally attached to at times such as feeding, to help it learn to separate at an elemental level from its mother (Winnicott, 1953). The blanket is both "me" (the child) and "not-me" (the mother); so the child, who has omnipotent control of the blanket, can learn gradually to detach emotionally from his mother. Initially she is someone who he can seemingly summon at will for a feed while clutching the blanket. Later he learns to relate to her realistically, instead, in the external world of reality where the blanket is a comforting substitute for her until she appears in person. The patient reassured herself of her relationship with her analyst by looking at her pentapointed diagram of her own mind which contained her analyst. It represented her mind's contact with him in his absence from her, and immensely helped her to tolerate the twenty-three hours of the day when she was not with him. Because it was an abstract concept she was able to summon it up at will and experience some comfort from its conceptual reality in her life at times away from her analyst.

The use of geometric shapes in the PPCC model

The PPCC model in its pentapointed form represents the patient's schizoaffective disorder in its neutral, paranoid-schizoid position during stable intervals between episodes of depressive, manic or schizophrenic psychosis. Over time the geometric pentapointed PPCC model was adapted to describe later structures and qualities of the patient's mind in forms that were recognisable visually, and thus was comparatively easy for non-psychologists to conceptualise and understand.

The author used the patient's creative, graphic approach in furthering her clarifying endeavour as she sought to elucidate the patient's mental changes over time. Geometric shapes seemed to the author to be an effective way of communicating to others what only psychologists, psychoanalysts and psychiatrists can readily understand about mental phenomena. A change to three dimensions from a planar, two-sided figure, for example, would seem a clear step towards containing something. In the case of the PPCC, it is the patient's past traumatic, psychotic memories which are now collected together within the pentasided pyramid and inoffensively orientated in time, place, and person and contained, rather than diffusively floating around in an unspecified manner in the patient's mind and frightening her. Closure of the vertex, when all five variables come together in a consolidation of the patient's representational world as this has been in all its forms since childhood, is one of the most major and significant changes that psychoanalytic psychotherapy can bring about in a psychotic or schizophrenic patient's mind. She becomes able to look back and review her life dispassionately, accepting its difficulties, ordeals, and hurdles without traumatised emotion or feeling unwell or threatened. Psychological treatments which do not attempt this endeavour are destined to allow further psychotic breakdowns because the memories and experiences giving rise to the psychosis remain misunderstood and can precipitate future psychological fractures. A psychoanalyst is able to shed a warm, bright light on such experiences for the patient's understanding. Meaningful understanding of experience is precisely what psychoanalytic treatments foster, and do so very effectively, enabling patients to reflect on the basis of their own initiative, to serve themselves as they endeavour to live their days independently. Learning to understand themselves is what all psychoanalytic treatments aim to help their patients achieve. The final phase of resolution is represented by a rounded sphere in the PPCC model, which describes the patient's now smoothly functioning and independent mind.

The psychotic and non-psychotic parts of the mind visualized through the PPCC model

The unconscious mind, when in the paranoid-schizoid position, tends to split good from bad aspects of other individuals and to experience anxiety. In the depressive position, the mind behaves more reflectively, recognises its own responsibilities, and tries to make amends to others for ways in which it may have hurt them. The PPCC construct, in its pentapointed, paranoid-schizoid position, illustrates how the non-psychotic Observations facility of the patient's mind is split from the psychotic Determining Orientation which characterises schizophrenic, depressed or manic symptoms; the patient may therefore be troubled by psychosis that causes difficulties independently of the sane Observations. The paranoid-schizoid position is comparatively normal for the schizoaffective patient, in that the patient is not overtly psychotic, but psychosis threatens the sane, Observing part of the patient. The division of the schizoaffective patient's mind into the sane Observations variable and the psychotic Determining Orientation variable persists when they are in the paranoid-schizoid position, and overwhelms the patient's state of mind when they are threatened by schizophrenic, depressive or manic symptoms, or when these actually break out. When the schizoaffective patient develops a depressive, manic or schizophrenic episode the pentapointed PPCC construct develops into its appropriate adaptation, which describes properties of that form of psychosis.

Bion (1967, pp. 43-64), Sohn (1999, p. 15), Lucas (2009, p. 6) and Murray Jackson (2001, p. 334) all held that psychotic patients have a non-psychotic, sane part of their mind which is the agency that therapists try to communicate with in treatment. During overt psychosis it is usually not possible to access this non-psychotic part. When the patient is in the comparatively healthy paranoid-schizoid position and is not psychotic, her mind may become even more healthily psychologically adjusted by conflating the Observations and the Determining Orientation variables, into the depressive position. Here the psychosis of the Determining Orientation no longer functions independently and potentially out of control; the Observations variable fuses with it and maintains it in a sane condition, unprovoked and calm. In the depressive position, the psychotic Determining Orientation variable is therefore no longer a threat to the patient's sanity; the patient can contemplate her existence much more broadly while she is communicating with her analyst, and this is why the diagram of the depressive position illustrates looser construing, enabling freer association and necessary learning during therapeutic sessions compared with the tighter, more limited construing of the paranoid-schizoid position.

The alternation of the paranoid-schizoid and depressive positions occurs quite normally in mentally healthy people, and in a schizophrenic or schizoaffective patient only when the analyst has become incorporated into the patient's representational world and has taken over the Problems variable. From this vantage point the analyst has full access to all the different parts of the patient's mind. The Internal Space at the centre of the PPCC construct contains all the parts and functions of the patient's mind that are not included within the representational world, and the analyst clearly has access to these other parts and functions also. The patient does not manifest the depressive position until she has been able to accommodate her psychosis upon a good-enough basis into a fusion between the psychotic Determining Orientation and the sane Observations variables. To sustain the depressive position, the patient must have been able to establish a sufficiently stable "internal good object" (Hinshelwood, 1994, p. 71), or close relationship. It is quite possible that the analyst may be experienced by a schizophrenic patient as her first internal good object that she has encountered in her lifetime. This allows the patient to encounter new "feeling states" (Sandler, 1972, p. 296), and consequently experience new thoughts with her analyst. Return to the paranoid-schizoid position would be expected in due course, in which state useful work can still be done. The patient's psychotic tendency would become latent under these circumstances, and as much learning work as possible is achieved in its absence. Psychosis may of course return at some point later in the treatment, before psychological resolution is arrived at.

Spatial correlations of the PPCC structure

The lines of communication in the PPCC model outline the margins of the therapeutic dyad within its environment. The lines of the structure also demarcate the directions of communication between the analyst and the different parts of the patient's mind. Outside the PPCC structure's lines exists External Reality, in relation to which the analyst tries to help the patient live equably. The outline of the PPCC coincides approximately with the boundaries of the consulting room; External Reality mainly relates to the external world beyond the relationship between the analyst and the patient, ie. the separate realms of the world known to the patient when away from the analyst, and the world known to the analyst. Within the lines of communication, at their centre, lies the patient's Internal Space. The triangles of the patient's Representational World occupy a position between External Reality and the patient's Internal Space, which is precisely the function of the representational world; it mediates between the external world and the patient's mind by representing aspects of the world that are meaningful to her, and acts as a guide to her as she negotiates through her life, interacting with her environment.

Emotions

Specific emotions do not influence the cognitive nature of the PPCC model, but occupy their place in the Internal Space of the patient and appear as components of the patient's past and present Experiences. The original schizoaffective patient whose mind's growth is described by the PPCC model was fighting for her sanity in the midst of her schizoaffective confusion, and so overlooked her own feelings in her understanding of her study's chapter headings. Once she had externalised her study's contents of her mind, she reflected and worked for many years on her emotional growth and balance. The internal life of the patient's emotions and internal objects, including her affect regulation and all aspects of her mind apart from her representational world, continued within her Internal Space (see Figure 2b).

Closure of the vertex

After a very great deal of work has been done by the analyst and patient working together, the fearful items in the patient's memory of experiences, perceptions, feelings, beliefs, and the way she has lived her life in illness thus far, may become understood by her at last, rather than being a source of fearfulness and excessive misery. If the patient concentrates on her work with the analyst, the conception of her past life as a series of encounters may emerge as something she is finally able to encompass and digest, as herself, as the person who has all this experience but who is now also able to reflect upon it. The experiences that have earlier frightened and disturbed her have now lost their capacity to terrorise the patient. Anger can be seen as having a source and sometimes an effect, rather than being a constant and debilitating memory or present general experience. The experiences now no longer limit the patient's wellbeing. The patient becomes able to re-orientate herself positively, rather than existing painfully as she was during past experiences; that is, she can adjust in time, place, and person, in a positive way that no longer threatens her. She may become able to identify her molester as an injurious, damaging internal object from her Internal Space, constructively adjust to it, and then tolerate it as an innocuous element of her past life within the closed PPCC vertex structure of her mind.

In the PPCC Theory, this event of becoming able at last to encompass her past life in all its contexts, described as "closing the vertex", is highly significant. The five variables converge to meet together at a very early point in the past, at the time of the earliest memories and the beginning of awareness, a point that is called the vertex. The PPCC becomes a physical, three-dimensional model that is able to contain all these past experiences in a realistic, non-alarming way that the patient can adjust to in her consciousness. Her past has a place in her mind that she can now explore and learn from, rather than being so afraid that she finds herself perpetually running away from it. Closure of the vertex is a profoundly significant stage in her therapy; it marks closure of the pathological process that was operating on the patient's mind, and becomes a measure of her determination to put her past behind her and move forward with energy and enthusiasm into what remains of her life. What remains now for her to concentrate on is to develop her personality and character, and to adjust to interchange and dialogue with other people on a social basis which may fulfil her and bring her the joys that healthy people enjoy, but sometimes without realising how fortunate they are.

Wellbeing benefits provided to the original schizoaffective patient by the PPCC

The original schizoaffective patient became so elated and happily celebratory after producing her beautiful transitional object that she filled her Internal Space with colour, music, light, flowers, and even her helpful medications, to assist her morale and sustain herself in her somewhat miserable situation of finding herself living long-term in a psychiatric hospital ward. Her Internal Space was where she kept everything abstract that she treasured. She kept her memory of sending baby garments to a friend who she heard had had a new baby son. Her sister brought her tea and biscuits to enjoy in the succeeding months with others on the ward. There was a record player on the ward where she played her favourite tracks, and a piano where she could express herself musically. All these memories remained in her Internal Space, connecting with the variables of Experiences, Observations and Representations, and with her analyst, and keeping her psychosis at bay.

The PPCC model and the three functional psychoses

The PPCC model is adaptable to the three functional psychoses that are suffered by schizoaffective patients: depression, mania, and schizophrenia (see Figures 8, 9 and 10). The Determining Orientation represents in turn Facts, Fantasies, and Schizophrenic Global Perspectives respectively in describing these illnesses. While they are threatening to hold sway the patient cannot adopt the depressive position or work as effectively towards closing the vertex. Much work has to be done to draw the patient away from her illness, to try to regain a sense of logic and reality, and to understand herself in terms of her improving representational world and current, ongoing relationships. Re-establishing the depressive position permits productive continuation of the analytical work, through stabilisation of the Determining Orientation by its conflation with the Observations variable and constructive interaction with the analyst.

Final stages of the PPCC model

The final form that the PPCC takes once the patient has developed healthily into an independent, autonomous individual is a sphere. Here the patient's mind has had all of its sharp, obtrusive corners rubbed off through diligent work by the analyst and patient alike, and the ward staff, working together. The patient has a balanced, mature identity which is able to move smoothly among other people without creating any impression other than the patient wishes to convey, through much improved confidence and self-awareness. She is capable, and substantially resilient, as a result of going through all the experiences that have been necessary to restore her true sense of herself in reality, something she might have dreamed about wishfully for many years prior to finding her transformative treatment. The patient during this concluding phase is invariably enormously grateful to her analyst, and to all the hospital staff who have nursed her through her extended psychological and sometimes physical ordeals, when she may have become lost or come to harm in the community or had to undergo unpleasant physical treatments. The hospital staff will have provided absolutely invaluable continuity for the patient throughout the different phases of her psychoanalytic therapy, in a place that really forms a refuge for the schizophrenic patient during her life-changing odyssey out into the unknown. The staff will have known all the patient's weaknesses that came to light during her admissions to the hospital unit, and familiarity with the staff who have this knowledge conveys a great sense of security to the patient. This secure environment permitted the patient to learn containment of herself, with all her personal difficulties, so that when she now tries to practise autonomy these difficulties do not break out into relationships and interfere with the patient's happiness and that of those she loves. The patient has developed internal security from her experience of security within the hospital, and from internalising her analyst as a steady, mature source of strength, self-protection, and ultimate common sense. All these influences are what the untreated but lively, alert schizophrenic patient desperately seeks from the wasteland that the world appears to her to be, in her initial completely disorganised and terrifying condition. Feeling strong and self-contained at the conclusion of her treatment seems, for this reason, to be a dream literally come true.

Overall structural sequence of the recovering schizophrenic or schizoaffective mind

The PPCC structure changes and adapts to the changing nature of the schizophrenic or schizoaffective mind in therapy (see Figure 7). The original nature of a schizophrenic patient's mind is represented by the schizophrenic triangular model. If the patient is now treated with warmth and kindness and encouragement, she may open up into the neutral, pentapointed, paranoid-schizoid-positioned PPCC construct that describes a schizoaffective patient's mind. In this position, engagement with the analyst becomes much more possible for the patient. In time, the patient may move between this paranoid-schizoid position and the loosely-construing depressive position in which mental state most of the useful analytic work is done. But eventually, when all the variables move backwards and join together at the vertex, the patient may progress from the pentapointed, neutral model to the closure of the vertex. When this has been achieved, the patient needs to become active socially and enjoy her new-found health with other people. Her personality and character now have a chance to develop, since she has achieved autonomy. She begins to flourish in healthy integration and independence of spirit; the angles on her personality become rubbed off and she gradually becomes smoothed, comfortable in herself as the person she is, and eventually mature.

CHAPTER 9

THE ADAPTABILITY OF THE PPCC MODEL

The pentapointed PPCC construct representing the relatively normal, healthy, neutral state of a stabilised schizoaffective patient can be adapted for each of the functional psychoses that schizoaffective patients are subject to, that is, depression, mania, and schizophrenia (in some cases of schizoaffective disorder mania is absent) (see Figures 8, 9 and 10). Well-managed patients spend most of their time in this comparatively healthy, neutral mental state, between the psychotic episodes which may involve different combinations of these three kinds of symptom. The patient upon whose case history the PPCC model is based realised she was on the cusp of wellness between a state that was as good as her illness allowed her and the excellent health and insight that her sessions with her analyst afforded her, when she studied her mind. She was, therefore, in very good mental form while regarding her representational world; and this mental state, as it turned out, actually was the psychological material described by the first pentapointed PPCC diagram. Dr Michael Robbins' schizophrenic patients, at the start of their therapy when first interviewed by him, may or may not have been frankly and overtly psychotically ill, when the triangular, blocked PPCC model of schizophrenia would have applied. They may have been temporarily suspended in the paranoid-schizoid state described by the pentapointed model where the Determining Orientation was latently active in producing mental symptoms such as splitting and hostility. At these times the patients were commonly very disturbed regarding their internal mental structure but were trying to relate to other people as best they could, and in this mental state may have resembled schizoaffective patients through the pentapointed PPCC construct. But, evidently, for long periods, especially early in their treatment, they suffered complete schizophrenic block as represented by the triangular PPCC model.

Depression

A schizoaffective patient who is experiencing Major Depressive Disorder symptoms would be represented by the PPCC with its Determining Orientation variable set at Facts, which would evolve into its adaptation for depression (see Figures 8a and 8b). This would describe the very depressed patient who is so emotionally flat that the bare, stark facts around her are all that she is aware of, in her state of utter dejection. Being utterly swamped by her misery, she takes little notice, if any, of her surroundings which appear as immutable, hostile, cold hard walls and floor, in an unresponsive world.

Figures 8a and 8b illustrate the development of the PPCC model describing depression. Sigmund Freud held that the origin of the process initiating depression was when "the shadow of the object [lost loved one] fell upon the ego" of the patient, and this shadow tormented the patient as an unkind effect of the bereaved patient's memory of her loved one. Freud believed that in the patient's memories, the lost loved one pathologically affected her, leaving her vulnerable to the memories' effects which could be very severe. The PPCC model shows how the "shadow", a Representation, translocates across the PPCC structure to join other variables, notably the Determining Orientation set at Facts, and sad Observations also based on Facts, to arrive at the Experience of Depression. On the way, it passes through Jerry Fodor's Relation R as a central mental function, which is a "functional or computational relation".

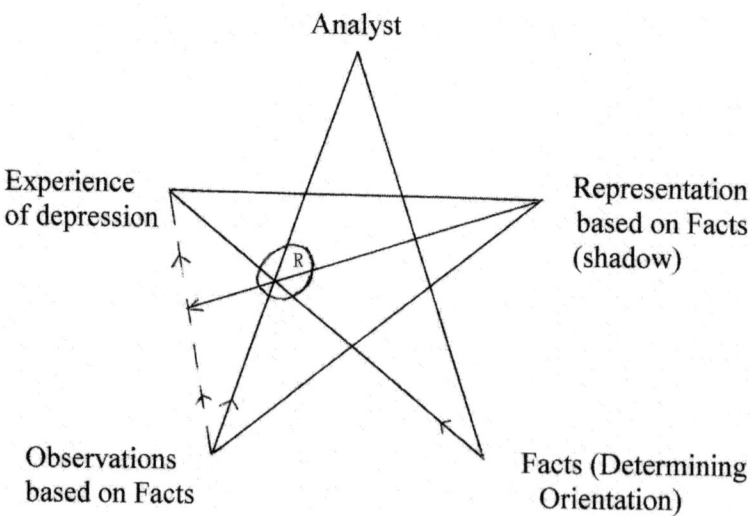

Figure 8a The development of the PPCC adaptation for depression
© BMJ 2017

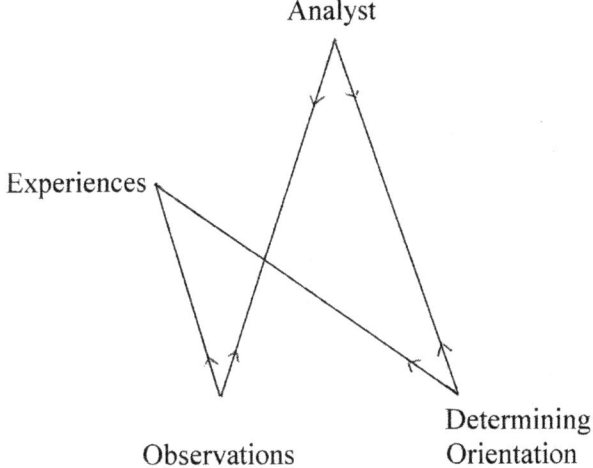

Figure 8b Adaptation of the PPCC construct for depression
© BMJ 2017

Mania

Similarly, mania can be illustrated by its adaptation of the pentapointed PPCC model in an obverse direction (see Figures 9a and 9b). Not enough research has been done to compare the PPCC's construction of mania with other theories, as was the case for depression. However, Freud believed that mania results when the superego fuses with the ego, which is an experience. Therefore, the PPCC model for mania shows the Experience variable translocating across towards the Dreams/Representations variable via the Manic Defence. The Determining Orientation manifests Fantasy, in line with the clinical finding that manic patients fantasise hugely about themselves, other people, and aspects of the world, ignoring their rational Observations and all the time rejecting friends' reasoned or calming appeals and attempts to steady them. The Determining Orientation set at Fantasy combines synergistically with the Experience of a fused ego and superego, and arrives at Dreams/Representations with manic omnipotent and grandiose self-representations. Reversal of this situation requires the analyst to strengthen the patient's sense of reality, patience, calmness, and rationality, which may take many days or even a number of weeks or months to achieve, and usually requires medication to take effect. Accompanying depression can take even longer to resolve, sometimes in the most unfortunate cases requiring months, and lasting at a low, albeit fluctuating, level for years.

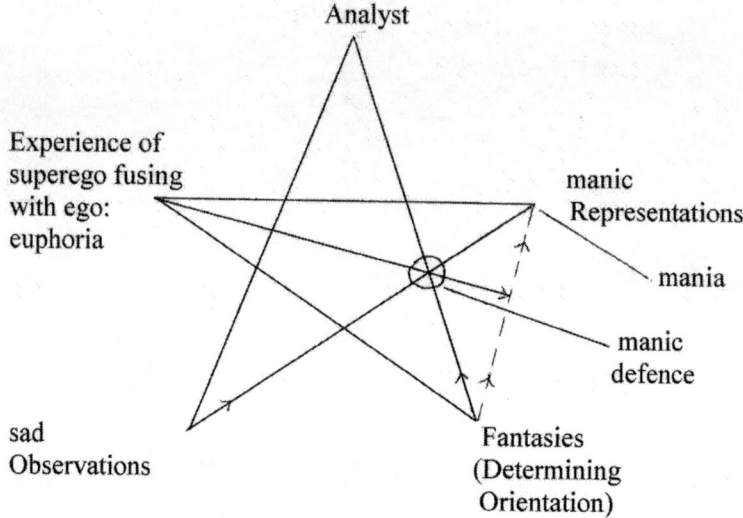

Figure 9a The development of the PPCC adaptation for mania
© BMJ 2017

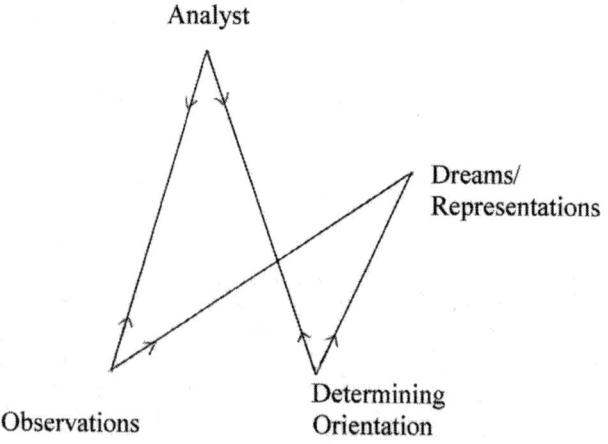

Figure 9b Adaptation of the PPCC construct for mania
© BMJ 2017

Schizophrenia

Schizophrenia can be described by another adaptation of the pentapointed PPCC model (see Figures 10a and 10b). In schizophrenia, parts of the mind close down and fail to function. The PPCC's variables on both sides conflate, so that Observations predominate on the left hand side, including bad

Experiences, and the psychotic Determining Orientation dominates the right hand side, accommodating Dreams/Representations. These two prevailing variables are blocked off from each other in the resulting triangular structure, and they do not interrelate in the patient's mind while she is suffering from schizophrenic symptoms. The analyst occupies his usual position in the patient's mind, but can only do his best to communicate with the patient's sane Observations capacity while both of them try to support the patient's struggle with the schizophrenic illness; or he may try to communicate with her "on the psychotic wavelength" (Lucas, 2009), depending on his psychoanalytic technique.

In his work with the patient, the analyst mainly attempts to connect with the sane part of the patient's mind, the part that knows she is undergoing therapy in order to overcome her illness. Awareness of herself is a feature of the patient's life that the analyst tries to enhance, leading to insight. Earning a kinder form of self-regard is a goal which helps this, when the patient on her own can accept the difficulties and sadder or more culpable parts of herself without blame or contempt. This is sometimes not at all easy to do, particularly if in the past the patient has reached contentious or hostile situations where she has been at fault, even if all of this was clearly a result of illness and not wilfulness. This is why the sooner a patient can receive remedial therapy when she develops a schizophrenic illness, the better; lives can be lost because of the patient retreating down the slippery slope, helpless to save herself from further harm.

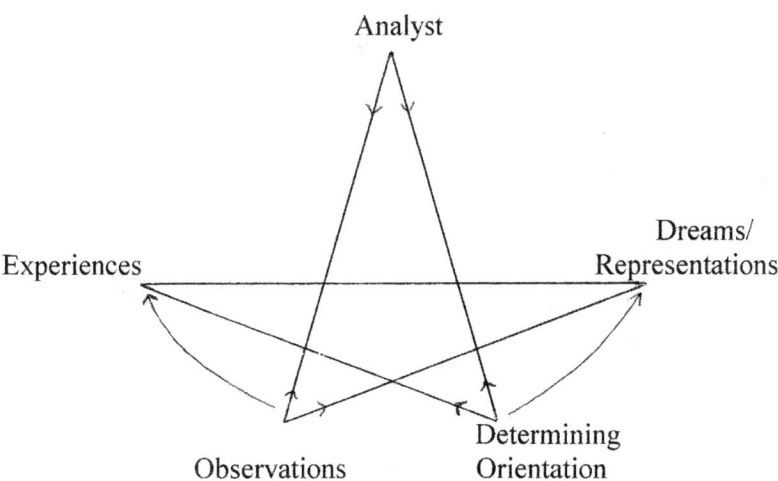

Figure 10a The development of the PPCC adaptation for schizophrenia
© BMJ 2017

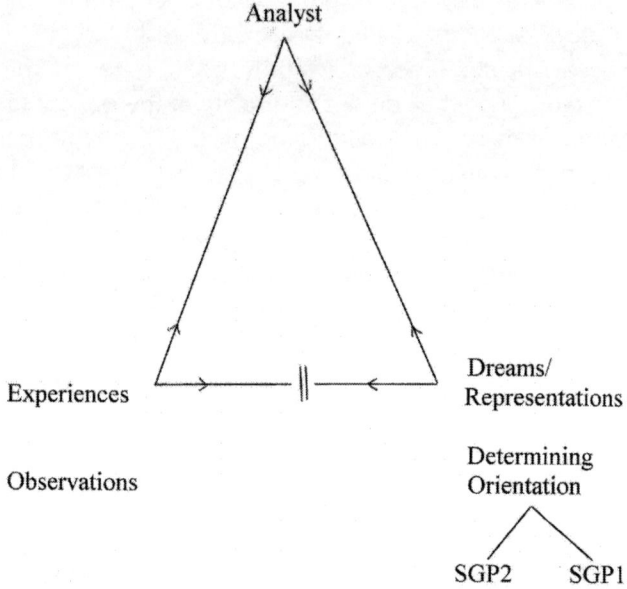

Figure 10b Adaptation of the PPCC construct for schizophrenia
© BMJ 2017

When the patient's mind is in the schizoaffective, pentapointed, paranoid-schizoid position and tending towards schizophrenia, or actually in the schizophrenic triangular formation, the Determining Orientation may manifest the two Schizophrenic Global Perspectives (see Figure 10b). These are mental states that the schizophrenic or schizoaffective patient may experience when she is developing her illness within her family. Schizophrenic Global Perspective 1, (SGP1), may evolve if, as a young person, the patient was molested by an adult in the family. The future patient may become full of hatred and resentment towards this person, and SGP1 may be quite intolerable. The other parent may never acknowledge the molesting event or broach the subject with the future patient, and the future patient's siblings may be completely oblivious to it, quite unaware that anything is, or has been, wrong. This perspective, barely tolerable for the future patient, is SGP2. The future patient is faced with these two options, SGP1 and SGP2, neither of which offers the slightest comfort or consolation, and together make the patient's position untenable, leading to illness. This kind of predicament is the situation that many schizophrenic patients experience. Without a third option, such as the attention of a kind, intelligent, and actively supportive psychoanalyst who can help the patient work out what her confusion consists of and suggest a way through the terrible difficulty it presents her with, the patient may be staring death in the face. A young person in a family may have no outside contacts who could help them. Patients in psychoanalysis have usually reached the age of young adulthood at least, with some practical access to independence, and scope to reach autonomy. Children do not have these benefits and are quite dependent upon their family, which in the case described is, of course, the source of the problems to start with.

SGP1 and SGP2 at the PPCC's Determining Orientation variable evolve into Peter Liddle's new classification of symptoms of schizophrenia (Liddle, 1987). These new classifications of symptoms are Reality Distortion Syndrome, Disorganisation Syndrome, and Psychomotor Poverty Syndrome, which supersede the earlier Positive and Negative symptom classification system. These symptom classifications comprehensively describe the symptoms that a patient suffering from schizophrenia is subject to. The analyst has to try to access the patient's non-psychotic, sane part of her mind, described by the PPCC's Observations variable, and to encourage fresh experiences, and images at the Dreams/Representations variable, so that the patient can return in the long term to a more normal mental state, represented by the pentapointed PPCC model. All of this work is very arduous, and therapeutic stalemate at Dr Michael Robbins' Therapeutic Stage 3 (see Chapter 14) is always a spectre in the distance to be avoided. The analyst's humanitarian endeavour for his patient is what keeps him going, and if this treatment has been deemed suitable for the patient then trust is held by both parties that the treatment enterprise will be worked at until it is successful. The patient is very, very fortunate to be given her chance in this way. If she has been prepared well beforehand then she will persevere, depending on her personal qualities and characteristics, according to her own best efforts.

If the analyst is able to establish a transference relationship with the very ill schizophrenic patient, the patient may begin to experience warmth and human contact again, as she learns to trust the analyst. The Experiences variable will separate from the Observations variable if this occurs, in the PPCC's description of the patient's mental state, and the pentapointed PPCC model appears again (see Figure 2a). The patient's sane, more agreeable faculty appears, represented by the Observations variable, and co-operation with the analyst develops on a surer footing. She is still in the paranoid-schizoid position, however, and may therefore be hostile to the analyst, possibly evacuating her aggression and hatred, because of her suffering, into the analyst through projective identification, making the analyst feel full of anger from which the patient has alleviated herself so that she, at least, can feel better. Eventually, after a lot of therapy, the paranoid-schizoid position may give way to the depressive position (see Figure 3). The patient's range of new experiences has allowed her to feel sufficiently accepting of the analyst so that the unpleasant side of herself, where the patient feels resentful or rejecting, is combined with warm, accepting feelings, and the analyst is experienced as but one, many-sided individual rather than in two contrasting forms, good and bad. In the depressive position, the patient feels aware of her own responsibilities for herself and other people, and tries to make amends for the consequences of all she may have done to the analyst while in the throes of illness. She may feel very guilty because of this, and quite sad; she tries to make reparation to other people who she may have wronged, and tries to heal psychological injuries.

If the patient returns to the pentapointed, neutral PPCC form of mind, her mind is able to become further modified, eventually by closing the vertex, when she can look back in time and, in an adjusted way, accept all her past experiences. A great amount of work needs to be done before this point can be reached, and the patient usually suffers as she re-engages with her past. Much stamina is needed for her to acknowledge these difficulties, which may impinge on her present. For example, people who have given her problems in the past may still occupy roles that are relevant to her present-day life, and wondering how to relate to them might be a constant source of perplexity. Sometimes it can be preferable not to see them at all, if this can be arranged.

The movements of the PPCC model from its pentapointed form to its triangular form in schizophrenia, which occurs when a schizoaffective patient has a schizophrenic episode, and, alternatively, from the pentapointed, paranoid-schizoid form to its healthy, three-dimensional pyramidal form, are shown in Figure 11. These are the changes demonstrated when a schizophrenic or schizoaffective patient becomes more ill, or achieves stages of healing, respectively. These mental changes are very unpleasant to experience for the patient, disconcerting her and making her feel very anxious. She is deeply dependent on her analyst for stability and reassurance.

The psychoanalytic psychotherapy of schizophrenia causes reversal of the development of the illness in the sense that can be illustrated in terms of mental events, as the PPCC model demonstrates. These changes in their most general sense can be shown by the PPCC to apply both in worsening illness and in improving health, which may be seen in Figure 11. This applies to the development and healing of depressive, manic and schizophrenic

THE ADAPTABILITY OF THE PPCC MODEL

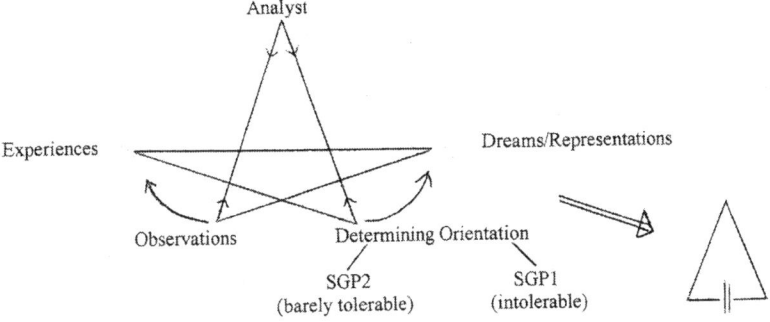

Figure 11a The PPCC tending towards illness in schizophrenia

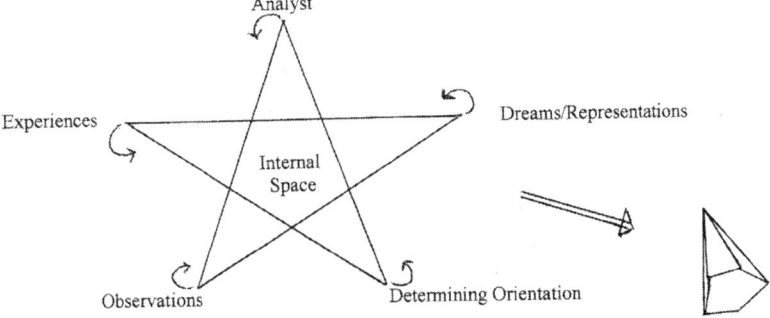

Figure 11b The PPCC tending towards resolution in schizophrenia

Figure 11 The PPCC illustrating the processes towards illness and towards resolution in schizophrenia
© BMJ 2017

illness in schizoaffective minds and to schizophrenic patients. The geometric designs present an overarching, most general sense of the changes, which are worked at in the finest detail and at every level by the analyst and the patient every day in the consulting room. Psychoanalytic theory developed by very many authors substantiates their work, describing, clarifying, and explaining the therapeutic process. The PPCC Theory simply outlines the overall changes in very simple terms so that the totality of this process can be recognised and understood for what it is, the healing of a schizophrenic or schizoaffective mind by a dedicated psychiatrically-trained psychoanalyst. The PPCC model and theory embraces very many psychoanalytic theories as an overarching, inclusive umbrella that outlines the general processes of recovery from schizophrenic illness through psychoanalytic psychotherapy (see Chapter 11).

Alignment of Freud's theory of depression, Bion's theory of cognition, and Fodor's representational theory of mind in the PPCC model

Figures 12 and 13 illustrate how three different theoretical constructions involving different features of mental life are each established as occurring through an element arising within the mind interacting with an element from the external environment. Freud's theory of depression links the lost loved one's external "shadow" to its falling upon the patient's ego, an internal mental component, to produce depression (Freud, 1917). Bion believed that a preconception within the mind, such as an image of a dog, "mates" or "coheres" with a sensory perception in the external environment such as sight of a real dog, produces a conception, such as the thought "I am looking at a dog" (Bion, 1962). In Jerry Fodor's Representational Theory of Mind (Fulford et al, 2006, p. 676), he considered that a Person O, if he adopts a "functional" or "computational" relation R (internal) towards a Mental Representation, MP, of a real (external) object with which it has a causal relation, he will develop a Propositional Attitude A towards the Mental Representation. The Mental Representation encodes the content of the Propositional Attitude and is its internal vehicle. If the Mental Representation is, for example, the statement "My friend's illness is serious", about a friend of Person O, then if the person adopts a Relation R of sadly believing towards it, he consequently sadly believes that his friend's illness is serious, which is his Propositional Attitude. All three of these examples show how an element in the mind can combine with an element outside the mind to produce a mental function. The PPCC model illustrates quite clearly their similarity. It also demonstrates graphically how Freud's theory of depression relates the patient's causative representational variable, ie. the "shadow", to their unsatisfactory representational world full of hard, cold facts; and it demonstrates how normal healthy attitudes, thoughts or observations arise from sensory perceptions and mental representations.

The versatility of the PPCC model

The pentapointed PPCC model can thus be adapted in several different ways. It is able to illustrate the functional psychoses, changes in the stance of the patient's mind to other people, commonalities in the functioning of the mind according to different theoretical approaches, and progress of the schizophrenic or schizoaffective mind as it heals in therapy.

Each instance of its adaptability illustrates visually qualities of the human mind's functioning, in health or illness. The PPCC model therefore offers a

THE ADAPTABILITY OF THE PPCC MODEL

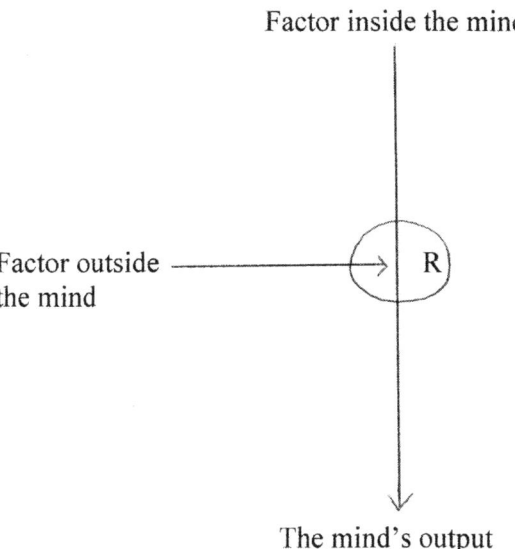

Figure 12 A combination of internal and external factors of the mind leading to a mental outcome
© BMJ 2017

```
                        Objective Facts eg. loss of loved object
                                        |
                                        v
                        Fodor's Person O making sad Observations
                        Freud: ego function
                        Bion: preconception
                                        |
                                        |
                              Fodor:    |    Fodor: 'functional/computational'
Fodor: Mental Representation MP: -----> (R)   Freud: 'falls upon'
       causal relation to very sad            Bion: 'mating', 'cohering'
       objective Facts (content)
Freud: 'shadow of the object'                 |
Bion:  sensory experience,                    v
       a negative realization
                        content-laden mental state (despair) ) Fodor: A
                        Propositional Attitude (helplessness))
                        conceptualization or non-tolerance of frustration)Bion
                                                            ie. psychosis)
                                        |
                                        v
                        Experience of clinical depression: Freud
```

Figure 13 Comparison of the mental processes of Bion's and Foder's theories of thinking with Freud's theory of depression
© BMJ 2017

conceptualisation of the mind which is usefully able to convey meaning concerning the progress of a patient's mental health when in psychoanalytic psychotherapy. The overall clarity of the psychoanalytic process can therefore be represented in an understandable language which may be particularly helpful for readers who are not familiar with psychological phenomena.

CHAPTER 10

THE OVERALL STRUCTURAL PPCC SEQUENCE OF THE RECOVERING SCHIZOPHRENIC OR SCHIZOAFFECTIVE MIND

Chapters 7, 8 and 9 illustrate how the schizophrenic or schizoaffective mind in therapy can be described by geometric structures. The changes in these structures, from being restricted by a limiting and unpleasant representational world, albeit a relief to discover its balance and beautiful potential when including an analyst, to a mature, rounded personality, may be seen as an overall structural sequence (see Figure 7). The fact that this sequence can be illustrated by the changing geometric PPCC model affirms perception that the pathology is being resolved, and reveals the nature of the process.

Each structure in the sequence actually represents qualities of the schizophrenic or schizoaffective mind at that stage. The pentapointed PPCC model illustrates that the analyst has been introjected, or internalised, into the patient's mind so that he or she can be related to psychologically by the patient, in their physical absence. It indicates that the representational world is an intermediary between the patient's internal world, their Internal Space, and External Reality. It includes all the variables that the Shorter Oxford Textbook of Psychiatry indicates provide the data during psychoanalytic treatment upon which psychoanalytic theories mainly depend (Gelder et al, 2006, p. 89). It illustrates Melanie Klein's paranoid-schizoid position where objects (people) that are the focus of attention are split between good, positive qualities and bad, unpleasant qualities; the PPCC illustrates the paranoid-schizoid split with limited permitted mental flexibility that the psychotic Determining Orientation variable causes when the non-psychotic Observations variable cannot be conflated with it. When these two variables are conflated, the marquise PPCC model demonstrates the broader flexibility and construing of Klein's depressive position.

Thus the PPCC's pentapointed construct and the PPCC marquise construct provide rich details about the schizoaffective patient's mind while it is in the early stages of psychoanalytic psychotherapy. These geometric constructs are exemplified in the two illustrative case studies (see Parts IV and V), where the wretchedness of the two patients' early environments, absorbed as their representational worlds, is plain to see. It really seems hardly any wonder that these two patients developed along unhealthy lines, becoming unable to cope in other environments because the impoverished life skills they did manage to acquire were less than good enough for their survival outside their homes. They succumbed to the dearth of opportunity they grew up with, their minds were unequal to their struggles to make sense of this, and finally gave way to the unhealthy conclusions and attitudes which defined their illnesses.

So the PPCC is well able to describe the minds observed by the psychiatrist upon meeting a newly-presenting patient suffering their first episode of schizophrenic or schizoaffective illness. This graphic illustration also describes for the benefit of non-psychologically-orientated readers the reality of distressed minds and what form this distress can take; for schizophrenic and schizoaffective patients the distress affects their whole mind and is acutely intense and painful. The case studies allocate features of the patients' environments to the four analysand variables so that their representational worlds can be observed as the entirety of the patients' perceptions; very unpleasant places to be at, psychologically. Non-psychologically-orientated readers might feel great compassion for schizophrenic patients and also great understanding if they were to read the details of these patients' representational worlds, and then see from the PPCC model that this is all a patient has to work with in trying to adjust her personal privacy, in her Internal Space, to the rigours of the world's reality surrounding her. The strength and energy of any individual, whether or not a patient, has limits; and growing up requires stamina. If the environment is hostile, a process of steady attrition may attain an ever-increasing stranglehold on the patient's life-force, her zest for living, or simply her abiding interest in it. Eventually, when seriously under-nourished and with inadequate positive response to it, her effort ceases, her mind implodes and a major mental catastrophe ensues. The PPCC model contains the material of these truths, as the patient's representational world, at the outset of the schizoaffectively disordered patient's therapy, in the form of the pentapointed PPCC construct.

If a patient is suffering from schizophrenia the initial model is the blocked triangular PPCC model, where the patient's few non-psychotic

Observations are completely separated from the prevailing psychotic part of her mind at the Determining Orientation variable. The analyst retains contact and communication but has to decipher and interpret the patient's psychotic communications (Lucas, 2009; Evans, 2016) while trying to understand her meaning in context. Long passages of time may pass while the analyst remains uncertain about the meaning being communicated by the patient. Stamina is required by both parties. Ward staff may be able to shed some complementary light for the analyst from noticing aspects of the patient's behaviour on the ward. But the patient may scarcely be able to help the ward staff at all to understand her by articulating via her non-psychotic Observations variable; in the throes of psychosis, she occupies her world of psychosis which is separate from the world of reality, and has been provoked into existence by her entirely unsatisfactory original representational world, the unpleasant environment in which she has been trying to develop as an individual.

Thus the triangular model remains blocked while the patient suffers schizophrenic psychosis. Warmth, encouragement and patience on the analyst's part may bear the fruit of attempts at meaningful non-psychotic articulations by the patient. The more this response flourishes, the further the psychosis recedes into the background, and meaning may gradually become established within the transference/countertransference rapport. Upon this foundation may be built the substance of the therapeutic alliance (Zetzel, 1970), and all the therapeutic dyad's endeavours towards insight. Eventually, the blocked triangular model modifies into the pentapointed, neutral form of the PPCC where communications may be much more freely exchanged between analyst and analysand (the patient). The patient's mind is still divided between its psychotic and its non-psychotic parts, in the paranoid-schizoid position, where good and bad aspects of another person are still perceived separately (Klein, 1946, p. 14). And this in turn may change into the marquise form of the PPCC which illustrates maturation into the depressive position, allowing much more learning and adaptation to occur from a perspective of gratitude and concern, as Melanie Klein outlined (Klein, 1935, p. 276).

When the patient has worked with the analyst in the depressive position for long enough, sometimes for quite a number of years, her perception of herself and her insight may have become so substantially enlightened that she is able to look back at her life without fear or anxiety. All the pain and distress encountered at the time no longer precipitates a feeling of losing control or psychosis itself. The patient can remember events and people and reflect that, if her attitude to these at the time had been different, maybe the bad reaction or difficulty or problem could have been overcome more effectively. She could try to "rewrite her history". The patient takes responsibility for her own past reactions and feelings, attitudes and behaviour. She is now orientated in time, place, and person to the whole of her earlier life. She can remember her past differently; and has now resolved her psychosis.

Resolution of the patient's psychotic tendency is illustrated by the five variables of the pentapointed PPCC model folding back and coalescing at a single point, the vertex; this phase is "closure of the vertex", and signals that the treatment is nearly complete. There may be psychotic "wobbles", and indeed this is quite likely, but the disease process itself has been halted, the illness' functioning mastered, the psychotic tendency recognised, and thereby the patient's fearfulness of the diagnosis and all that it implies has been overcome; the patient now has her own awareness and insight of herself as an essentially integrated and intact person. Any hint of psychosis is remedied by reflection upon the stability of her now-insightful past life, lived and coped with, retrospectively, with support and her own courage. The three-dimensional, five-sided pyramid physically contains all the events and people of the patient's past life, securely and stably, and the patient is no longer afraid of it.

This is followed by an ongoing period of socially mixing and interacting with other people, friends and fellow-residents or work acquaintances. The possibly-sharp "corners" of irritabilities or impatience or, indeed, shyness, or anxiety or grief that may remain in the patient's personality, after all the endured years of illness and distress, need to be "rubbed off" or soothed and smoothed until the patient feels as comfortable, socially and congenially companionable as she wishes to be. This stage is described in the PPCC model as the pentasided pyramid evolving into the balanced sphere, which is smoothly finished in all its aspects and is able to roll steadily on its course without internal disturbance. The patient who has completed her psychoanalytic psychotherapy has a wealth of fresh insight that she can take with her into all her new relationships, smoothly adjusted to herself and to other people as she is. Even if she encounters difficulties she will have internalised her analyst (a very early step illustrated by the PPCC model), which will companionably strengthen her efforts through improved self-regard and self-confidence and, most importantly, self-understanding; her analyst, as an internal object, remains present in the patient's awareness, and the patient may imagine what the analyst might say in any situation she finds herself addressing. The analyst in this sense can continue to guide the patient even after treatment has terminated, by his constant presence in the patient's mind as an internal good object.

The sequence of diagrams that form the PPCC's description of the overall process of resolution of schizophrenia and schizoaffective disorder (see Figure 7) is the original series of concepts that the author of this book found to illustrate the changes which occurred in her original schizoaffectively disordered patient. The individual PPCC shapes each describe exactly the nature of the patient's mind during one phase of psychoanalytic treatment. The connections between them show the changes that the patient's mind has undergone, so that the PPCC model continues to describe the mind in this way. The case studies in Parts IV and V of this book illustrate equally clearly the details of the two clinical histories that the individual graphic models describe and represent in each case. The two histories can be compared in the completeness of their recovery. They share this overall resolution in common, and the PPCC is as relevant in one as in the other; its shapes represent the common stages that each case undergoes, and the two patients' minds are equally validly illustrated by the same PPCC structures as they move towards recovery. Within each case study, the variations in the two patients' progress are illustrated by variations within the PPCC sequences; but the overall pattern of progress remains consistently illustrated by the PPCC model.

The fact that schizophrenic and schizoaffective patients' illnesses may be resolved through psychoanalytic psychotherapeutic treatment may be a surprising fact for some clinicians. It may be considered that schizophrenia is an organic disease that can only be resolved by medications that affect the dopaminergic and other functioning brain connection systems. Heightened reactivity to stressors has also for a long time been accepted as a cardinal feature of schizophrenia (Larkin and Morrison, 2006, p. 37). Over-reactivity and dysregulation of the HPA axis is found in abused children (Read et al, 2001). These adversely functioning, physiologically-mediated features of psychosis are established beyond doubt. Their physicality may justify remedial medication being prescribed to try to reverse them.

This approach is clearly valuable. But equally important to the schizophrenia sufferer is their experience of schizophrenia. They are in dreadful distress. One look at the representational world they have tried to grow up within (see Case Studies 1 and 2 in Parts IV and V herein) illustrates the basis for their unsurprisingly disturbed psychology. The symptoms they manifest can be aligned with the equivalently demonstrated PPCC stage, thus demonstrating the place that these symptoms occupy on the patient's personal journey from schizophrenia to mental health. This is irrefutable because of the reality and truth of the PPCC model's demonstrable veracity. These patients undeniably had schizophrenia and now do not. The psychological features of the patients' minds have been taken seriously by their psychoanalytic psychotherapists, and adjusted during years of therapy. The patient's experience of schizophrenia has been accepted as all and everything except funding and, importantly, hopefully also an irrepressible determination to be well, that the patient can bring to the table of their future recovery, with their doctors. Medication can facilitate healing. But it cannot affect the details of the patient's memories and experiences, which need to be shared with another human being so that the interpretation returned by them to the patient facilitates the patient's adjustment to their own experience of themselves. When the patient knows what is true within themselves they begin to gain confidence and to act from a sense of integration and confidence. With schizophrenic illness this can take a long time, usually a number of years. In this way, everything the patient is, ie. their experiences and their memories, together with their individual brain physiology, medicated as required, and their determination, has been taken into account and assisted to develop. As a person, they have required the details and facts of their life to be taken into account, registered, recognised, and interpreted, and then that this history be used to organise how best they may be helped to pick up the healthy, strong parts of themselves and move forwards in their life. Medication simply is not enough on its own; far more attention needs to be paid to the patient's experience of life before they have any chance of relinquishing dependence, or becoming less dependent, on psychiatric services. If independence can be achieved then a substantial component of NHS resources can be saved. And if this treatment were rolled out for suitable schizophrenic patients universally, that is in every psychiatric practice, then suitable patients would be found far more frequently and helped eventually to move out of psychiatric care.

Many ancillary therapies for schizophrenia and schizoaffective disorder are available, for example CBT, family therapy, social skills therapy, and many others besides psychoanalytic psychotherapy. Only those patients who are bright enough, determined and forgiving and patient enough, and, at present, those whose families are able and prepared to pay for psychoanalytic psychotherapy, are likely to be able to benefit from it (see Chapter 3 for a discussion of costs). But, in a National Health Schedule for Schizophrenia, every patient with schizophrenia would be assessed for their suitability for it. In this way, none would be overlooked as potentially becoming able to find their mind and take part fully in life. The idea that inside schizophrenic patients lies a versatile, energetic, determined, possibly creative mind that has not received sufficient resource to emerge into normality is one that makes all therapists shudder from the horror of the patient's experience of entrapment. All therapists desire that their patients emerge into being the person they are trying to become, through their mutual efforts. Patients simply cannot do this solely by accepting medication. The fault lines in their psyches need to be reflected upon with the help of their therapists, whether psychoanalytic psychotherapists, cognitive behavioural therapists, family therapists, or therapists in any other psychologically based specialty. Psychiatrists are in a strong position to be able to recognise when a patient requires skilled therapy. Medical psychotherapy may help some, who have capacity to think for themselves at a level consonant with outpatient work, not requiring hospitalisation. Deeper psychological work is required to help more afflicted patients. Plumbing the depths of schizophrenia, as has been done by Dr Michael Robbins and others through psychoanalytic psychotherapy, is the way to alleviate schizophrenia in carefully selected sufferers who possess observed indications of aptitude for hard psychological work and so might be expected to decrease both psychiatrists' patient lists and social services expenditure. The PPCC illustrates the psychological processes involved in the alleviation and resolution of schizophrenia. If CBT or other therapies are able to match psychoanalytic psychotherapy's ability to remedy schizophrenia then they should be employed to help suitable patients, as happens at present. But every patient, in a National Health Schedule for Schizophrenia, should be given the opportunity to be assessed for psychoanalytic psychotherapy on humanitarian grounds in case they have inside them the germ of a life which could save health services large amounts of money and be truly fruitful.

PART III
SUCCESSFUL PSYCHOANALYTIC PSYCHOTHERAPY FOR SCHIZOPHRENIA

....

DR GILLIAN STEGGLES

CHAPTER 11

THE PSYCHOANALYTIC CONCEPTS OF THE PPCC THEORY

The PPCC Theory is an observational theory based on careful observation and recording of the psychological states which a schizoaffective patient moved through during the psychoanalytical resolution of her illness. The psychological processes that she underwent may be explained by existing psychoanalytical theories that underpin the processes of change she demonstrated. Schizophrenia affects all parts of the mind, and the relevant psychoanalytical theories described below illustrate in an explanatory way how these different parts of the patient's schizophrenic or schizoaffective mind begin to adopt more mature functioning under the psychoanalyst's influence. The lines with arrows in the PPCC structure indicate the lines of communication between the analyst and the analysand, or patient, and imply the transference relationship (see below) and the dynamic nature of the therapeutic dyad (see Figure 2a).

The PPCC model is a structural representation of the patient's schizoaffective mind. It forms one example of a dynamic presentation compatible with Sigmund Freud's structural model of the mind, ie. that conceptualisation of it which purports to show different structural parts of it working in relation to other parts (see Figure 6). In the PPCC construct the ego, superego and id lie within the Internal Space, the ego bounding it as Jaak Panksepp's SELF on the PPCC's inner pentagon (see below). The PPCC construct thus clearly delineates the interface between the patient's Internal Space, where many of her mental processes continue, and External Reality, which forms the context for most of the patient's personal relationships and is the area where everything relating to "not-me" is based. The PPCC model describes structural psychological positions adopted by psychotic minds in response to different experiences as the patient moves from developmental pathological helplessness to adjusted, smoothly functioning psychology. A number of different structural and functional psychoanalytical concepts explain some of the positions, features, and changes described by the PPCC Theory.

Joseph Sandler's and Bernard Rosenblatt's Representational World concept (Sandler and Rosenblatt, 1962) was conceived of as a structure that a young child develops in response to its experiences of successive environments which it must adjust to in order to be able to cope successfully with future encounters. The representational world thus acts as an intermediary in the child's psychological development between its inner self and External Reality; External Reality is represented in part, ie. those parts that are significant for the child, by the representational world, which can be seen visually to be positioned between the Internal Space and External Reality in the pentapointed PPCC construct. The representational world changes as time passes and the child matures. The PPCC's graphic representational world illustrates all these points visually. Each analysand PPCC variable includes all those parts of External Reality which fall under its aegis in the patient's mind.

Thus the PPCC pentapointed construct relates the patient's Internal Space to External Reality via her Representational World. These divisions also, but broadly and in a general way with some overlap, reflect the patient's unconscious relating to her conscious via her preconscious. Appropriately, they differentiate the patient's consciousness, largely using which she negotiates her way through External Reality; the patient's unconscious, which is housed largely in her Internal Space; and her preconscious, which is the part of the original schizoaffective patient's mind from which she accessed her Representational World and then drew it out for the first time in her original pentapointed diagram. In the PPCC model the patient's consciousness, preconscious and unconscious are largely sited in the Internal Space, but her preconscious extends to her representational world and her consciousness extends to External Reality. The three divisions are clearly connected, quite certainly functioning through interactions with each other via the lines of communication between analyst and patient. Her analyst has full access during the patient's sessions to all three parts of her mind, and is able through his interpretations to inform subtly, stimulate carefully, and modify the patient's mind gradually into improved mental habits, kinder experiences and gradually more hope, as her therapy sessions progress.

The four analysand variables, viz. Experiences, Dreams/Representations, Observations (thoughts), and Determining Orientation (Facts, Fantasies or Schizophrenic Global Perspectives), embrace the material that the Shorter Oxford Textbook of Psychiatry (Gelder et al, 2006, p. 89) identifies as the data obtained in the course of psychoanalytical treatment that psychoanalytic theories are mainly derived from. The PPCC model thus contains the patient's personal information and psychological features comprehensively as it sets out to show what happens to the patient's mind as therapy progresses. Whatever occurs during the course of treatment may be attributed and located to a destination within the structure of the patient's mind, where it may, or may not, affect the structure itself. Changing as it does, in accordance with Sandler's and Rosenblatt's concept, the PPCC's depiction of the representational world faithfully acts as a repository for the patient's initially distressing connections with, and experiences of, her early environments. Peter Liddle's schizophrenic syndromes (Liddle, 1987), for example, are located at the paranoid-schizoid pentapointed PPCC's psychotic Determining Orientation variable, as the patient's Schizophrenic Global Perspectives 1 and 2. As the nature of her responses changes once the analyst is in the representational world as an internal object, so the quality and shape of the patient's mind changes. Her capacities change, eg. she becomes better able to construe loosely and freely in the depressive position, or she is enabled to address her past experiences orientated in time, place, and person without fear or anxiety of triggering a psychotic episode. The representational world forms a visual, structural framework in the patient's mind, described by the PPCC, and analogous to the conception of a guiding, dependable structure in the mind of a child growing up.

Neuropsychoanalytically, parts of the PPCC construct (A) may be considered to represent salient functional parts of the mind (B) which locate to specifically active parts of the brain (C). Such functional parts of the mind (B) include the Extended Reticular and Thalamic Activating System, or ERTAS, (Solms and Turnbull, 2002), that modulates internal arousal and governs aspects of the patient's internal world such as wakefulness, consciousness and dreaming; these functions are involved in the emotional drives of FEAR, RAGE, LUST, SEEKING, PANIC, CARE and PLAY (in capitals for specification purposes) that constitute Jaak Panksepp's SELF, a "Simple Ego-type Life Form", or primordial self-scheme (Panksepp, 1998); and then the mind's executive function modulates the SELF in relation to external reality.

Corresponding parts of the brain (C) include for the ERTAS the brain stem reticular formation proper and the thalamus, as well as other nuclei such as parts of the hypothalamus, the parabrachial nuclei, the locus coeruleus and the raphe nuclei; the mesopontine tectum and the dorsal tegmentum, in the periaqueductal grey of the upper brainstem, localise the origins of the SELF which "forms the foundational ego upon which all our more complex representatives of our selves are built" (Solms and Turnbull, 2002, p. 110), (Panksepp, 1998); and the prefrontal cortex, especially the ventromesial cortex, monitors all the internal and external sensory and motor activity focused in the SELF in relation to the patient's memory and current thoughts and emotions and needs, acting as "the crowning glory of the human brain" (Solms and Turnbull, 2002, p. 281) through inhibition of what is not currently required by the patient to relate effectively to External Reality.

Three parts of the PPCC construct may be described in this way:

(i) The PPCC's Internal Space (A) encloses the ERTAS (B) among other functions; and this mechanism may be located in the brainstem reticulum and the thalamus, parts of the hypothalamus, the parabrachial nuclei, the locus coeruleus and the raphe nuclei (C);
(ii) The inner pentagon of the PPCC (A) represents the SELF or ego which relates a) parts of the internal world in the Internal Space such as the ERTAS to b) parts of the outside world represented by the patient's Representational World (B); and the SELF's mechanism is located in the mesopontine tectum and the dorsal tegmentum, in the periaqueductal grey (C);
(iii) The corners or nodes of the PPCC's pentagon where the Internal Space is in contact with External Reality (A) are where internal (viz. The ERTAS) and external (viz. the patient's Representational World) representations of the SELF relate to External Reality through executive functions in a practical way (B); and the mind's executive functions, integrating all the patient's internal and external sensory and motor activity in relation to external reality, are located in the prefrontal cortex, especially the ventromesial cortex (C).

The PPCC's facility for representing the functionality of the patient's mind in its relatively healthy, neutral state may be seen here, even relating to brain structures, to be consistent with many aspects of their relativity, thus graphically, psychologically, and physically.

Biological aspects of the patient's mind when it manifests pathological features may also be represented by parts of the structure of the PPCC construct. The Determining Orientation variable may house in its triangle what are widely understood to be the biological processes underlying depression and schizophrenia; the biological processes of mania are not well understood. In this triangular area of the PPCC are located the NMDA receptors that are excited by glutamate and inhibited by GABA. Hypofunction in the NMDA receptors accompanied by decreased stimulation by excitatory glutamate leads to inhibited dopaminergic activity in the mesocortical neurones between the A10 nucleus in the ventral tegmental area and the prefrontal cortex, and thus also in the prefrontal cortex, which in turn leads, as is widely held, to the negative symptoms of schizophrenia, and Peter Liddle's Psychomotor Poverty Syndrome. Hypofunction in NMDA receptors on inhibitory GABA-ergic interneurones leads to increased activity in the mesolimbic dopamine neurones between the A10 nucleus and the nucleus accumbens, causing excessive dopaminergic activity in the nucleus accumbens and, it is thought, to the positive symptoms of schizophrenia, or Peter Liddle's Disorganisation Syndrome and Reality Distortion Syndrome.

These functions are found in the preconscious Determining Orientation variable's triangle in the PPCC model because the patient is partly aware of how they are being affected by their schizophrenic illness. The patient's original, deprived Representational World is in the patient's preconscious, in broad contact with External Reality in the PPCC model. The author's (GS) case study patient was able to access it from her preconscious to produce her abstract transitional object which satisfied her need so substantially while apart from her analyst. The low 5-HT blood levels commonly found in depression are also located in the Determining Orientation variable triangle. The patient's manic symptoms as a defence from depression are located here, too, but with few clear indications at present of its underlying biological mechanism.

Almost none of this neuroscience was available to Sigmund Freud in his day. And yet Eric Kandel stated in 1999, when describing his New Intellectual Framework for Psychiatry Revisited (Kandel, 1999), that "psychoanalysis still represents the most coherent and intellectually satisfying view of the mind". This is highly complimentary towards Freud's monumental canon of work and that of subsequent authors. Kandel threw down a gauntlet for neuroscience and psychoanalysis to synergise. This has been wonderfully picked up by Mark Solms and colleagues, from whose work in neuropsychoanalysis, elucidating the neurophysiological origins of mental phenomena, the above reflections on the PPCC's representations have been derived.

Developing his own theories clinically, Sigmund Freud believed that a schizophrenic patient is unable to develop a transference, or close relationship with the analyst that is similar to the particular kind of relationship that a given patient tends to develop with people generally; and the schizophrenic patient's relationships are all adversely affected by her illness. The countertransference relationship, the analyst's feelings for the patient, is also strained because the patient is so difficult to communicate with and her responsiveness tends to be so limited. Freud thought that a schizophrenic patient's narcissism, or inward looking preoccupation, is so intense that it prevents her being able to communicate feeling outwards in this way to other people. But Melanie Klein, Wilfred Bion, Herbert Rosenfeld and Hanna Segal all demonstrated that positive transference relationships can indeed be established with schizophrenic patients. Today's analysts find that, if they persist in their efforts, they can establish useful connections with the patient that can form a life-saving bond, and break down the isolation commonly suffered by schizophrenic patients. Sara, Case Study 2 as described in this volume, exemplifies this function of the analyst, in this case Dr Robbins, very vividly. For several years, Dr Robbins persisted in sitting with Sara while she worked through her extreme psychological difficulties during her sessions without knowing what the outcome of her treatment would be, and while she experienced the emotional support he was giving her. Eventually, Sara learned to trust Dr Robbins, to allow him to help her move out of her existing psychological attitudes and mistaken ideas, and instead adopt ways of thinking that would be more helpful to her in the real world outside her family. Dr Robbins' patience and Sara's persistence were rewarded, and after eleven years of therapy Sara emerged well and strong. Transference and countertransference relationships are implied in the PPCC construct by the lines of communication between the analyst and analysand variables, which are indicated by arrows. Over time, in a successful psychoanalytic treatment, the transference relationship tends to grow stronger, and allows all the psychological growth that the patient needs, to take place.

Initially, at the start of treatment, a schizoaffective or schizophrenic patient's ego is commonly fragmented and has vague boundaries; that is, the strength of her personal identity is weak. These failures of development occur because the experiences lived through by the patient from birth have not been satisfying to her and have not reinforced her sense of herself as an individual. She really doesn't know who she is. She has not received a clear impression in the eyes of another about aspects of herself that she really needs to know. In these important areas her psychological needs have not been met. In psychosis there is an uncertain boundary between "me" and "not-me". This gives rise to the basic anxiety that all schizophrenic and schizoaffective patients suffer from, as one source of this anxiety, and it contributes to the patients' overall experience of distress at their illness.

Psychotherapeutic help, amounting to psychologically nourishing support, may strengthen the patient's ego over time. These ego changes are represented within the Internal Space and at its boundary in the PPCC model; the superego and id are also located within the Internal Space.

"Good enough containment", reflecting both Winnicott's views on a mother's good enough parenting for her baby (Winnicott, 1965) and Bion's concept of an analyst's supporting role or containment of the patient's feelings in the same way as a mother contains her baby's feelings (Bion, 1962, p. 90) permits the patient to feel understood and protected, and provides her with the opportunity to grow into greater differentiation and individuation. The ego bounding the Internal Space gains scope from the psychoanalytic psychotherapy for better tolerance and endurance, allowing it to respond increasingly effectively when it is exposed to instances of imposition upon it by adverse circumstances. Eventually, improved assertiveness from a strengthened ego structure, and more confident decision-making, may follow.

Another ego function, located within the bounding of the Internal Space by the SELF in the PPCC model, is affect regulation. Normally, this develops from the stable bond between a baby and its mother through "mirroring". The mother "mirrors" and contains the baby's raw emotions as these arise, and the baby learns to experience these emotions safely, in this context. Gradually, the baby recognises its feelings when away from Mother, and learns to manage and control them on its own. Figure 2b illustrates in simple terms how affect regulation may function. This is one illustration of the unconscious activities that are represented as occurring in the PPCC construct's Internal Space. Affect regulation is an early challenge, and may be one of the last functions to be achieved during recovery from schizophrenia or schizoaffective disorder. It proceeds once cognitive resolution is well under way and may reach mastery only when the Time, Place, and Person orientation of the pentasided pyramid has been achieved, in the last stages of the PPCC model.

Adults in therapy sometimes have difficulty containing their emotions. The analyst "contains" the patient's emotions in just the same way as a mother "contains" her infant's feelings, as described above. Schizophrenic patients are subject to rage and anger, especially early in treatment, and sometimes subsequently, when the realities of their unnecessarily painful past experiences become apparent to them. Indignation and outrage can rise to the surface, and the patients need to master these with self-control. Depression, also, can be overwhelming. The analyst is tasked with helping to stabilise the patient in her distress, identifying as far as possible specific elements that might be contributing to the depth of the patient's suffering, and offering helpful insight through interpretations. Acting-out of emotions is not encouraged, and self-control is advocated, especially on a hospital ward. The PPCC models for depression, mania, and schizophrenia illustrate

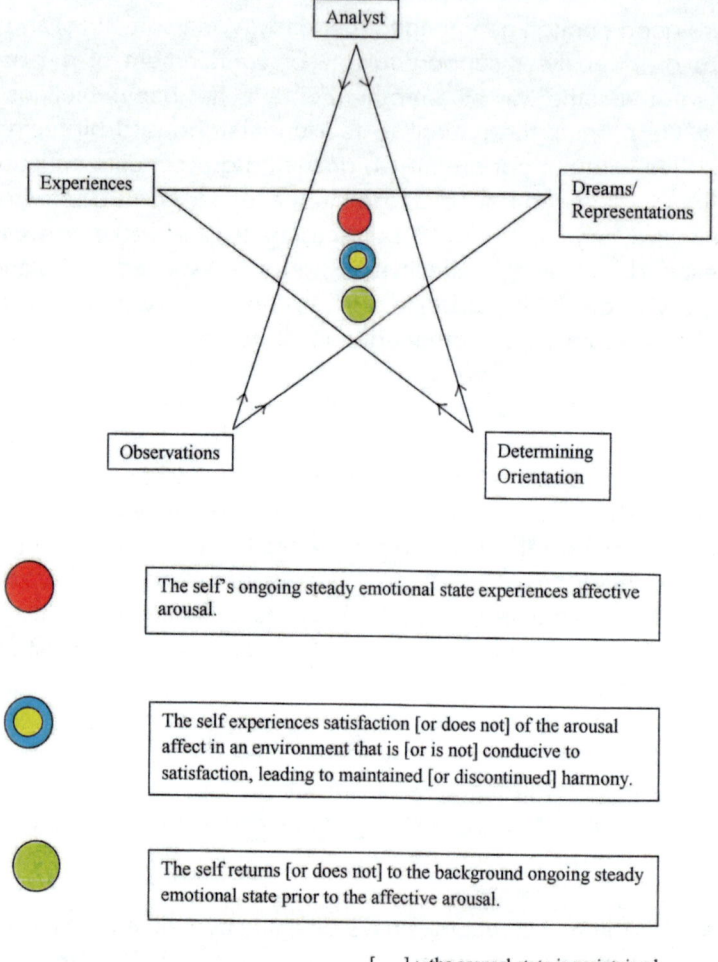

Figure 2b The PPCC model illustrating affect regulation

the absence of an Internal Space with its pentagonal representation of the ego; and self-control develops when the patient's mind regains its Internal Space and a stable representational world under the influence and subsequent inclusion of the analyst within itself, initially in the paranoid-schizoid position.

Ego boundaries improve with learning through the therapeutic transference. The analyst's boundaries are set firm, and this enhances the patient's own identity as she relates though time to the clear margins of the analyst as another individual. When she becomes psychotic the margins may blur again, but consistency throughout the therapy helps the patient to see herself as the analyst manifestly sees her, and encourages her to find out about herself so that her identity becomes clearer to herself as an individual person, with clear margins to her personal, experienced sense of herself, and thus a stronger ego.

In treatment the patient experiences maturation of autonomous conflict-free ego functions (Hartmann, 1939) such as coping with the demands and restrictions of external reality; thus mediating between the drives of hunger and sex through the id, and reality, and between the drives and the superego, becomes increasingly possible after engaging in a healing transference with the analyst. This process helps to enable her to live independently following her treatment. An important aspect of this is satisfaction of the need for safety, another idea expounded by Joseph Sandler (Sandler, 1987). He suggests that seeking safety is a primary goal for a young child, and that unless this is achieved development will be held back. In his view, finding safety is at least as imperative as finding food or a mate. And in 1989 (Sandler, 1989), Sandler opposed the safety and drive concepts, demonstrating that the urge to gain feelings of wellbeing and safety has to be stronger than instinctual gratification, in order to keep a close check on the latter when its expression implies danger. He advocates "feeling states" (Fonagy and Target, 2003, p. 99):

> *"While drives, needs, emotional forces, and other influences arising from within the body are highly important in determining behaviour, from the point of view of psychological functioning they exert their effect through changes in feeling."*
>
> (Sandler 1972, p. 296)

Unconscious fantasies associated with wishes for safety predominate in a child, and influence all adults' mental life. These activities all continue in the patient's Internal Space, in the PPCC model.

Improving the strength and range of unconscious defence mechanisms is a later phase of treatment, once the corrosive, pathological schizophrenic process has been halted and the patient is becoming able to reflect upon her past without fear of breakdown. Reviewing alternative ways of interacting with events and incidents may create possibilities for the patient's responses to the external environment and other people. The PPCC vertex closes (see Figure 4) when the patient's repertoire of self-defence and style of self-preservation mechanisms are sufficiently robust. The Internal Space becomes three-dimensional, enclosing all the matured ego functions, in the PPCC model.

Within the Internal Space, in both its planar and three-dimensional forms, are carried out the ongoing underlying mental functions of the patient. Cognitive and mentalising functions take place here and are linked to, and update, the Observations variable ie. observations that the patient makes, via their common boundary. Similarly, reflective functioning and experiencing occurs in the Internal Space and is connected to the Experiences variable at this side of the Internal Space. Symbolic and narrative aspects of the self relate to Dreams and Representations, and when these parts of the self become active in the Internal Space, the Dreams/Representations variable of the representational world is updated. The Variables of the representational world are constantly revised according to the patient's continuing mental activities which progress inside the Internal Space. The functions connected with a particular part of the representational world involve the ego which, as the SELF on the Internal Space's boundary, mediates between that part of the representational world which is active and the rest of the patient's mind in the Internal Space. When the patient is psychotic, however, normal mental processes cease and the Internal Space loses its form and identity so that only confusion is manifest in the patient's mind.

The patient needs to adjust to External Reality as an ongoing task, once she has internally adjusted to her past interactions and to her personal difficulties with it. The analyst usually keeps an eye on the patient's life outside her sessions, and his references to the outside world will be constructive and positive to try to help his patient adopt a meaningful stance towards it. Not being afraid of it is a very helpful approach for the patient to pursue, since unforeseen difficulties in fresh encounters can otherwise prove daunting for the patient's further explorations. Managing personal relationships and the need for instinctual gratifications of different kinds may be difficult at first, when the patient starts to explore after beginning to feel stronger within her therapy. Sometimes new relationships can interfere with the treatment's progress. In these circumstances, the analyst can only concentrate on monitoring how the patient's therapeutic changes are affected, and do what he can to oversee these.

The analyst becomes an internal object for the patient in a successful treatment. The PPCC construct shows how the analyst is incorporated into the patient's representational world in place of the variable "Problems" (see Chapter 7). Melanie Klein developed the concept of Internal Object from its origins in Karl Abraham's writings (Abraham, 1924), which at the time were contemporaneous with her early work, although she never used the term herself. As an internal good object, the analyst is able to strengthen the patient's functioning as an individual, through decreased anxiety, improved interpersonal communication, and decreased isolation. This author's PhD Thesis (held at the University of Essex Library) demonstrates that internal objects can coexist with mental representations within the same mind. Thus the patient's internal object relating to the analyst can function as this within the patient's own representational world, which may be clearly illustrated visually by the PPCC construct.

Melanie Klein developed her concept of the depressive position, and later with Ronald Fairbairn her concept of the paranoid-schizoid position, to describe two different resting states of the normal mind. The paranoid-schizoid position is a state of mind where the patient regards another person as all good or all bad, as extremes of perceptual experience which bear no relation to each other. The depressive position is a second state of mind where both these good and bad perceptions are appreciated as being attributable to the same person at the same time. Wilfred Bion has shown (Bion, 1963, p. 3) how the two positions may relate to each other in an alternating fashion separated by a bidirectional arrow. John Steiner has discussed the interchange between the two positions in terms of the development of a pathological organisation where neither position can be tolerated by the patient (Steiner, 1987). As he says, "it is common to observe that a patient will make contact with depression position experiences and then retreat again to the paranoid-schizoid position as if he could not tolerate the mental pain he encountered (Joseph, 1981; Steiner, 1979). He then meets the disintegration, fragmentation, confusion and persecutory anxiety of the paranoid-schizoid position and if these too become unbearable the patient has nowhere where he feels safe unless he can find or construct a defence against both positions." Steiner suggests that this defence could consist of a pathological organisation, a narcissistic one which is a structure defending against both the paranoid-schizoid anxiety and the depressive one, with great importance attached to which one predominates.

Ronald Britton refers to John Steiner's 1987 paper, and has elaborated the alternation between the two positions into a model which "describes the movement through each position in turn as part of a continuous, lifelong, cyclical development and limits the term 'regression' to descriptions of a retreat to a pathological organization", ie. that described by Steiner (Britton, 1998). Britton develops elaborate constructive sequences of paranoid-schizoid and depressive positions which vary from each other depending upon which precedes the other and in what form.

The PPCC Theory only engages with Melanie Klein's paranoid-schizoid and depressive position concepts in their basic forms. But these are important, as it is important to recognise in the patient which position or mental state prevails at a given time so that responses and interpretations may be appropriately applied; or, indeed, if a psychotic episode is imminent, so that appropriate care can be instigated.

In moving through the seven therapeutic stages which a successfully treated schizophrenic or schizoaffective patient undergoes, the final two stages are eventually reached, where the patient differentiates and integrates into her final, evolved condition and then separates from the analyst. She has differentiated, ie. she has become more clearly her own self, who is different from other people; and she has integrated, that is, she has grown into a more solid, internally consistent and self-contained individual. Margaret Mahler describes (Mahler, 1971) how a very young infant, who is bound up in a single conscious awareness with its mother, eventually achieves a separation of identity from her and develops its own attributes which give it a personality of its own, ie. it individuates into its own self. In each case, the individual becomes a self of their own, separate from the mother and separate from the analyst, after a lengthy period of containment by the supervising adult which has enabled the differentiating and individuating processes to take place. These two processes occur as a result of the totality of the baby's development thus far, or of all the prior therapeutic stages visualized by the PPCC model, and in the therapeutic case represent the schizophrenic or schizoaffective patient's ultimate achievement of her own mental health.

In these ways, it may be seen how the PPCC Theory incorporates different elements of psychoanalytic theory according to the changes that succeed each other in the patient's schizophrenic mental state as she evolves through her therapy. The understanding of schizophrenia provided by psychoanalysis includes the concepts of narcissism, disturbed object relations, ego boundaries that are vague and afflicted by excessive projective identification, negative tendencies regarding other people and withdrawal from the world, and the psychological deficits associated with these. The PPCC Theory embraces all of these features of schizophrenia; and, in the PPCC construct, locates these changes, which are not associated with the patient's representational world but rather with her internal psychodynamic functioning, collectively in the Internal Space, without further description. Aspects of the functional illnesses, ie. depression, mania, and schizophrenia, which distinguish their features from each other and which are involved with relating these illnesses to External Reality, are represented by changes in the PPCC construct's outer structure, ie. to the triangular variables of the patient's Representational World, and by the disrupted shapes of the adapted PPCC structures which do not include an Internal Space.

The PPCC Theory is a descriptive and representational concept which displays relations and connections between different parts of the schizoaffective and schizophrenic minds in terms of established psychoanalytic theory. In this way it tries to connect psychiatric concepts with psychoanalytic concepts so that therapy based on psychoanalytic understanding may be understood and implemented by the agencies upon whom the burden of treatment for schizophrenia mainly falls, ie. clinical psychiatrists. By understanding as far as possible the non-psychotic elements of the patient's mind which may have survived the schizophrenic illness process, as well as recognising the elements of her mind which have been damaged by the illness, the psychiatrist may be in a good position to identify whether or not a particular patient might respond well to psychoanalytic treatment. For example, a patient's psychotic illness could be due to childhood molestation and subsequent years of disturbed relationships, and if this could be identified early then a large amount of psychiatric resource could be saved, as well as improvement in the experience of many years of that patient's life. Not very many cases have as simple an explanation as this, but examination of a schizophrenic patient's mind in terms of detailed internal structure does help to open a door for that patient's improved quality of life, rather than simply providing an antipsychotic prescription and social work care. Patients undergoing psychoanalytic psychotherapy should be studied in minute detail as their treatment progresses, so that any general trends among patients may be observed; and all possible lessons that can be should be learned from cases that do not proceed well, and from cases of mistakes or unusual events, so that the treatment schedule improves for future patients. Enlightenment is such an important gift for successfully treated schizophrenic patients that efforts to produce it really should be seen as very well worthwhile indeed. Careful patient selection, ensuring maximal cooperation and initiative from the patient, is essential for success, and if the preparatory requirements are all fully met by a committed therapeutic hospital team working with the analyst, then the treatment environment should prove to be one where patients and staff alike enjoy working together, towards some greatly-desired and valuable results.

CHAPTER 12

ASPECTS OF PSYCHOANALYTIC PSYCHOTHERAPY THAT ARE HELPFUL FOR SCHIZOPHRENIC AND SCHIZOAFFECTIVE PATIENTS

Common patient presentations

Patients with schizophrenia present in a number of apparently contrasting ways which are all, however, psychotic mental states caused by a complex aetiology of disturbance in the patient. Young patients, especially, may be angrily aroused and resentful towards the world in general and towards those in their vicinity in particular. At times such as these they are impervious to reason, and require continuous supervision at a distance until they have calmed down. While really angry they are not able to make use of psychoanalytic sessions. Anger may be a long term stance during this phase, and when they are able to attend sessions it may be apparent to the analyst that it needs to be explored, which can be done in due course when this becomes manageable by the patient.

By contrast, sometimes a patient presents in a dependent, complacent, inert, helplessly "parasitic", as Dr Michael Robbins describes it, state (see Figure 14). In this condition the patient can do little for herself. She tends to agree with everything that anybody suggests to her, with little individual perspective on any matter. She is quite likely to be depressed, sometimes only mildly, but to be unaware of this. She may appear to be unarousable, saying little, with impoverished thought and initiative, leading to therapeutic impasse. Dr Robbins spent much time with his patient Sara in this state (see Chapter 18). The analyst can make a few strong, clear points to the patient, and then await a response. Or perhaps the analyst may feel he has to be somewhat provocative, starting with physically irritating behaviour such as periodically vigorously scratching his arm (if bare) to stimulate the patient into saying something. If this is ineffective he might try asking direct questions or leading his interpretations into areas of known interest to the patient. Much patience is needed for the analyst to sustain the intensity of the relationship and indeed increase it so that the patient becomes increasingly involved with what is being said. The analyst's hard work may be rewarded by improved participation by the patient; if he cannot engage the patient in "pathosymbiosis", as Dr Robbins terms the process (see Figure 14), after many months of effort without some response then the treatment should be prematurely terminated in therapeutic stalemate.

Patients with schizophrenia typically have episodes of psychosis, when they are very confused and unable to communicate meaningfully with others, and may be distracted by hallucinations or florid delusional states. It is not possible to conduct psychotherapy sessions with them when they are distracted by psychosis. Medications can usually be found which subdue the positive and, to some extent with some medications such as flupentixol, the negative symptoms, to reach a point where the patient's disturbance is sufficiently unobtrusive to allow her to follow logically normal conversation. This may not happen for several weeks after commencing the medication. Relapse is to be expected, during which time ward care and ward groups can be used to address the patient's experiences, sometimes enhanced by visits to the ward by the analyst, who has this chance of observing the patient on the ward while particularly vulnerable. Such contact strengthens the therapeutic relationship, since trust is deepened, although this may not be immediately apparent. While psychotic, the patient may reveal aspects of herself which in her sessions in the analyst's consulting room may be buried more deeply in her psyche and not so evident.

Transference

The patient's transference of her style of existing relationships on to the analyst develops gradually. First impressions are made, but the therapeutic relationship develops steadily, and on a continuous basis with successive ups and downs, over months and years, because of the severity of the patient's problems.

The transference can be strong eventually, even in schizophrenic patients. Freud thought that it could not be developed in schizophrenic patients, but Melanie Klein, Hanna Segal, Herbert Rosenfeld, and Wilfred Bion all showed that this can be achieved, and used it to good effect with their patients.

It changes with time, depending on many factors such as the patient's temperament, her changing situations in different areas of her life, the analyst's personality, external events, changes on the ward involving other patients, and unconscious elements emerging during the treatment. Overall, with successive stages of the treatment process identified by Dr Robbins, the therapeutic relationship and the transference both change accordingly.

Countertransference

The analyst's countertransference of feelings about the patient can indicate useful information. It can impart information about the patient's progress, for example. If the patient is not progressing as she should, this can encroach irritatingly on the analyst's frame of mind until he becomes aware of this reality. Perhaps the patient is not being active enough in her sessions, lazily waiting for the analyst to speak without attending sufficiently to what he has already said and framing a response. The analyst may be unaware of this pattern that has developed, until the irritation in his countertransference draws to his attention that all is not well in the sessions. He may be puzzled until investigation provides his answers.

The countertransference also can positively indicate the patient's progress, for example when the patient responds well and the analyst feels pleased at the result of their mutual work. The countertransference should not intrude into the therapeutic relationship if it amounts to a satisfactory and balanced general approbation of the patient.

Countertransference needs attention if it becomes stressful or unpleasant, or if it does intrude into the analyst's awareness. In this eventuality the analyst should duly investigate his feelings about his patient in detail until he locates the crux of the difficulty, its source from within his own personal experience. Dr Michael Robbins has written that "success in the treatment depends upon attitudes and techniques of therapist self-analysis, which are a unique aspect of psychoanalytic training and practice" (Robbins, 1993, p. 266). It is only when the analyst understands himself thoroughly that he becomes sensitive to small nuances in his response to his patient that indicate changes in the therapeutic situation. He can then use this as a sensitive gauge when cognitive discernment or diagnosis of the change is not possible.

Symptoms

Medication should suppress symptoms as far as necessary to enable the patient to express herself as freely as she needs to, in order to make full use of her sessions. The patient who is unduly troubled by symptoms is not in a position to respond to her analyst. If she has suffered generally from psychotic symptoms at the time of diagnosis then these may take several weeks rather than days to subside under the influence of antipsychotic medication. She will have been shocked and distressed by what has happened to her, and unlikely to be willing to talk about herself to anybody. Any degree of confidence in herself requires time to become re-established. Mild approaches by ward staff are the best way to encourage her to feel more comfortable being the person she is, symptoms and all, and to reconcile herself to the possibilities of talking treatment with an analyst. Intrusive demands should not be made by staff or others into the psychotic patient's private world when she is very disturbed, since confusion militates against secure communication or increased understanding. It is far better to nurse such a patient through her distress in a generally supportive way, leaving information collecting to a later time when this may be more fruitful. When she is somewhat recovered, the patient may be quite willing to report her experiences and describe them in some detail. Analytic investigations into their nature may reflect aspects of her everyday real life which have not been apparent previously, especially of some of her relationships. Symbolic representations of those well known to her are not an uncommon presentation of psychotic symptoms. In particular, if a family member has been giving the patient problems then they may appear in a disguised form among her symptoms (see Chapter 2, 'Psychotic delusions', and Chapter 6).

It has been said that a mental state examination should be done every five minutes on a psychotic patient who is receiving psychoanalytic treatment. This is because the psychotic mind is very unstable and can switch and oscillate between different states instantly as a response to circumstances or simply because of its intrinsically unstable nature. Psychiatric training is required to manage potentially psychotic patients for this reason. The psychiatrically-trained analyst should be prepared to anticipate fluctuating mental states and to remain vigilant throughout the sessions for substantial change in the patient's perspective. This unfamiliar experience can be disconcerting for the analyst unused to treating schizophrenic patients. Referring to well-established and milder aspects of the patient's world is one way of keeping the patient steady and grounded within the session if she is flitting from one idea to another psychotically, or the session could be terminated early.

A delusional system should not be challenged, since it provides the psychotic patient with one form of reliable, even if very faulty, reassurance within which she retreats habitually from the world. Challenging her is nearly always ineffective: it upsets the patient, and it can be dangerous if the patient feels threatened (the delusional system can represent, to her,

her one lifeline). Individual delusions may be rationally questioned when the patient is calm, and safe on the ward or settled in a session. It is not a good idea to challenge her lack of realism directly unless the clinician is prepared to contain a likely backlash of aggression or disturbance in susceptible patients. Hallucinations may be more readily addressed with psychotic patients who suffer from them, especially between symptoms; less disturbed patients may be ready to discuss their hallucinations when calm. Avatar Therapy (Leff et al, 2013) has shown considerable initial success in reducing the distress caused by auditory hallucinations. Other kinds of psychotic symptoms need duly sensitive nursing; apathetic patients need much encouragement sometimes to speak at all.

The question of whether or not to continue a session if the patient becomes distressed sometimes raises itself in a session where the discussion has moved into an area where the patient's strong emotions are embedded. If the therapeutic bond is a strong one, what the analyst says may of itself be able to contain the patient's reactions during the session and permit continuation of the therapy. The patient must, after all, learn to contain her emotions for herself; but this does not happen early in the treatment. Premature exploration weakens rather than strengthens her ability to contain herself, and if it proves disruptive then it can instigate discouragement rather than providing helpful information.

When psychotic symptoms re-emerge during therapy there is a case for an interval out of therapy and stable maintenance on the ward while the symptoms quieten. When the patient is too ill for sessions, the analyst may be able to visit the patient on the ward to deliver sessions there. It is therapeutically sound and strengthens the therapeutic relationship for the patient to know her analyst cares enough to see her there. And seeing the analyst in a different setting gives the patient an alternative perspective on her treatment, seeing him in a rounder, more personal way. The analyst in no uncertain way can seem more approachable to the patient, having made this extra approach towards her.

Dreams

Antipsychotic medications tend to suppress dreams. But the dreams of a schizophrenic patient which do occur should be interpreted as for any other patient. Equally, the analyst should as usual ask the patient whether or not his interpretation is consonant with the patient's thoughts and feelings. If it is not, this should be explored with the patient, and corrections and elaborations made. The patient may not be able to explore her dreams with the analyst, simply from lack of understanding; and she may not be interested in doing so. In this eventuality the analyst must make the best use he can of what the dream reveals to him about the patient's state of mind.

Recurring dreams are, as always, significant. The question of why a particular dream recurs should be asked and explored with the patient. She is more likely to be able to contribute a probable answer to this than the analyst. Her hypothesis should be tested in relation to her past life and her hopes: how the figures in the dreams, if approximating to real figures in the patient's' life, influence the patient like the real people they represent.

The patient's narrative

The psychotic patient may be quiet and withdrawn due to negative symptoms. In this eventuality, the analyst should continue to present a cheerful, kind, patient stance long term, of evenly suspended attention. The patient may gradually relax and begin to communicate. Simply hearing her analyst speaking, kindly and reassuringly, may go a long way towards healing the patient's wounds from long ago. The analyst may have to speak for a long time, over weeks and months, before the patient feels secure and encouraged enough to make her own contributions at the level needed for her illness to be resolved. Her ability to freely associate usually improves with consistent effort and practice over time. But schizophrenic language can be halting and stilted and difficult to follow. The analyst may only be able to pick up individual words to begin with. And if he follows these leads sometimes he can coax out of the patient some meaning that lies accessibly in the front of the patient's mind, ready to be externalised. Frankly confused and nonsensical language indicates that the medication has not been adequately prescribed to stabilise the patient, who is still suffering psychosis. The fact that the patient has attended the session shows that she is putting effort into her own healing, and that she connects to this extent with the analyst. It is kinder on these occasions simply to send the patient back to hospital in a taxi and for the analyst to attend her there. The ward needs to reassure the patient as much as necessary for the patient to continue to feel stable. And then the staff and the analyst have to wait for the patient to recover and to start working again with her own narrative.

Interpretations

These should be kindly framed whenever possible. Sometimes they need to be direct and challenging if change is required in the patient concerning the point at hand.

As much material as possible that currently is occupying the patient should be brought into the interpretation, because the analyst's familiarity with what the patient has been saying greatly reassures the patient. The analyst should make his interpretations generally positive, and always constructive even if not altogether palatable to the patient.

His interpretations should be confined to the patient's material. But occasionally, judiciously introducing new features connected with the patient's narrative which open up awareness of thinking or a perspective that the patient might find helpful can be a useful tactic; these fresh concepts are likely to be remembered by the patient, sometimes long-term, and help her with her later life, after therapy has been completed.

Accuracy of interpretations

Schizophrenic patients have had a very unpleasant experience of life. They feel cowed by life itself, by the misfortunes they have met with, by whatever unkind words have come their way from family members or others, and they are sensitive, even hyper-sensitive, to whatever may befall them in the future; anxiety abounds in patients with this illness.

So nearly always they are somewhat wary, even suspicious, of a new contact, such as their analyst. Ward staff can do much to allay these preliminary fears and anxieties about treatment.

The patient will nonetheless experience great anxiety in her new situation, in an unfamiliar consulting room, with a stranger. The best way the analyst may allay these fears, in addition to exercising his qualities of kindness, patience and cheerfulness, is to pay the greatest attention possible to the sense the patient is able to make in her free association, and to include these details in his interpretations. Alluding inconspicuously to the patient's previous statements is a good way to gain the patient's confidence. Referring discreetly to facts volunteered by the patient is another. Accurate familiarity with the patient's case and with her history goes a long way towards validating the patient's presence in the consulting room, in the patient's mind: she feels recognised, welcome, and understood. Under these conditions her psyche may comfortably expand, grow, and develop through absorbing the richness that the analyst indirectly delivers as a good and recommended possible new approach for the patient's perspective, for the patient to think about. If the facts in the analyst's interpretations are correct, the patient is more likely to try out alternative methods, broached in the treatment, of thinking about her personal issues and of organising herself with regard to external reality.

Emotional outbursts

When controlled behaviour is required at all times on the ward and in therapeutic sessions, but strong emotions are both aroused and discussed during treatment and on the ward, it is only to be expected that tensions involving other people will rise to the surface from time to time.

As long as physical aggression is not intentionally enacted, these outbursts can be dealt with by the ward staff through addressing the feelings directly with the patient in an atmosphere of kindness and firmness. This ambience should be sufficient to keep all thoughts of weapons or dangerous aggression out of conscious awareness. If outbursts are relatively uncommon they are more readily addressed as unique events for which an explanation must be found.

If several occur, and each outburst is investigated, a pattern may be identified as occurring in a predictable manner for a particular patient. Care plans may be a suitable method of identifying clear sequences of actions that prevent feelings escalating to the point of loss of control. The patient, as much as the staff, may be very grateful to have her "explosions" brought back into the realm of her recognisable and regular emotional range, from being alarming events outside her voluntary control. Trigger events, topics, associated feelings, sensitive cognitive associations, difficult relationships or experiences of undue stress or fear may then be watched out for and duly avoided. Associations to earlier life events or previous relationships, if identified, may bring meaning to bear on phenomena that otherwise may appear merely frightening and potentially dangerous. Everyone benefits when the cause is located and the outbursts become understood and then prevented through insightful anticipation.

Violence

The priority if a patient becomes violent is the analyst's safety. He should have an emergency button near the chair where he works; and staff or family nearby ready to assist if difficulty arises. He could keep a walking stick nearby for self-defence, and possibly a button to contact the police, like a medical emergency neck pendant.

If the ability to summon help has been enacted, keeping the patient talking until help arrives is the next priority. If she is kept engaged in conversation her mind will be distracted away from violent actions as such. Maintaining composure and concentrating on the present moment are the analyst's greatest aids in this situation.

The ward staff should be informed of the incident and the patient asked to give an account of herself shortly after arriving back on the ward. No violence is acceptable in the mental health system, as is the case everywhere else; suffering and difficulty are not excuses for overt aggression.

Monitoring

Close monitoring is essential while supervising the progress of a schizophrenic patient undergoing psychoanalytic psychotherapeutic treatment. At times it needs to be continuous, like that for a bone marrow transplant patient in the physical medicine sphere.

The reason for this is that the minute-by-minute experience of a schizophrenic patient whose mind is just beginning to be changed by the therapy, and which she is just starting to become aware of in light of the analyst's observations, can be very disconcerting and difficult for her to manage. The patient may frequently, now, be becoming aware of aspects of herself, her relationships, and her situations in not-always-favourable ways. She may feel dreadfully inept, helpless, ignorant, angry, frustrated, miserable, or afraid. The human presence of ward staff can help immeasurably to comfort the patient once she has learned to trust her individual nurses and care workers. The staff's caring concern can preserve the progress made by the patient and prevent any retrograde sliding if the patient is distressed.

Close monitoring is also essential when patients are using public transport to reach their analyst's consulting rooms and to travel back to hospital. Every journey should be registered at the time of departure and at the time she arrives back on the ward, so that if she is delayed this is noticed early, and steps may be taken to look for her when either the hospital or the analyst becomes concerned about her lateness in relation to her mental state when last seen. If the hospital staff are worried, the patient should not be allowed to leave the ward; if the analyst is concerned, he should send the patient back to the hospital in a taxi with instructions not to say anything to the taxi driver on the way there.

Boundaries

Boundaries need to be kept crystal clear. This is especially important for schizophrenic patients, because their sense of themselves and their ego boundaries (their awareness and sense of themselves as an individual person) in practical terms are not at all well-established (even if they do not understand the technical nature of this), but within which they are trying to exist.

Predictability in the analyst is greatly welcomed by the patient, since it relieves her of some of her work in defining her own stance: if relating to the analyst is easy (appointment times, fees, holiday periods, location, and a clear arrangement regarding whether or not the analyst visits the patient when in hospital) the patient does not have to concern herself or think about matters other than her own self and her own issues.

External reality

In the early stages of the psychoanalytic psychotherapy of a schizophrenic patient, the patient's psychosis will be under the control of medication, sufficient at least to allow her conscious mind to relate fully responsively to the analyst. At first the majority of the patient's responses to the analyst will be cognitively-based. The patient may demonstrate some idiosyncratic emotional responses to the analyst's words, some aspect of the consulting room or an intrusive memory. But she will be trying to understand what the analyst is saying to her.

All this time, the patient will be trying to keep her grip on "reality", the reality of her own words, her own experience, her own appearance and behaviour, possibly her appearance as the analyst sees her, the reality of the consulting room, of the bus that brought her there, of the busy ward she has left behind, of her own misery and her miserable predicament.

At this time there is little point in the analyst's trying to enhance the patient's appreciation of the reality of any other aspects of external reality except for occasional references to it; all the patient's energy should be encouraged to focus on her internal world, the analyst, and the consulting room. Only later should external reality be embraced, and usually only in appropriate terms when the patient has first broached it in a specific context.

Relatives

The caring families of younger patients always appreciate an opportunity to meet the therapist or analyst. If family therapy is not contemplated, then it is usually appropriate only to try to bring about small changes in the family if these become desirable. Reviewing the manner of their addressing the patient, for example with less aroused emotion, allowance for the patient to have more time doing certain activities, and choice over issues such as different activities or foods or friends, for example, can be conducive to better harmony in the setting of the patient's life at home.

If the family is uncaring, or if the patient is older and has had a measure of independence in her life, there is not usually a need to meet the family or her partner unless a specific request has been made. But it is useful for the analyst to have met the important figures in a patient's life before therapy commences, so that he has an opportunity of understanding the patient's relationship dynamics. It is also useful for him to be able to envisage those to whom the patient refers in her narrative during sessions.

Sexuality

At least initially, schizophrenic patients' problems usually overwhelm them so fully that they have little energy remaining after addressing their own difficulties. Once the patient has stabilised in her therapy, even still at the level of "pathosymbiosis" (see Chapter 14 and Figure 14), she may sometimes manifest some of the character she has shown freely as herself in her family. This may have been to some extent cheerful or playful; and, if so, the same traits may be exhibited in therapy. Or the patient's natural sexuality may have been adversely affected by family dynamics.

The patient may be taken by surprise at her sexual feelings for the analyst during therapy. This scenario would only develop once the therapy was well under way, and the feelings might have been present for a considerable time before being given expression by the patient. The analyst's role is best preserved by resolving the matter verbally rather than allowing any physical contact. Schizophrenic patients, because of their prevailing confusion, may easily misinterpret any physical exchange, so physical contact is not at all to be encouraged.

Calm reference to the patient's feelings of this kind in previous relationships, to her prior experiences and to her hopes for the future, are good ways of deflecting her focus away from the analyst and back on to issues relating to the patient and her psychic needs where these can be better explored. It is not helpful to explore the patient's sexual feelings for the analyst, and indeed this can adversely affect the remainder of the therapy, sometimes leading to disappointment, guilt, shame, or premature termination. A kind but firm approach is often all that is needed to reassure but not encourage the patient in this direction.

The analyst's patience

Preserving patience, needless to say, is mandatory practice for the analyst treating a schizophrenic patient, at least as much as for others. Sometimes it may seem that no progress at all is being made, and that the patient's words do not make much structural sense.

However, with patience the transference and countertransference may develop, when cognitive progress seems to be stalled. Preserving a kind demeanour is a key goal, for it is this stance that the patient may remember when all the words passed between the therapeutic dyad have been long forgotten. The patient's memory of her kind analyst may inspire her for the rest of her life, as she builds on the better mental habits, novel perspectives and newly discovered motivation uncovered within herself as a result of the analyst's interventions. Her analyst's steadiness and unflappability during times when the patient feels most unsteady, faltering, and afraid, lacking any objectives or direction, preserves the patient's sense of self in a reassured continuity. During long periods of silence the analyst's patience gives the schizophrenic patient time to reflect and grow in the analyst's terms, time to adopt in trust what the analyst has drawn attention to, and to gather strength in this new stance.

The analyst's ability to bear with the patient her pain and the depth of her distress extends beyond mere patience. Schizophrenic patients do bear terrible distress for much of the time. And as they begin to progress along the path towards distant better health they initially have to address the realities of their original psychological stance in the representational world from which they started out in their life, derived from their home of origin. The truth of its reality can come as a very rude awakening and shock, leading to deep resentment, anger, hatred, and distress. For years this may continue as very hard times for the patient in therapy. Bit by bit she must acknowledge the awfulness and dismal truths of her life and of herself with her vulnerabilities and bad habits, and her own limited capacities that have not had a chance to grow.

By sitting with the patient, hour after hour, session by session, the analyst shares the experience of the patient and offers enlightenment where he can. The countertransference may be so frustrating or unpleasant that he may feel an inclination to turn away completely and simply drift off to sleep. This may well not go unnoticed by the patient, who could unconsciously be trying to be unpleasant and to have this effect on her therapist. To endure such experiences is the role of the analyst, however, and to keep going through difficult times to bring the patient through to clear perceptions of herself in the light of reality. Choices will have to be made by the patient eventually, and in helping her to address the most difficult issues concerning herself the analyst enables her to do so realistically.

Encouragement

Giving encouragement can have the opposite effect to that intended, by unwittingly making the patient relax too much and not continue to concentrate on the therapeutic process.

But if the patient becomes secondarily depressed, or even just slightly more miserable, an occasional kind word of oblique encouragement can sometimes permanently stick in the back of the patient's mind, unconsciously supporting her darker moods towards the perspective of hope. If possible, the analyst's tone should habitually be positive as well as kind. If this is the regular pattern, the patient may on a continuous basis find herself glad to be in her analyst's consulting-room, glad to have made the effort to be there, and pleased to hear what he or she is saying. On occasions when the patient feels simply too weak to talk, she may find listening to her analyst in itself quite satisfying. Compassionate enriching of the patient's world is the outcome objective of close monitoring once safety issues have been met: close monitoring keeps the patient accessible to the compassionate enrichment of therapy, and encouragement or psychological enrichment sustains the therapeutic process itself, especially when combined with the patient's desire to be well.

Patients quite often encourage one another on a ward that successfully preserves a supportive and cheerful ambience. The staff have a major role in maintaining every patient's mental state in a condition of openness and contentment as far as possible between therapeutic sessions; and this promotes tacit encouragement.

Ill feeling, sourness in the patient

Feeling fed-up, sour and miserable is common in most people when faced with predicaments they feel scarcely able to deal with effectively. The schizophrenic patient's challenge caused to them by their illness is a huge one, which at times may realistically seem to have no answer, no solution. Bearing up under such a load demands great stamina, and can easily lead patients to feeling miserable, even to clinical depression itself.

Kindness, patience, a welcoming stance and a degree of cheerfulness are all virtues in the analyst that the patient responds to best. The patient may take a session or two, or indeed several months or years, to thaw out from a miserable feeling, but while she is discomfited the analyst may learn something of what disturbs his patient by identifying the issues raised in this miserable state. These difficult issues may be unconsciously causing repression of aspects of the past that the analyst needs to know about, or may be caused by them. Exploring them, as far as the patient permits, is essential for building an accurate clinical picture and ideally learning later what had been repressed. Returning to them at a later date, when this can be done subtly but effectively, is a good idea for completing the details. If this is done when the patient is in a more cheerful state of mind, she may accept the analyst's more positive suggested associations of past events in place of her own previous miserable ones; or the analyst may simply imply these so that a newly appraised reality is gradually assimilated by the patient.

The patient's hopes

The patient may have high hopes for the resolution of his or her illness. Sometimes these are quite unrealistic, and the analyst's task is to supervise the patient's progress into as much realism as possible without dampening their hopes flatly. Some symptoms, such as hallucinations, may be very persistent, although Avatar Therapy (Leff et al, 2013) may help, sometimes achieving resolution of this symptom.

The patient's hopefulness may be associated with considerable motivation, which the analyst can most effectively utilise in the patient's interests to achieve real progress. Application of this motivation towards good timekeeping, interest during the sessions, development of insight, use of new knowledge gained in the patient's life outside the therapy sessions, and general enthusiasm for the possibilities that might open up for her as contingent benefits are all to be encouraged.

Channelling the patient's hopes into reality is the analyst's responsibility. It is more likely, however, that the patient will be depressed and unable to see or think beyond the immediate session she is attending. Here again, the analyst should try to bring reality to bear on the patient's situation, pointing out obvious facts that the patient may have overlooked, such as good progress that has been made, the positive side of an event the patient is worrying about, or a valid and true aspect of the patient's character that vindicates her stance within a difficult situation. If the patient cannot on her own apprehend these positive attributes, the analyst could draw her attention to them, and so reinstate or reinforce the patient's positive sense of herself. It is, however, more effective in therapy for the patient to work out for herself reasons why she should feel positive. Thus therapy is directed towards her using her own mind, and her own self-motivation may be tapped into, or may be unconsciously absorbed from the analyst's own positive attitude.

Curiosity

The analyst's curiosity is one of his most powerful and useful tools. It sustains the therapy even when this seems to have ground to a halt or impasse.

Patients vary in the amount of information they impart within their free associating during sessions. Some can hardly speak, they are so troubled. Others talk but without making much sense.

In all cases, the analyst's aim is to understand the patient's perspective, and how her background impinges on her psyche, and how to bring about the changes in the patient that would best serve to alleviate her impaired functioning. Listening to the patient, asking her to elaborate on a point, gently probing and trying to explore areas potentially offering useful knowledge about these matters, form the basis for the analyst's understanding of his or her patient. Intense reflection on the information gleaned thus painstakingly allows formulation that will help further tentative exploration and interpretation, and also shapes the countertransference; sometimes more compassion is demonstrated, sometimes firmness, so that the patient is caused to take responsibility for his or her attitudes and decisions.

Curiosity is the analyst's stimulation that keeps a therapy alive, given compassion and concern as the basis for the therapeutic relationship itself. Judicious probing, after deep reflection upon the therapeutic material, is one way of bringing answers to light when stalemate threatens. The analyst's confidence is then more likely to extend as he or she gains a stronger position from which to appraise the patient and produce a formulation.

Regard for the patient

Sustaining evenly suspended positive regard for the patient is what the analyst aims for. Generally this may be attained, since the patient's plight in having to address schizophrenia renders her piteous, suffering, and seemingly helpless, and it is difficult for the analyst not to feel deeply compassionate. The patient's best chance of eventual thriving is served by this positive, enquiring, kindly stance in which she feels psychically warmed from her state of frozen helplessness.

It may be difficult for the analyst to maintain this stance if the patient is aggressive or chronically resentful or casts blame about, or if personal hatreds are expressed; or, worse, amoral behaviour such as thieving, or lying, or threats of violence emerge. But these are highly unusual, and if they do occur the ward staff should be informed if they are not already aware of them.

Laziness and rudeness and aggression do occur and should be registered and dealt with at the time, with a non-punitive but cautionary remark and a query, to draw out more detail or an explanation if these might be forthcoming. The human condition applies to us all, and patients generally try not to reveal their worst characteristics to the analyst, as does everyone else, interpersonally. The analyst is in a very privileged position, having the access that they do to their patients' innermost selves. Recognising a patient's foibles and helping her to accept herself as she is in order to address her adverse mental habits can facilitate working on these to correct them, and so permit greater freedoms and possibly some happiness later in her progress. There is sometimes much to admire in a patient as she struggles with herself to adapt to life's demands. It is very important, however, for all parties to adopt proper attention to ethical principles throughout the treatment, and for these to be firmly established also on the psychotherapy ward in the hospital.

CHAPTER 13
SOME PSYCHOANALYTIC PSYCHOTHERAPISTS OF SCHIZOPHRENIC PATIENTS

A number of clinicians since Freud's time have worked with schizophrenic patients through a psychoanalytic approach, with increasing degrees of success, all dedicated to the patients' progress, and all contributing to our knowledge and understanding of schizophrenia and psychosis.

Sigmund Freud (1856-1939)

Until about 1920 (Klein, 1952, p. 53), Sigmund Freud and others considered that the narcissism shown by schizophrenic patients, their inward-looking tendency, prevents them from being able to develop a transference relationship with their analyst, and that consequently they cannot be helped by psychoanalytic treatment. Melanie Klein and her followers subsequently found this not to be the case, and that they could establish both positive and negative transference relationships with schizophrenic patients (see below). Freud observed that while schizophrenic patients give up their object-cathexes (emotional attachment to objects or people) so that, as far as he saw, they cannot develop a transference, they retain their cathexis of an object's "word-presentation" (a word considered as the abstract constitution of the information being received). This observation is interesting to consider in relation to Hanna Segal's later identification of "symbolic equation" in schizophrenic patients, where a symbol such as a word is so equated with the object symbolised that the two are felt to be identical (see below). Freud was interested to observe that in the dreams of schizophrenic patients there is no free communication between their preconscious word-cathexes (emotional attachment to a word) and their unconscious thing-cathexes (emotional attachment to a thing). Thus a word may become a thing in itself. So Freud mainly approached the treatment of schizophrenic patients by trying to understand the structure and use of their language and studying their dreams rather than by observing or utilising a transference in them.

Carl Gustav Jung (1875-1961)

Carl Gustav Jung founded and practised analytical psychology as a direct contemporary of Sigmund Freud's contributions to psychoanalysis during the late nineteenth and early twentieth centuries. C G Jung's work as a psychiatrist and psychotherapist contributed to psychiatry, psychology, philosophy, and other branches of knowledge such as anthropology and religious studies. He met Freud, and found that Freud's published studies on hysteria and dreams "threw light on schizophrenic forms of expression". He published his own book "The Psychology of Dementia Praecox" in 1907, which interested Freud, and for a time they agreed enthusiastically about the subject, although following different directions of interest subsequently. Jung believed that individuation was central in human development, and was reached by reconciling and then assimilating opposites, including the conscious with the unconscious. He conceived of by now well-known psychological concepts such as archetypes of conceptual imagery, and universal phenomena such as the collective unconscious, and psychological traits such as introversion and extraversion. So his work latterly became entirely independent of Freud's thinking, although early on in their careers they had discussed the unconscious and psychotherapeutic work in relation to schizophrenic patients together.

Melanie Klein (1882-1960)

Melanie Klein continued Freud's work on schizophrenic patients and schizophrenia and made her own contributions. She was, for a long time until her position became untenable, eager not to dissent from Freud's positions on his psychoanalytic discoveries. For example, she confirmed Freud's identification of splitting (Freud, 1940, pp. 271-8), which is a tendency to separate good from bad aspects of a person (Hinshelwood, 1989, p. 433), and developed his and Karl Abraham's ideas of mechanisms of defence, or ways that the normal mind can protect itself in its relations with the outside world. She believed, and her students later confirmed, that mechanisms of defence, such as splitting, particularly intensely, afflict the schizophrenic mind, another example being pathological projective identification. When too intense and aggressive, these defence mechanisms are harmful to the mind and contribute to schizophrenic illness.

Some followers of Melanie Klein

In her 1946 paper "Notes on some schizoid mechanisms" (Klein, 1946), Melanie Klein related her own discoveries about the paranoid-schizoid (conceived of together with Ronald Fairbairn) and depressive positions to the development of schizophrenia; the paranoid-schizoid position consists of a split between good or loving and bad or hateful, and the depressive position enables remorseful acceptance of both at the same time. She found that splitting is closely related to the paranoid-schizoid position, and is an important part of the development of schizophrenia. In 1952 (Klein, 1952) she stated that schizophrenic patients are capable of both positive (agreeable) and negative (antagonistic) transferences ie. relationships with the analyst. Wilfred Bion, Herbert Rosenfeld, and Hanna Segal, who were all students of Melanie Klein, confirmed this discovery in their relationships with their patients. They learnt new information about schizophrenia through persevering with treating their schizophrenic patients, and some of their patients clearly benefited from this. For example, Hanna Segal wrote about her schizophrenic patient Edward (Segal, 1981) (see below). Bion, in particular, wrote at length about new understandings that he had reached from his clinical work. A later generation of therapists, notably Richard Lucas, Murray Jackson, and Leslie Sohn, continued to work with schizophrenic patients, using in particular this knowledge that true connection can be made with schizophrenic minds in therapy.

Bion (1897-1979)

Bion believed that schizophrenic pathology develops as a result of poor interaction between the personality and the environment, although later he thought that physical factors might be responsible for the illness (Bion, 1967, p. 37). There are four features in the personality that he thought are characteristic of schizophrenic patients: (i) an ongoing conflict between life and death instincts, or a person's tendencies to yearn towards life or death; (ii) a preponderance of destructive impulses; (iii) hatred of external and internal reality; and (iv) a frail and tenuous kind of psychotic transference in therapy. These characteristics cause schizophrenic patients to become overly dependent upon projective identification, which is mentioned below and is a way of causing one's own ill feelings to be felt by another person.

Herbert Rosenfeld (1910-1986)

Herbert Rosenfeld also worked with schizophrenic patients (see below), and especially with a view to understanding the narcissism that they manifest and which Freud had believed precluded analytic treatment. In particular, he found that schizophrenic patients use the defence of projective identification as a means of communication; it is also used by them as a denial of psychic reality (Steiner, 2009, pp. 134-5).

Hanna Segal (1918-2011)

Hanna Segal was interested in artistic creativity as well as schizophrenia, and relates that through her work with a schizophrenic patient, Edward, he experienced at least 20 years of useful life, marrying, having a family and working at professional life (Segal, 1981) (p.119). She identified the phenomenon of "symbolic equation", where a schizophrenic patient may mistake a symbol for the real thing. This relates to Freud's observation that, for schizophrenic patients, a word may become a thing in itself.

Followers of Klein supported by the PPCC model

The PPCC model illustrates some of the processes outlined by Melanie Klein and her followers. Bion, for example, held that, due to the characteristics he describes that distinguish schizophrenic patients from healthy people, they progress differently from healthy people through the paranoid-schizoid and depressive positions due to a "massive resort to projective identification" (Bion, 1967, p. 38). The PPCC model can usefully describe some of these changes. It illustrates the main process of the movement from the paranoid-schizoid position to the depressive position, and vice versa, and also illustrates the analyst's sustained vigilance in his maintained position within the PPCC model as he supervises the patient's mental functioning while this process occurs, receiving their projective identification.

Bion holds that their own perceptive apparatus is destroyed by the schizophrenic patient, resulting in a mental state that is felt to be neither alive nor dead. The projection, through projective identification, of conscious awareness of internal and external reality into other people and the consequent stifling of verbal thought is what distinguishes the psychotic patient from non-psychotic people. Moreover, there is an ever-widening divergence between the psychotic and non-psychotic parts of the personality until the gap between them cannot be bridged by the patient. This gap is seen in the triangular PPCC model for schizophrenia, where conflated Experiences and Observations, the normal variables on the left hand side of the model, are blocked off from the conflated Dreams/Representations and psychotic Determining Orientation variables on the right side of the model.

Considerable work has been achieved, as in the examples shown above by Freud, Klein, and Bion and her other followers, in understanding the mind of the schizophrenic patient. The challenge faced is in how to ameliorate the situation in the mind itself. A start was made by Melanie Klein when she discovered, countering Freud, that schizophrenic patients could, indeed, develop a transference relationship with the analyst and so open up access by him to tend the patient's illness. Bion learned much about the fragmentation and consequent vulnerability of the schizophrenic patient. These elements of knowledge about schizophrenia indicate the need, if treatment is to be successful, for the analyst to foster as strong a bond as possible with his patient, and to work hard to uncover meaning attached to feeling within the patient's internal world. Hanna Segal's dedicated, early work with her patient Edward (Segal, 1981) was an early example of this kind of demonstrable success. Herbert Rosenfeld treated a schizophrenic patient, Mildred, quite successfully using only pure psychoanalytic interpretations (Steiner, 2009, p. 43), which at the time had not been thought possible.

Practising psychoanalysts use this kind of knowledge to understand their schizophrenic patients and to try to encourage more appropriate activity in their minds. The PPCC may illustrate some of the processes constructively. Consider, for example, an analyst making use of these few basic principles of psychoanalysis in addressing a hostile, helpless, despairing schizophrenic patient. He may enable the patient to recede from the narcissism of frank schizophrenia (the triangular form of the PPCC model, where normal Observations has been completely blocked off from the psychotic Determining Orientation, and psychosis is predominating), because of contact the analyst has succeeded in making with her, and the patient can relate better to the analyst. Suppose the patient has emerged into the comparatively normal pentapointed, paranoid-schizoid PPCC model, and the analyst is in an influential position regarding the patient's mind (he occupies the Problems variable at the top of the pentapointed PPCC). Here, the patient is in the paranoid-schizoid position, and has split off her bad, hateful feelings and through projective identification has projected these into her analyst. In herself she does not like being nasty, but is helpless in her behaviour driven by her illness. She is holding on to as much that is good and loving as she has in herself, and she has turned outwards all her split-off anger and passed this on to her analyst, who must look after himself and sustain his own integrity. The analyst may even then succeed in guiding the patient into a more integrated state, the depressive position, through further work with him. The PPCC structures describe clearly several characteristic properties of these psychological states.

Bion's idea that the patient's sense of reality and conscious awareness gives rise to verbal thought indicates that if the analyst can improve the patient's conscious and unconscious awareness of him, with kinder feelings, then her verbal thought might be enhanced. The patient's perception, conscious awareness, and verbal thought are enhanced by the analyst reaching out towards her, offering stimulating connections with what the patient has already said, trying to integrate what is apparently in the patient's mind at that point. The analyst helps the patient move from the paranoid-schizoid position to the more integrated depressive position. Effective interpretations can only be made once the patient's mind has become more integrated (Robbins, 1993), but the work of the analyst in enhancing the patient's connections with him, by improving her perceptions of reality and in helping her to feel more comfortable through their relationship, continues throughout the progress of the therapy, and is described graphically by the PPCC model.

Frieda Fromm-Reichmann (1889-1957)

Frieda Fromm-Reichmann was a psychoanalyst who escaped Hitler's Anschluss in 1935. She became a staff member at Chestnut Lodge in Maryland in the USA, and there worked with psychotic patients. She sometimes entered the figurative and symptomatic world of the patient, observed the conflict and guilt underlying symptoms which she saw as metaphors and smoke screens for the actual experiences of the patient, and presented reality to the patient as an alternative to their symptoms. She practised eminently humanely, with broad empathy, flexibility, courage, and special understanding.

Harold Searles (1918-2015)

Harold Searles trained in medicine at Cornell University and obtained his MD at Harvard Medical School in 1943. He worked as a psychiatrist and psychoanalyst at Chestnut Lodge, Maryland between 1952 and 1964, and became a psychoanalytic supervisor and therapist, and a prolific writer. Through his personal honesty he was able to be a particularly skilled clinician to his patients, often being able to elicit significant events or turning-points in their lives, and enabling thereby their subsequent better adjustment to life.

Harry Stack Sullivan (1892-1949)

Harry Stack Sullivan's psychoanalytic approach to treating schizophrenic and schizoid young men and women was practical and humanist. His interpersonal relational ideas are gradually becoming integrated with contemporary systems of psychoanalytic thinking, although his relational principles differ from classical, non-relational approaches such as ego-psychology.

Sullivan conceived of the analyst's role as being a participant in a shared activity. Objective truth becomes replaced with subjectivity; the intrapsychic is replaced with the intersubjective; fantasy gives way to practical considerations or descriptions of experience or of events; concepts of truth and distortion are replaced by appreciation of perspective; strong theories are avoided (Fonagy and Target, 2003).

Sullivan believed that schizophrenia originated in interpersonal anxiety so great and so early that the dissociative component of the personality could not be overcome. He considered that fear in acute schizophrenic episodes was so severe because it originated in infancy's fearfulness (Fonagy and Target, 2003).

Henri Rey (1912-2000)

Henri Rey was interested in identifying the common ground between psychiatry and psychoanalysis, the core material of this present book. He was influenced by Melanie Klein, and was given his training analysis by Herbert Rosenfeld. Joan Riviere, a colleague of Melanie Klein, supervised him, and Hanna Segal constructively helped him towards his own unique perspective.

As a psychiatrist he was sensitive to the sufferings of psychotic patients. He conceived of the mind as representing objects, or other people, in a spatial sense (for example the self residing in another object) as does the pentapointed PPCC model. Aspects of this paradigm led him to an understanding (Rey, 1994, p. 27) of the young woman who rang his flat's telephone and let the phone ring and ring because she derived comfort from "being in his personal space". He quotes Guntrip's (1968) observation that "the schizoid person is a prisoner:... He finds himself enclosed in a dilemma, enclosed in a limited space, and with limited objects and limited relationships" (Rey, 1994, p. 9). Rey had an imaginative view of the relationships between the ideas of time and space, destruction and reparation.

Elvin Semrad (1909–1976)

Elvin Semrad worked at the Massachusetts Mental Health Center in Boston, USA, for four decades, and taught trainees how to sit with schizophrenic patients and bear their pain and suffering with them. Michael Robbins, who specialised in, and was very successful in delivering, psychoanalytic psychotherapy to schizophrenic patients, articulated his great debt to Semrad in his book "Experiences of Schizophrenia" (Robbins, 1993).

Gaetano Benedetti (1920-2013)

Gaetano Benedetti joined the psychiatric staff at the Zurich University Clinic, Burgholzli in Switzerland in 1947, and then at the University of Basle. He worked with schizophrenic patients, concentrating on psychoanalytic psychotherapy and observing that they "have an intellectual and emotional life as do normal people". He tried to break through their isolation and alleviate their suffering.

Richard Lucas (1943-2008)

Richard Lucas wrote about "the psychotic wavelength", a way of communicating with patients when psychotic which allows the clinician to clarify his understanding of both the psychotic and the non-psychotic parts of the personality (Lucas, 2009). Lucas emphasises that therapists connect therapeutically with their psychotic patients through accessing the non-psychotic parts of their personality. But the patient's non-psychotic mind is not always accessible, for example when the patient is distracted or resistant to contact while psychotic. If communication is attempted "on the psychotic wavelength" when managing the psychotic patient on the ward, the clinician is better enabled to help the psychotic patient adjust to reality. Strengthening therapeutic relationships with ward staff through communicating in this way is always a good objective, and can improve the chances of subsequent sought, and helpful, non-psychotic communications with the patient. Through the therapist addressing the patient both when psychotic and when non-psychotic in these ways, the patient is better enabled to understand and to feel understood, and so begin progress towards improved insight.

Murray Jackson (1922-2011)

Murray Jackson specialised his psychoanalytic practice in the analytic psychotherapy of psychosis. Two of his books, "Unimaginable Storms"

(Jackson and Williams, 1994) and "Weathering the Storms" (Jackson, 2001), describe case studies of psychotic patients. His book "Creativity and Psychotic States in Exceptional People" (Jackson, 2015) sensitively draws pictures of four outstandingly artistic people who were prone to psychotic states of mind. He draws attention to the emotional pain they each experienced early in life, but shows how they used this as a source of powerful forces inside themselves which propelled them to make some sense of the world they found themselves in; in each case this sense was an artistic interpretation of reality, and each of the four became widely known for their creative personal response to life.

Murray Jackson supervised the psychoanalytic psychotherapy of patients on his Psychotherapy Unit, Ward 6 at the Maudsley Hospital, and was clear that the long-term view had to be adopted where psychotherapeutic treatments were concerned. This wisdom is apparently becoming lost in today's rushed and cramped treatment facilities. Murray Jackson held that "psychoanalysis offers an indispensable source of knowledge for the understanding and treatment of psychotic disorders" (Jackson and Williams, 1994, p. xviii). Professor Peter Fonagy, the Freud Memorial Professor of Psychoanalysis at University College London, and Professor Alessandra Lemma, also of the Psychoanalysis Unit at University College London, jointly declared to the British medical profession in the British Medical Journal in February 2012 (Fonagy and Lemma, 2012), "If psychoanalysis is thrown out, these aspects of the mind will have to be rediscovered – just like Greco-Roman culture was rediscovered after the dark ages." If skills like those of Murray Jackson are lost to the psychiatric and psychoanalytic professions then many psychotic patients will lose their best lifeline towards mental health.

Leslie Sohn (1919-2013)

Leslie Sohn, a psychiatrist and Kleinian psychoanalyst, worked with some of Murray Jackson's patients from Ward 6, and had a special interest in unprovoked violence and the relationship between psychosis and violence. He was Honorary Consultant in the Academic Forensic Psychiatric Department of the Maudsley Hospital, and at the Dennis Hill Unit at the Bethlem Royal Hospital, where he worked for many years. He was also Honorary Consultant Psychotherapist at Broadmoor Hospital, Crowthorne, UK. He wrote four papers displaying his interest and expertise in understanding psychotic features of his patients.

He taught psychoanalytic techniques to clinical staff supervisors, including Marcus Evans at the Tavistock Clinic, and passed on his instinctive ability to understand the meaning of psychotic communications; Marcus Evans subsequently wrote his book of his own astute observations on the psychoanalytic understanding of psychotic communication (Evans, 2016).

David Bell (contemporary in 2018)

David Bell speaks and lectures on the relationship between psychoanalysis and literature, philosophy and politics from a perspective of the psychoanalytic theory and technique of Melanie Klein. He fights for the survival of the psychoanalytic perspective in the public sector.

He is Consultant Psychiatrist in the Adult Department at the Tavistock and Portman NHS Foundation Trust where he leads the Fitzjohns Unit, and he was President of the British Psychoanalytical Society 2010-2012.

He has written many papers and book chapters, eg. on hysteria, projective identification, paranoia, the concept of the death drive, and on narcissism. Recently, he has written on the deterioration in the care of the mentally ill. Clinically, in the Fitzjohns Unit, he cares for seriously ill psychotic adult patients through psychoanalytic understanding of their predicaments.

Andrew Lotterman (contemporary in 2018)

Andrew Lotterman MD is a training and supervising psychoanalyst and Associate Clinical Professor of Psychiatry at Columbia University, USA. He has three areas of special interest: psychoanalysis and psychoanalytic psychotherapy, psychological research, and psychotherapy with severely ill patients. He has published widely in each area, and is a distinguished teacher on the psychotherapy of patients diagnosed with schizophrenia.

Paul Williams (contemporary in 2018)

Paul Williams worked with Murray Jackson at the Maudsley Hospital. Initially trained as a social anthropologist, he studied Ward 6 patients there and had a close interest in trying to extend the psychoanalytic technique of understanding and assisting psychotic patients; he recorded and videotaped sessions as teaching material for later use with trainee analysts (Jackson and Williams, 1994, (pp. viii, xix and xiv), and taught at University College London Hospital. Currently he works in private psychoanalytic practice in Hampshire.

Bent Rosenbaum (contemporary in 2018)

Bent Rosenbaum, a psychiatrist and psychoanalyst, together with others in 2005 (Rosenbaum et al, 2005), demonstrated, through the Danish National

Schizophrenic Project, that supportive psychodynamic psychotherapy in addition to integrated treatment as usual may improve outcome after one year of treatment for people with first-episode psychosis compared with only treatment as usual; and that this tendency continued after two years. Rosenbaum described the dynamics of the psychotherapy process for schizophrenic psychosis (Rosenbaum and Harder, 2007), and identified three phases of therapy: an initial phase, a middle phase, and a termination phase (Rosenbaum, 2009).

Brian Martindale (contemporary in 2018)

Brian Martindale is a psychiatrist and a psychoanalyst who has worked extensively in South Tyne and Wearside, Sunderland, leading Outreach and Crisis Resolution teams especially for young people experiencing psychosis for the first time. He made a generous and dynamic contribution to the International Society for the Psychological and Social Treatment of Schizophrenia and other Psychoses (ISPS), by developing the organisation from being a small one that had an international conference only every three years, to becoming an even more active one meeting every two years, and that has branches in twenty-one countries, culminating in becoming its first Chair, a position he held for five years. He is the first Series Editor of the ISPS Book Series, which has now assembled at least eighteen titles. He also founded the European Federation for Psychoanalytic Psychotherapy in the Public Sector, an organisation which grew from his determination to make psychoanalytic psychotherapy more easily available to the general population within Europe and not to only a privileged few. He retired from NHS work in 2012, and now works in private psychoanalytic practice.

Johan Cullberg (contemporary in 2018)

Johan Cullberg is a Swedish psychiatrist and psychoanalyst whose approach to psychosis is to emphasise crisis as a potential starting point for a process of maturation and normalisation that opens up insights not otherwise accessible. He is interested in environmental effects on mental health, and argues for a reduction in both antipsychotic medication and compulsory treatment wherever possible, and for more humane psychiatric care, although he acknowledges firmly the necessity for medication in adequate doses in the management of schizophrenia. He believes that cultural and environmental anomie can lead to psychiatric illness. He has written several important books on psychiatry which manifest his special interest in psychotherapy for psychosis; here his compassion for the psychotic patient is evident, and manifested by his concern to tailor each treatment to every patient's individual needs.

Manuel Gonzalez de Chavez (contemporary in 2018)

Manuel Gonzalez de Chavez is a former Professor of Psychiatry at the Complutense University of Madrid, and a former President of the International Society for the Psychological Treatment of Schizophrenia and other Psychoses. He is an Editor of "Psychotherapeutic Approaches to Schizophrenic Psychoses: Past, Present and Future", in the ISPS Book Series. He is interested in group analytic therapy for outpatients diagnosed with schizophrenia, and runs courses of workshops in Madrid which help patients and their families to better understand and manage the illness in all its many symptomatic aspects.

Michael Robbins (contemporary in 2018)

Dr Michael Robbins, the author of the two case studies included herein, has tried hard to engage his schizophrenic patients in therapy with himself, building a strong transference relationship, and a loyal commitment in them to their treatment. It may be apparent to the reader that it is not easy, indeed it is not possible, to be certain which patients will choose to work with the analyst, and which ones will fall away from commitment to a purpose that would save their life. The psychoanalytic psychotherapist can never state that a particular patient will be cured by opting to engage in therapy. There may be mental factors which preclude this, even if therapy continues for many years. But for as long as the analyst is able to oversee the direction of treatment, that is, to continue building reflective ability, self-scrutiny, and initiative by maintaining interest by the patient in their own self in therapeutic dialogue, the patient will be growing stronger by the day even if this is not readily apparent. Fresh ideas brought by the analyst may feed the patient's impoverished mind on some occasions when the patient appears stultified, while at other times the analyst must wait for the patient to contribute to the session, particularly if the patient's mind remains lazy, possibly as a result of excessive pain. It is important for resource conservation that patients are carefully selected for personal characteristics such as patience, tolerance, initiative, determination, and a capacity for insight as well as personal application, in order to receive psychoanalytic psychotherapy. While none of these qualities will reliably predict success, they are all required for a successful outcome to this treatment.

The accounts that Dr Robbins has written up of several of his patients' therapy exemplify and validate many psychoanalytic and PPCC principles. The history of Emily, a patient suffering from paranoid schizophrenia, who underwent a successful psychoanalytic therapy with him and whom he describes in his book "Experiences of Schizophrenia" (Robbins, 1993), demonstrates many psychoanalytic principles, and follows closely the PPCC sequence of therapeutic gains leading to resolution (see Part IV, Case Study 1). Here the patient's progress has been written up in detail by Dr Robbins, and then illustrated by the PPCC model's graphic steps. The changes in the patient's mental perspective are clearly evident from the narrative text, and have been translated into graphic form so that they are registered incontrovertibly as shifts in the mental state of the patient during psychoanalytic psychotherapy. This process has also been carried out for another of Dr Robbins' patients' case histories, Sara (see Part V, Case Study 2), whom he describes in his paper "The successful psychoanalytic therapy of a schizophrenic woman" (Robbins, 2012). This patient's case study is as readily adaptable to the PPCC model as is Emily's. Every step of the patient's clinical progress can be translated into its graphic stage which illuminates it as part of the whole therapeutic process, from her early quite unsatisfactory representational world and the triangular, blocked state of her mind to rounded self-understanding and self-sufficiency. The PPCC illustrates the progress that Dr Robbins achieved for his patients, and which they achieved for themselves, working together, while all of them sustained their determination to resolve the illness and overcome every obstacle in their path. These case studies have been included herein by very kind permission of Dr Robbins.

From Freud's first dismay at schizophrenic patients' narcissistic apparent resistance to properly relating to him in treatment, to Dr Robbins' successes in nine out of his series of eighteen patients, clinicians have sought to help patients with this most serious of mental illnesses. Melanie Klein's interest in schizophrenia, transferred to her students, and the recent generation of clinicians, up to Dr Robbins and notable others, have all contributed to the progress established today when in expert hands: up to half at least of analysands might hope to emerge out of their schizophrenic illness. This is progress indeed. Many factors must obtain before such a result becomes achievable, however, with no slackness in maintaining them. Careful patient selection, clinical vigilance for fresh onset of psychosis at any time, acute psychoanalytic observation of the patient in the consulting room, skilful medication prescribing, and every care for the patient's safety on and off the ward where they are being supervised while not well enough to look after themselves, including in sheltered accommodation while they need it, are all measures which must be in place for success to be achieved. Dr Robbins has found that female patients are more likely to succeed in therapy for their schizophrenic illness than male patients, while his overall success rate is as good as any that has ever been achieved in his field. Much of the hope for future work of this kind depends on the skills and training experience that remain available for therapists who are in training to do it. The pool of skills will shrink unless energetic individuals join forces with the earlier pioneers to continue their efforts, which especially in the case of Dr Robbins have seen such excellent results. His patients have been deeply appreciative of what he has done for them, in full awareness of their own input but also acknowledging his lead in guiding them through the stages of their recovery. At every stage he knew what they were suffering, and took steps to guide them through it. There is no reason why training should not continue in active professional centres, or why current and future schizophrenic patients should not be treated like their very fortunate predecessors. Financial considerations would be greatly assisted by confidence in the treatment process. Once clinicians become confident about what can be expected in treatment, based upon the knowledge that Dr Robbins has produced and what has been confirmed by the PPCC model relating validly to a schizoaffectively disordered patient, they will find it easier to move forward into the pioneers' shoes. When a critical mass of activity has emerged, the probability of receiving appropriate treatment will be greatly increased for highly intelligent, motivated, tolerant, and determined schizophrenic patients who will do everything they possibly can in order to be well. This should be a minimum expectation for these determined patients in the community who thoroughly deserve treatment on the same basis as every patient with an equivalent physical disease.

CHAPTER 14

THE SEVEN THERAPEUTIC STAGES OF SUCCESSFUL PSYCHOANALYTIC PSYCHOTHERAPY FOR SCHIZOPHRENIA

(IDENTIFIED BY DR MICHAEL ROBBINS MD)

The successful psychoanalytic psychotherapy of individual schizophrenic patients has been found by Dr Michael Robbins to have similarities between one patient and another. He treated a series of eighteen patients, and some further patients, and then wrote up their case histories in detailed clinical accounts. One of these accounts, about his patient Sara, he wrote up as "The successful psychoanalytic therapy of a schizophrenic woman". This account is included for scrutiny in this book (see Chapter 18), followed by this author's (GS's) analysis of Sara's progress according to the PPCC's understanding of changes in a schizophrenic patient's mind when undergoing psychoanalytic psychotherapy (see Chapter 19). Dr Robbins' account is highly detailed, and the PPCC's analysis includes as many as possible of Sara's symptoms in the context of her changing mind. This author is privileged to include Dr Robbins' account, with full permission, because of his immense clinical acumen and skill, and because of the insight into the clinical condition of schizophrenia that his writing affords. Moreover, his observations about how he countered his patient's symptoms provide so far unparalleled evidence about how schizophrenic illness can be made to subside in patients.

Dr Robbins' account of his patient Emily's treatment, also included herein (see Part IV), similarly illustrates the therapeutic process he used to resolve his patients' illnesses.

7 THERAPEUTIC STAGES OF SUCCESSFUL PSYCHOANALYTIC PSYCHOTHERAPY

Once he had treated a substantial number of schizophrenic patients with psychoanalytic psychotherapy, Dr Robbins observed that their treatments followed a general, recognisable pattern amid all the digressions and vicissitudes of their individual therapies. He identified seven therapeutic stages (Robbins, 1993, p. 259) which have direct parallels in the PPCC's description of the patient's perspective (see Figures 14 and 15). Not all of the patients who he treated were able to complete their therapy. Those patients who prematurely terminated treatment still followed, however, the early pattern shown by the successful patients. The difficulty of Stage 3, when the patient must accept the views presented by the analyst in his interpretations even when these are at odds with what she herself thinks, can provide such an obstacle that the patient is unable to overcome it. These patients are less strong than those who will emerge successfully, or else are unwilling to make the necessary changes that would enable them to continue in treatment. The unsuccessful patients leave therapy at Stage 3 when they are no longer able to co-operate with the analyst in what he is broaching with them as the way forward. They relinquish effort in the direction of their own salvation, and fall away from the enterprise they had embarked upon to become healed from their faulty mental structure.

Dr Robbins observed seven clearly identifiable stages that all his successful patients reached and moved through during the course of their therapy with him; and these stages are mirrored in the PPCC's graphic illustrations of the patients' experiences. Dr Robbins' identified stages of psychoanalytic psychotherapy of schizophrenia have also been aligned (as shown in Figures 14 and 15) with the phases experienced by the patient as outlined in verbal terms by the PPCC Theory. The therapeutic stages and those experienced by the patient coincide definitively, although some overlap inevitably occurs between successive stages.

The first stage is "Protopathosymbiosis", or "parasitism" as Dr Robbins describes it, where the schizophrenic patient exists within the limits of her psychotic mind and relates to the analyst on this basis, not fully comprehending what he says to her and unable to respond very constructively to him. She is dependent upon him for their relationship's existence, and contributes little to its maintenance. All she is able to do is to attend her sessions daily, and to sustain her responsiveness to him as well as she is able, within her limitations. The PPCC model of this stage describes the patient's unhappy and unfulfilling representational world, which is what the patient's unconscious awareness consists of, and what constitutes the basis for her weak and insufficient mental engagement with regard to the real, external world. Realities that the patient is not aware of

Stages of Psychological Therapy of Schizophrenia: Dr Michael Robbins	PPCC Model of patient's mind: Dr Gillian Steggles	Stages in the patient's experience
1. Protopathosymbiosis (parasitism): patient's identity is invested in her psychotic state.	Patient is unable to function healthily using her impoverished representational world.	Patient feels alienated in her environmental world, suffering from painful schizophrenic confusion.
2. Engagement: patient's sense of individuality is threatened.	Patient unconsciously includes analyst in her representational world.	Patient attempts to engage with analyst: she may be well-defended.
3. Pathosymbiosis: may lead to collusion and Stage 3b: Therapeutic Stalemate.	Patient's 'blocked' schizophrenic mindset may prevent insightful interaction with analyst.	Tendency towards comfortable (but false) assumptions with analyst: reality cannot be contemplated.
4. Disengagement from pathological symbiotic collusion.	Patient succeeds in rejecting her previous maladaptive relationships and unhealthy engagements in her representational world	Patient works at reviewing her relationships and contemplating reality.
5. More Normal Symbiosis: growth-promoting.	Patient is awakened to the reality of her life in all its (painful) aspects of Time, Place and Person in context.	Patient is able to address reality with her analyst; she suffers intolerable experience of herself; she begins to understand her conflicts; she absorbs good feelings from the analyst; she begins to experience her own self-identity positively.
6. Psychic Differentiation and Integration.	Patient evolves into a discrete, integrated individual.	Patient can contain her own emerging integrated mental life successfully as a discrete individual, relating well to the analyst and individuating from him. Patient evolves into her own independent autonomy.
7. Therapeutic Termination.	Patient's mind is self-sufficient.	Patient leaves therapy with her difficulties resolved.

Figure 14 Dr Michael Robbins' 7 Stages of the resolution of schizophrenia by psychoanalytic psychotherapy, illustrating the coinciding of Dr Robbins' therapeutic perspective, Dr Gillian Steggles' PPCC model, and the patient's perspective

act as inhibitors to her comprehension in conversing with the analyst, and restrict her knowledge and understanding in her sessions. If she cannot understand, she cannot respond adequately. As described in Chapter 13,

1. Protopathosymbiosis
   (patient helpless in representational world).
2. Engagement with analyst pathologically
   (patient includes analyst in rep. world).
3. Pathosymbiosis
   (patient tries to communicate with analyst); then
3b. Potential therapeutic stalemate
   (patient cannot accept analyst's truths); or
4. Disengagement from pathosymbiosis
   (patient rejects her previous stances).
5. More normal symbiosis with analyst
   (patient orientates in time, place and person).
6. Psychic differentiation and integration
   (patient becomes integrated and autonomous).
7. Therapeutic termination from therapy
   (patient becomes self-sufficient).

Figure 15 Summary of Dr Robbins' 7 Stages of the resolution of schizophrenia by psychoanalytic psychotherapy, paralleled by changes in the PPCC model: Robbins (and PPCC)

Bion held that schizophrenic patients demonstrate projective identification of their own conscious awareness, and of the associated inchoation of their own verbal thought, into other people. That is to say, they give up their ability to make sense of what their senses are actually presenting to them, and subjugate themselves to other people's influence over themselves. They then are unable to think clearly or verbalise anything in their own defence. Dr Robbins is saying that when the patient is in this state, at the start of her treatment, she cannot initiate any sensible or helpful or meaningful conversation with her analyst. The PPCC Theory identifies the patient's unpleasant, perhaps threatening representational world as being a large part of the origin of this debilitating state of mind, within which the patient has become unable to draw enough impetus to interact energetically with the external environments around herself. Figure 14 relates that while in this Stage 1, the patient therefore feels alienated in her environments, and therefore confused and full of pain. It is no wonder that simply filling her with pills or injections does not resolve her experience of illness.

If the patient is able to tolerate this painful and confusing stage, she is faced with having to address the next stage of treatment. In Stage 2, she has to engage with the analyst and not simply remain passively in his company for the therapeutic hour. Her individuality, to her, is threatened by having to accept his statements, whether about herself or as general points about reality, and adopt them for herself: truths that are about realities which she must endorse and use as part of herself. The analyst's opinions might be unpleasant to her; they may feel threatening in some way; she may initially even feel that they are untrue, and she may feel miserable in accepting them. However, she has to internalise them and adopt them as her own beliefs. These ideas may contradict what she has been brought up with, in her family, and in thinking them she may be flying in the face of a decades-old existence, learning a different system of norms and principles. She may be aware that she is rejecting family relationships with those senior or respected individuals in her family whom she may love and enjoy rapport with, if only "for old times' sake". Her thinking during her development was embedded in these relationships, however, and within them she developed her schizophrenia. So reject them she must. This can seem truly cruel to her. However, she has to make her choice. Schizophrenia is a terrible illness and makes enormous and cruel demands and limitations on sufferers, so emerging out of it inevitably involves great sacrifice, in order to cut away and make a clean break from influences which have instigated it and impinged on healthy thinking in the patient. The PPCC model at Stage 2 describes the analyst assuming the problems variable at the top of the pentapointed construct, in his influential position within her mind. He has become her internal good object, a person who means a great deal to her, and in some cases he may be the first helpful adult male person she has successfully adopted into her life in this way. Other internal objects tend to remain in her Internal Space, present in her life but not instrumental in ameliorating her mind's disorders. In the patient's experience at Stage 2, she is described in Figure 14 as attempting to engage with the analyst even though she may be well-defended and resistant to change due to strong family ties.

Stage 3 of the psychoanalytic therapy of schizophrenia involves the possibility of the therapy terminating prematurely. The pathological nature of the therapeutic relationship that is due to the patient's psychological restrictions may have subliminal or unintended benefits for the analyst. He may unconsciously enjoy the patient's dependence on him, or he may for other unspecified reasons wish the treatment to continue indefinitely. These scenarios are not very likely to occur, but if they do influence the relationship then he would be acting in collusion with the patient's dependent, unhealthy mental condition. If he is unwilling or unable to assert truth and reality to his patient, the patient may slowly decline in her contributions to the treatment and the therapy will grind to a halt. This would be the end of the therapy due to therapeutic stalemate. The PPCC holds that the patient's blocked mind-set is unable to permit insightful interaction with the analyst, who may or may not be engaging in collusion with the patient; but communication between the therapeutic dyad fails either way, and the patient thereby becomes unable to progress. If collusion does occur, the two participants in the treatment may make comfortable but false assumptions together, and both fail to deliver due regard to reality: they cannot contemplate it. This is very serious for the patient, and represents the loss of her chance of happiness and wellbeing in the whole of the rest of her life.

The next stage, Stage 4, consists of the opposite choice of the patient, that is, to disengage not from the analyst but from the pathological symbiotic collusion that threatened the therapeutic dyad due to the patient's adherence to her past values. To adopt Stage 4 is a choice that the patient must make, independently of the analyst. The analyst can help the patient by consistently reiterating objective truths and adhering to reality, but the patient must decide for herself to turn away from her previously mistaken views. She must also cease regarding the analyst as being, himself, the salvation of all her woes, and begin to regard herself as an independent agent. The PPCC model describes the position of the patient successfully rejecting her previous maladaptive relationships and unhealthy engagements in her representational world, through active functioning of the paranoid-schizoid-positioned pentapointed construct alternating with the marquise-shaped depressive-positioned construct, with the analyst as the variable at the top of both structures. The patient works at reviewing her relationships and contemplating the realities presented to her by her analyst. This Stage requires motivation in the patient, with a real effort towards reviewing herself in relation to the environment around herself, including especially observing objectively her family and unhealthy ties to her deficient representational world.

Stage 5 consists of a more symbiotic, growth promoting relationship between the analyst and his patient. Having detached from her original, restricting representational world, the patient is awakened to the reality of her life in all its painful aspects. The pain is the result of seeing much more clearly how past circumstances and situations contributed to her mental deficits, and that she must now leave all of these behind if she is to become truly herself. She can now adjust to and relate to her past events and experiences in terms of Time, Place, and Person so that they no longer tend to cause her confusion, unhappiness, and psychotic illness. This is illustrated by the PPCC model becoming three-dimensional and containing all her past experiences and memories in a five-sided pyramid, and the patient adding constructively to these as the model moves forwards in time. In clinical terms, the patient is able now to address reality with her analyst. She suffers painfully upon learning that she is who she is, faults and all. She can now see, upon looking back at her past, what her own contributions to her illness have been; if she had responded differently to previous situations and circumstances then perhaps she might have been able to process them differently and caused them to have a different effect upon her, the same effect on her as she now remembers them. As it is, she can now look back upon them quite harmlessly and experience no drive towards psychosis from them. Absorbing good feelings from the analyst helps the patient tremendously to progress from day to day as she relives her memories differently: previously very painfully but now somewhat philosophically. In doing so, she begins to experience herself as a discrete person, with her own identity and in a positive light.

When psychic differentiation and integration come about in the patient she has reached Stage 6. She has learned to rely upon herself in bad times as well as good times, and to hold her own opinions based on reality and solid experience. She has her own distinct personality and holds herself together, integrated and with her own identity. Unlike her early family influences, the people she now spends time with do not cast expectations upon her that warp and distort her view of herself. She probably has little exchange with her family by now, and her mind and representational world are peopled by individuals who recognise and accept her as she sees herself, not seeing her through an overwhelming and mistaken lens. Among similarly evolved, integrated individuals like her friends, the patient can contain her own emerging integrated mental life successfully, relating well to her analyst and differentiating from him. The patient individuates and evolves into her own independent autonomy. The PPCC shows all of this in its representation of her as a sphere, a solid individual with "all her corners rubbed off" and able to move smoothly in her life without crises, difficulties or obstructions any more than the usual untoward events that are to be expected.

Therapeutic termination is the final stage, at Stage 7. The patient is able to use her mind to help herself through life's difficulties when these occur. She is self-sufficient and can determine her own goals and progress, and leaves therapy with her difficulties resolved.

Staging psychoanalytic psychotherapy is helpful because it allows closer comparison between different patients undergoing the same treatment than if comparison remained based only on overall progress. The seven stages relate to the changing relationship of the patient to the therapist, as shown in Figure 14. The PPCC's evaluation of these differing relationship types describes the changes in the patient's mind at each stage. Figure 15 then outlines succinctly the patient's experiences at each stage. Changes in the illness of schizophrenia as it affects the patient are thus elucidated, and it is helpful to know how the mechanism of therapy of schizophrenia brings about its results.

With all of this knowledge firmly based, there is a real imperative to reproduce Dr Robbins' results with fresh impetus in newly-diagnosed schizophrenic patients. Knowing in general terms what the mental state of a patient is likely to be, and how the patient is likely to be feeling, should at any stage in treatment be of great help to today's psychiatrically-trained psychoanalyst tackling schizophrenia in his or her patient. Understanding what to expect, as a guide to the course a successful therapy might take, could also be very useful to them. Clinical experience is, of course, of the greatest assistance, but until it is acquired, ascertained clinical structures and processes operating in the treatment of the illness may prove, in their way, helpful to the analyst unfamiliar as yet with this work.

PART IV
CASE STUDY 1

....

INCLUDED HEREIN BY KIND PERMISSION OF
DR MICHAEL ROBBINS MD
AND OF THE GUILFORD PRESS

CHAPTER 15

CASE STUDY 1: " EMILY: AN UNUSUALLY SUCCESSFUL TREATMENT"

THE WORK OF DR MICHAEL ROBBINS MD

Acknowledgements: This case study is entirely the clinical and literary work of Dr Michael Robbins MD, of Massachusetts, USA, who is a psychiatrist and a psychoanalyst, and a Member of the Boston Psychoanalytical Society. It is reproduced from Chapter 4 of "Experiences of Schizophrenia", by Dr Michael Robbins MD, published in 1993 by The Guilford Press, with the kind permission of Dr Robbins and of The Guilford Press.

Dr Robbins has, since his clinical work described herein, developed a fascinating new concept of the unconscious mind, described in a number of original works, particularly "The Primordial Mind in Health and Illness: A Cross-Cultural Perspective" (Robbins, 2011).

All aspects of this case study are entirely Dr Robbins' work. None of the case study material is connected in any way with Dr Gillian Steggles, Professor R D Hinshelwood or Dr Miomir Milovanovic. Dr Robbins and his publishers, The Guilford Press, retain all rights and copyright to this Case Study.

This case study is included herein by permission only to demonstrate how the PPCC model can permit visualization of, and a clear conceptual pathway for, successful treatment of schizophrenia using psychoanalytic psychotherapy, thus conclusively describing the process and illustrating sequentially the efficacy of the treatment.

Disclaimer: Dr Michael Robbins MD is in no way associated with the PPCC Theory, the PPCC structures or the PPCC model.

History

Emily was raised in a depressed, nonverbal family. Her mother, who was from a rural background, had wanted to become a doctor but became a nurse instead. She met Emily's father while he was in medical school. She worked throughout most of Emily's childhood, and shortly after she divorced Emily's father, when Emily was around puberty, she changed careers and gained considerable success as an executive in the entertainment industry. She was a chronically depressed person, and her masochistic life was testimonial to her articulated belief that life was painful. Emily's father came from a socially prominent family. His own father was a very successful physician. By contrast, Emily's father's accomplishments as a physician were marginal, and he suffered from chronic feelings of inadequacy. By the time Emily was born, he was a depressed, suspicious, isolated general practitioner who had come to specialize in performing vasectomies in his office.

Mother wanted a boy for her third child. The delivery was difficult. Emily was said to be unhappy from the very start of life. She was breast-fed for three months and switched to the bottle because of colic. Emily was separated from mother for a time toward the end of her first year because mother became ill and required hospitalization and surgery.

By all accounts Emily was an irritable and isolated child. She was acutely sensitive to loud noises and would cringe and hide when airplanes passed overhead. She had nocturnal phobias and eventually a school phobia. She had temper tantrums that escalated in intensity. At such times her parents would ignore her or put her in her room. As a small child Emily began a pattern of scratching her abdomen until it bled, which got her much attention from mother. Father took her on some hiking and canoeing expeditions with him, but for the most part ignored her except when she hurt herself and required medical attention. He sutured several of her wounds, and gave her physical examinations until the time of the divorce. Attention from mother consisted of being dressed in outfits that were frilly but rather inappropriate in relation to her peers, and being forced to participate in mother's causes as a civil rights crusader. When mother was not pushing Emily into difficult situations she tended to leave her alone a great deal. When mother would return home from an absence she would ask Emily if she had missed her, and would be delighted if the answer was no. Like many things mother did, this response reflected her philosophy of life, namely, that children had to learn to accept reality (that is, suffering) and learn to be strong.

But Emily became quite fearful of separating from mother. This was most pronounced when she began school; mother had to take her there

CASE STUDY 1: "EMILY: AN UNUSUALLY SUCCESSFUL TREATMENT"

and remain with her. Because of mother's crusade against the required pledge of allegiance in school, Emily was required, as early as kindergarten, to walk out of the classroom when the other children saluted the flag. Mother's philosophy about this was that the needs of the individual (in this case, Emily) had to be balanced against the needs of society. As one might expect, Emily was soon perceived as strange and tended to be scapegoated by her peers. When she was eight, other children referred to her as "piggie girl" and ostracized her. When she was beaten up by some boys on her way home from school, mother's response was "Don't worry about it; they did it because they love you."

Emily's parents' marriage, which was never happy, deteriorated gradually. When Emily was nine or ten her parents separated, and as she entered adolescence they divorced. A year or two later mother began an affair with a successful professional man who was also divorced. This man, unlike Emily's father, was quite extraverted and very fond of Emily; his attraction to her contained a latent sexual element, and the attention made Emily most uncomfortable. Emily's menarche, at eleven or twelve, was celebrated with champagne by mother.

Though she tended to be isolated from peers, Emily was academically successful at school, and tended to be teacher's pet. When Emily was fourteen, mother and her lover were married. As mother became increasingly preoccupied with her growing career and her new marriage, she tended to leave Emily alone. Emily was manifestly naive, and tended to get herself into potentially dangerous situations through such behaviours as hitchhiking, frequenting locations where there was potential for her to be assaulted, and acting passive and compliant when she was mistreated by others.

Emily was sent to boarding school, where, though she remained quietly depressed, and apparently began to hallucinate robed figures advising and admonishing her, it appears retrospectively that she radiated a kind of charisma that attracted the attention of her teachers. She obtained glowing reports for her achievements, which included painting. During her senior year her male English teacher, who seems to have been depressed, took to calling her "Virginia Woolf". Emily began secretly to think of herself as van Gogh.

After graduation Emily began college, but she was unable to concentrate and dropped out after a semester. She began to hallucinate. Her dress and hygiene deteriorated. She wandered from city to city like a bum. Her judgment and ability to care for herself were obviously impaired, and it is a wonder she escaped serious injury. She went to live with her father (who had also remarried), held several menial jobs briefly, and got entangled in a sexual relationship with a foreign student from a culture that tends to devalue women. Finally, even her ordinarily inattentive father was moved to express his concern about her, which led to a quarrel and caused Emily to return to her mother and stepfather. There she spent most of her time in the attic, writing in her diary and painting, but destroying anything mother seemed to like.

Emily had fits in which she smashed things, and she ingested several overdoses of pills. She began to cut and burn her body in symbolic patterns. In her diary she spoke of despair, suicide, and her belief that she was a possession of mother's; the writing, which I eventually saw, was often incoherent and even bizarre in content. Finally, mother became alarmed and arranged for her to see a psychiatrist. About a year before I met her Emily attempted to kill herself after completing a picture of a princess looking out on the world through the window of a castle battlement. She slit her wrists and overdosed while mother was away from home, but was discovered and hospitalized for almost a month. After her discharge she ran away. When she was found and rehospitalized, her psychiatrist recommended long-term treatment; Emily was transferred to the hospital, distant from her home, where I met her.

At the time of Emily's admission to the hospital psychological testing revealed a person who did not experience herself as autonomous and whose defences were unstable. Emily was delusional and her logic was autistic. She tended to make arbitrary, grandiose, global syntheses of information and to engage in paranoid thinking.

Treatment

Year One

Emily was nineteen when our therapy commenced, and twenty-five when it was completed. She was attractive and slightly overweight. She chain-smoked and showed not even ordinary anxiety about meeting me. She was friendly and obviously intelligent, but there was a vacant, mechanical, compliant quality about her. She spoke softly and without affect, and the content of her remarks was vague and abstract. She said she felt adrift. She did not understand her feelings or the reasons for her actions. I tried to empathize with what she must have been feeling, and restricted myself to attempts to rephrase what she was telling me and to find out whether she thought I had comprehended. She seemed to feel understood, and expressed some surprise and relief.

CASE STUDY 1: "EMILY: AN UNUSUALLY SUCCESSFUL TREATMENT"

At our second meeting, around Easter, Emily's head was bandaged and she was much more distant and suspicious. She did not look at me as she recited an elaborate delusion about killers and victims involving herself and the ward staff, a delusion that had culminated with her carving a cross in her forehead. She fell silent, then gradually became agitated. Rather than commenting about the provocative content of the delusion I asked her about her immediate state of mind. She felt she was avoiding something that she experienced as dangerous, though she could not say what. She became quite disturbed, and I thought she was upset with me; in fact, she thought my question was important, and we concluded by deciding together that we would have a try at therapy.

Our third hour followed a similar pattern. Emily described extreme and disparate states of consciousness or mood, "good" states and rageful paranoid states, but her speech was flat, she chain-smoked, and she did not look at me as she talked. Again, rather than comment about the content of what she told me, I wondered aloud about her immediate state of mind, and again she seemed pleased. During the fourth hour she more or less enacted contrary states of mind; in one of these she claimed she wanted to relate to others and have constructive goals while in the other she was enigmatic, withdrawn, prone to tantrums, and preoccupied with her mother. When she spoke in one of these states of mind, she tended to attribute the motivation for the other to outside influences, which she then proceeded to attack and devalue. After helping her clarify what she was saying, I commented that it was hard for me to know what she wanted and that it was therefore difficult to make any kind of treatment agreement with her. In the fifth hour it became clearer that her meaningful communications were not so much verbal as behavioural; these were in the form of destructive, attention-getting enactments that were somehow related to her mother.

In my condensed presentation of Emily's treatment, you will mercifully be spared her long, tedious periods of silence and withdrawal, sometimes lasting a month or more, in which she would say but few words to me. You will have to imagine her affective cycles, including fits of rage during which I occasionally sensed – and she much later confirmed – that I was in danger of being attacked (not an inconsequential danger, as Emily was tall and solidly built). It will also be difficult to convey her disintegration. Her speech would say one thing, her behaviour another, and her affect yet another, often seemingly unrelated. The repetitive back-and-forth movement between progress and self-destructive regress also can only be hinted at. This report unavoidably conveys a false sense of coherence and continuity.

Emily was verbal and compliant, but it soon became apparent that the person who spoke with me had no contact with her feelings or with the person who was episodically out of control on the ward where I met with her. She hallucinated mystical robed figures speaking to her critically or seductively. From time to time she became enraged and panicked, convinced that the ward staff were about to execute or poison her – or had already done so. At these times she smashed objects, assaulted staff, and burned and cut herself in patterns associated with a private symbolism. The staff experienced her as frighteningly out of control. These gross psychotic episodes led to her restraint and seclusion, and they were a constant counterpoint to our work for the first fourteen months. I soon sensed that Emily obtained some gratification from the attention she got from staff for this behaviour. After two weeks of therapy her ward administrative psychiatrist placed her on trifluoperazine, on which she remained for three years. Initially, the dose was 10mg daily; it was raised to as much as 40mg in the subsequent tumultuous months.

Emily found life intolerably burdensome: she had to satisfy relentless internal and hallucinated critics, she felt obligated to make mother feel good, and now I was forcing her to learn to be intimate. She had attended a rural private school, and she told me she preferred goats to people. She punished herself and her mother by being self-destructive, which also served to get her taken care of and to make mother feel needed.

Emily became more self-destructive during my first vacation, after five months of therapy. When I returned, her posture was robotic. She laughed hysterically and informed me that three white-robed figures were ridiculing her. She told me she had wanted to kill herself while I was gone. She expressed fear that she might become involved with me and lose her specialness, which she associated to her relationship with mother and to the belief that she was Vincent van Gogh (in fact, Emily had a considerable but undeveloped interest in art). After telling me this she doubled over, shrieked with pain, and said the three robed men were laughing at her.

After seven months of work together I told Emily that our meetings would be interrupted while I underwent knee surgery. She was initially sad but then said she wanted to go home and be a great artist while living in mother's attic, where she envisioned mother taking care of her unconditionally. She then imagined me tearing a baby from its mother's breast. She became withdrawn and paranoid, hallucinated more, looked menacing, told me everything was connected and had special meaning, and sat on the floor of the seclusion room (where we were then meeting because of her uncontrolled destructiveness), tracing womblike patterns in the dust with her finger.

CASE STUDY 1: "EMILY: AN UNUSUALLY SUCCESSFUL TREATMENT"

When we resumed meetings after my surgery, Emily sucked her thumb, rocked, talked baby talk, and maintained that she was six years old. She wanted me to take care of her and wanted mother, who was visiting, to take her home. After mother left she sadly told me that no-one in her family knew how to love, and she asked for my help. The night of this striking revelation, in a state of terror because her hallucinatory men were threatening to kill me, she called me at home. I suggested that she might be angry at me; although she confused the feeling with physical ugliness, she admitted she was enraged that I had "made" her need me and then was not always there to take care of her. The following hour she denied anger at me, but after I left the ward she had a rage reaction, bloodied both hands and had to be placed in restraints (a condition in which she now spent much of her time, including her therapy sessions). The dose of trifluoperazine was raised to 40mg. During this period Emily told me two dreams: in the first, she was trying, unsuccessfully, to get a tiger into a car in which she was having therapy. In the second, she was trying to build a world with pipe-cleaner men but failed, and a woman came to take care of her.

At Christmas, during the ninth therapy month, she presented me with a gift: a beautiful painting. Long afterward, she informed me that it represented a fetus trapped in a teardrop womb inside a tree trunk, but at the time she could tell me nothing about it. Then she decided to give up and go home; she began an active campaign to leave the hospital. I suggested that her plan to live in mother's attic and be a famous artist was a womb fantasy. I added that she was enraged that I did not treat her like an invalid. She promptly forgot what I said but decided she would remain at the hospital, adding that her mother thought she was perfect just as she was.

In the eleventh therapy month Emily took to her bed (in her single room) and refused to see me. She stared at the ceiling and was mute. After a month of being almost totally bedridden and mute and in response to pressure from the ward staff, she called and asked to see me again. She told me, without affect, that she was very angry that she had let me "get inside" and that she had been trying to get rid of the world. The month had been quite comfortable, she added, and she reported a dream of walking tirelessly and effortlessly through beautiful woods. But, she concluded, she knew no-one would take care of her the way she wished.

Year Two

Though she attended her sessions, Emily remained virtually mute with me for more than a month in the early part of the second year of treatment, and she seemed quite untroubled about it. Over the first four months her trifluoperazine was gradually reduced from 40mg to 10mg as she was no longer perceived to be such a destructive menace on the ward. I cast about for ways to relate to her, and tried to enlist her in a discussion of "my problem" by asking her what one does when rejected and left alone. She suggested, without any manifest concern, that I could daydream or read a book. She remarked flatly that she wanted to stop therapy, but when I asked if she was going to do anything about it she remained rooted to her chair.

Emily began to tell me how her mother never seemed to recognise that she (Emily) had problems and how she treated her as though she were perfect. She told me how she played along, by laughing and being superficial, and how, during mother's visits, the two of them would blame the hospital and me for the fact that she was still there. Emily used these interactions as "fixes" in order to feel "high", and mother would leave perplexed about why Emily mutilated herself and required seclusion between her visits. Emily then made an unconvincing, hence unsuccessful, effort to tell mother how upset she was. I suggested that I might join the meetings that were being held between Emily, her mother, and the social worker in order to assist her to communicate with mother. Soon after, Emily came to therapy, in the heat of summer, dressed in a red ski cap and long red socks with holes. Her expression was wooden, her affect flat, and she was very agitated. She voiced fear and anger that my participation in family meetings might disrupt her relationship with mother. Suddenly, Emily removed her cap, remarking challengingly that she had made it herself and that mother would like it but she believed I did not. I responded that she thought mother would like both her creativity and her crazy behaviour, whereas I distinguished the two, and that what she made was nice but wearing it here was inappropriate. In the following hour her leg shook uncontrollably, she smiled bizarrely, and described silly behaviour and a conversation in which she had participated on the ward as though it were profound. I expressed my concern that her condition was worsening. She wanted me to comfort her and reassure her that everything would be all right, but I responded that I could not.

Emily told her mother and stepfather what I had said about her condition, but they responded that she seemed better to them. Regarding the question of my participation in family meetings Emily reported, "Mother thinks you are too blunt; you must not let your kids get away with anything!" After her parents left, the staff discovered that Emily had severely mutilated herself. When I came to the ward for her next appointment, I found her in the quiet room, spread-eagled on a mattress on the floor in four-point restraints, laughing and singing loudly and bizarrely. I could not hide my

CASE STUDY 1: "EMILY: AN UNUSUALLY SUCCESSFUL TREATMENT"

distress at her degradation. At the time I looked upon my show of emotion as a breach of neutrality, however unavoidable, but years later Emily informed me that my involuntary response had been a turning point in her treatment, and I have learned over the years that the success of many treatments, particularly of more disturbed persons, seems to hinge around similar therapeutic "mistakes". I think it was the unplanned, out-of-character nature of this therapeutic event, which was "beyond" technique, that contributed to its value. In any event, Emily told me that she had carved NO HOPE on one arm; I subsequently learned from a letter that her mother sent me that she told mother that she had carved HELP on the other.

Emily remained in restraints for the next two weeks, acting bizarre and euphoric. I decided it was time I began to attend family meetings, and the social worker reluctantly agreed, although she thought my presence would be disruptive to Emily's mother. I met with mother, stepfather, Emily, and the social worker every other week for the next five months, and our work was extremely productive. Around the time we commenced, Emily's behaviour explosions permanently ceased, but she began a month-long fast, accompanied by the delusional conviction that she did not require food.

My first discovery in the family meetings was that it was mother and not Emily who experienced the distress of being hospitalized. Mother felt all the physical and emotional pain that Emily seemed not to, down to the sensation of being cut and burned. Stepfather cried when I pointed this out, and said that their marriage was deteriorating, but he was quite willing to make the sacrifice "for Emily's sake". We began to uncover a multiplicity of ways in which family members conspired to deny Emily's separateness and to avoid overt expression of anger and conflict. The parents tended to soothe Emily, to cut her off when she tried to speak, and to speak for her, asserting that they knew her thoughts. This was sometimes an invitation for her to act out their feelings, and at other times, as Emily later put it, a way of "stealing [her] thunder". That is, if mother knew about Emily's anger and understood and accepted it before Emily expressed it, then they were one and there could be no conflict. Parents also tended not to take Emily seriously. When Emily first began to tell mother how angry she was at her, mother became confused and refused to believe it. I pointed out that it had more impact on mother when Emily mutilated herself than when she expressed her feelings verbally. Stepfather's response at this point in the meeting was to give Emily a very sensual hug because she was "bleeding". I had to point out that this was an instance where she had not cut herself!

After several family sessions Emily reported two dreams: in the first, she and mother were guarding their house against an enemy attacking from the rear. In the second, Emily was preparing for her coronation, to succeed mother as queen. The coronation turned out to be a disappointment, however, and mother got all the attention. I wondered, in response, whether she perceived me as the enemy and whether that meant I should stop attending the meetings. Emily said she hoped not, and told me how important my participation had become to her. I suggested that, if this was true, perhaps she could begin to verbalize the negative feelings about me that her dreams suggested, and she began to do so. Gradually, the intense anger Emily and her mother felt for one another also emerged in the meetings, despite the belief each held that the other was too depressed and fragile to deal with that anger.

All was not well, however. Emily continued to fast; she lost twenty-five pounds over the month and became visibly gaunt. The staff became concerned she might require forcible feeding. In response to my concern Emily insisted she did not need to eat because mother was taking care of her. I told her I did not believe this, and she cried and responded that I had helped her to understand things about herself she preferred not to know. Then she said she believed that by fasting she could shrink herself and become mother's little baby.

Eventually, Emily began to express excitement that the family meetings were providing the first new direction in her life, and she decided to resume eating. She told me she wanted my help to learn to be more grown-up. Emily's subsequent feelings of depression, loss, and helplessness suggested some separation from mother and the loss of her illusion of security, and she began for the first time to take part, with some pleasure, in hospital relationships and activities.

After sixteen months of treatment trifluoperazine was reduced to 10mg. In anticipation of interruption of treatment for my summer vacation Emily first became enraged that she did not possess me and then confused, with paranoid thoughts and self-destructive urges. On my return she was withdrawn and did not make eye contact. First, she said, she had tried to control the separation by acting like me and encouraging other withdrawn patients to relate. Then she had smeared spaghetti over her entire body and had turned to a staff member who had helped her. She told me matter-of-factly that she guessed she didn't need me anymore. She had also gotten involved with a young man who, she asserted, was brilliant; she believed this was so because she couldn't understand a thing he said. He had told her not to look at anyone else; he also told her that if she didn't look at me, then I didn't exist. We realised that she, like her mother, had trouble distinguishing genius from psychosis.

CASE STUDY 1: "EMILY: AN UNUSUALLY SUCCESSFUL TREATMENT"

I made a slip and called her by the first name of another withdrawn patient of mine. With some embarrassment I acknowledged that she had succeeded in making me feel rejected the way she must have felt while I was away. She, in turn, cried and raged at me, but she began to realise, in connection with my habit of taking vacations, that nothing is totally satisfying and everything has limits.

Emily began to express dissatisfaction with the preoccupation with suffering, depression, and unreality that characterises hospital patients in general, and her family in particular, and to wonder if there might be a more positive world "out there". Her interests and activities blossomed, and partly in response to impending limitations in her hitherto generous insurance coverage she began to make discharge plans. She still wished for an endless womblike existence in the hospital, and she reported dreams in which she wanted to scream, masturbate, and otherwise let go but was unable to. She tearfully identified herself with a movie hero who achieved greatness through hard work.

Meanwhile, I gradually became aware that the attitude of ward staff and other patients had become rather hostile toward me as I came on the ward for Emily's appointments. My surmise that Emily was presenting distorted versions of our conversations to them in order to elicit their anger at me was subsequently confirmed by talks with her and with staff. When confronted with this, Emily began to express rage at the idea that I might be experiencing success as her therapist, wishes to mutilate me and reduce me to her "size", and doubts about my sanity. She told me, and I subsequently confirmed, that a junior staff member had said that a remark Emily told him I had made to her was crazy. Coincidentally, her administrator reduced her trifluoperazine to 5mg. Rather frightening outbursts of rage at me from Emily alternated with maniacal laughter associated with ideas of being a fairy in flight and a prostitute whose body was literally not her own and with the belief that someone was trying to poison her.

Things seemed out of control, and I finally shared with Emily my feeling of powerlessness to reach her, and remarked that she seemed convinced that one or both of us had to be destroyed. We agreed to increase the frequency of her sessions from three to four a week, a frequency we maintained throughout the balance of the treatment process. Emily became somewhat calmer and was able to review her hospitalization and illness reasonably appropriately, say good-byes, and prepare for discharge. She decided to rent an apartment with a chronic schizophrenic male patient whose acquaintance she had made in the hospital, and with whom she had a casual relationship, despite her administrator's suggestion I had once again colluded with Emily's grandiosity, but at the time I felt constrained by the financial pressures that her family reported.

After twenty-three months of hospitalization and twenty months of therapy Emily was discharged, her hair in pigtails and dressed like a little girl, in gauzy white (particularly inappropriate as it was a snowy day). I gave her a gift, a small book of walks or hikes of exploration one could take in the city area where she would be living, with an inscription saying that I believed there was a world outside the hospital and I hoped she would find it. Emily was touched and felt she should give me something in return. Perhaps I would be ill, she said, and she could take care of me, or she could give me sex, she continued, but that would be prostitution.

Emily became upset because her parents failed to respond emotionally to her discharge. She wrote them an angry letter and proceeded to gorge herself with food, to become paranoid, and to want my understanding without talking. She dreamed of being mother's sliced turkey and of messing her body but having her art work praised; then she dreamed of a phone call in which mother misidentified her and hung up, leaving a "dead line". However, she proceeded to plan a holiday trip home. Then she dreamed that since we could not find an office to meet in for therapy, we went to her parents' vacation home. We were in a car and I was trying to drive but she was blocking my view of the road and of her parents. Stepfather took over and almost hit a little car, which she associated with herself. Mother said "Don't hit the little car", but gleefully she proceeded to smash it. The dream ended with Emily thinking that I was caressing her, but looking up to discover that it was her mother.

When she returned from her short holiday Emily had to face her roommate's regressed behaviour as well as the fact that her trip home had been an effort to live out mother's fantasies and to believe that she was not only cured but perfect. Emily became disorganized and paralyzed with ambivalence and could not leave my waiting room; I arranged for a brief return to the hospital. There I discovered that Emily had secretly stopped taking trifluoperazine before her trip home, and a 10mg dose was resumed. As we began to talk about her poorly planned discharge, Emily expressed both her expectation that I would take perfect care of her and her rage at me for failing to do so. Although Emily began to feel enthusiasm about her life again, it was now accompanied by new feelings of vulnerability and dependency. She dreamed I was a bull-dozer filling in a great hole so she wouldn't disappear and also that she had purchased a defective outfit of clothing and was trying, in the face of a variety of obstacles, to return it. She realised that her mother's denial of problems, infantilization of her, and grandiose beliefs about her had kept her from learning to face and resolve problems. Emily arranged to separate from her schizophrenic roommate and to move to more suitable living quarters, which took several weeks. She enrolled in a literature course in preparation for starting college in the fall, joined a partial-hospitalization program, and began an important friendship with a woman who was able to be remarkably realistic, persevering, and resilient despite major physical handicaps and ill fortune.

When Emily told me with dismay that she had had a horrible weekend because she had fought with her schizophrenic roommate over his inconsiderate behaviour, had gone to the hospital to sleep overnight, and, as a result, had not done as much work as she would have wished on a course paper, I pointed out all the thinking, struggling and coping that had been involved, and added that coping with problems like these was a part of everyone's life.

As my vacation approached, Emily again experienced the rageful wish to eliminate me, but after she came at the wrong time for her appointment she remarked that she was finally understanding what she called my "lectures on limits", namely, that if you love someone you allow them to be separate. She wanted to let me go, but in return she felt entitled to whatever thoughts and feelings she might have about it. These turned out to include wishes to mutilate me and cut off my legs so I could not leave. Emily feared these wishes might come true, and she recognised that this, in a sense, was what her mother had done to her.

Year Three

My return after my vacation marked the beginning of our third year. Emily burst into tears when she saw me and told me how well she had done. She was beginning to value her body. She cried over the scars from her self-mutilation and attended a weight control group. As she struggled with her familiar sense of herself as a mess needing to be fixed, she began to talk about her father, a doctor who had specialized in performing vasectomies in his office at home. She recalled how he had sutured wounds on her scalp and knee poorly, and without anaesthesia, and she remembered the numerous physical examinations he had performed on her before he left the family around the time of her puberty. She began to wonder if he liked to hurt people.

Emily's hallucinations diminished, but one night while in the city she became paralyzed with terror and a sense of impending attack. Literally unable to move, she called me at home, and I drove into the city and brought her back to the hospital. In our next therapy hour she told me she was discovering sadistic wishes toward father. Emily scratched absent-mindedly at her scars and appeared to be bandaging her finger with tissues as she recalled the pleasure father seemed to take in doctoring her. She laughed inappropriately as she talked about her wish to have him "fix" her, and she acted as though she were being tickled as she scratched at herself. In the days that followed she began to binge eat and talked angrily of wishes to castrate father, eat him, and excrete him. A sense of gratitude toward me alternated with hatred that I made her aware of pain; perhaps, she thought, I had even inflicted it on her. To her surprise she realized that, however perversely he had treated her, she had loved her father, and this realization provided her with an impetus to separate from her mother.

I was away for two weeks. Again Emily stopped trifluoperazine. On my return I found her huddled in a corner in protection against some imagined assault, sobbing convulsively; she seemed to be living out a memory or fantasy (much later she concluded that it was probably the latter) of her father doing a vaginal examination on her to remove some "bumps" when she was eight or ten years of age. She remembered how mother had palpated Emily's breasts early in adolescence and worried that she might have cancer. As Emily became aware of her wishes to be father's neutered daughter, mother's cancerous patient (before her marriage mother had been a nurse), and my psychotic patient, she became paralysed with rage at herself and at others, and filled with paranoid terror and self-destructive wishes. Again Emily was discharged.

I told Emily I would be taking some time off in about two months when my wife gave birth. Emily reported more positive feelings about her body and new insights, which she felt she had gotten from me. She had a fantasy that I had impregnated her. After a gynaecologic examination she was enraged and disappointed that the doctor had not wanted to sleep with her, and she all but propositioned me. I remarked that some of her recent interest in her body was healthy, but that her notion that there were no limits or boundaries in the relationship between parents and children and between doctors and patients was a destructive one.

Emily got a job and planned to take college entrance examinations. At the same time she withdrew from me and began a pattern of nocturnal adventures; staying out late, frequenting clubs and bars, drinking heavily, and acting quite seductively, though it was my impression that she did not actually become sexually involved with anyone. During the day she did not want to wake up, missed therapy appointments, and felt much disappointment and rage. Gradually we began to reconstruct her memories of nocturnal excitement and fantasies about father, which had been stimulated by such things as his bedtime back rubs; these were often followed by sleeplessness, and fears of animals and intruders, against which she would rouse father from bed to "protect" her. In the morning father would "flash his penis" in the bathroom while he groomed himself, then leave for the day; Emily would have a tantrum and rejoin her mother.

Emily's full realisation of father's hurtfulness, seductiveness, and rejection happened to coincide with the birth of my baby and a weeklong separation. She felt rage that my wife and not she had gotten the penis and the baby. She talked of her confusion between sex and hurting. Her skin itched, her knee had "arthritis", and the chant "Kill, kill" went through her head.

Gradually Emily concluded that it might be better to put her energy into new activities and relationships rather than into lost causes. She enrolled in an acting class, where she learned she had talent, got a better job, and even wrote to father to suggest he provide some money for her education (he had provided no financial support since the divorce). She dreamed she got married and father killed himself on the steps of the church. Nevertheless, there was a resurgence of diurnal acting out, and an intensification of her hallucinations. Emily called people "cunts" and "pricks", and I think that is literally how they looked to her. She recalled, with excitement, how she would sit on the hospital ward and laugh as people literally turned into monkeys in front of her eyes, and how she could hallucinate psychedelic wonders and experience great highs. She felt entitled to skip her therapy hours, but when I pointed out that she would not want me to treat her that way, she raged at me. Then she began to control her behaviour again. She recalled her hospital discharge almost a year earlier, when she had dressed in white; she told me how she had believed that she was about to "marry the world" and how enraged she was that she hadn't found the great seductive, infantilizing presence she had been seeking.

At holiday time Emily visited her brother, whom she described as much like father, and his wife. She felt imprisoned and enraged in an environment she described as angry, nonverbal, action-oriented, and infantilizing. Shortly afterwards she had severe back spasms and had to be hospitalized for a week and immobilized. Before and after this hospitalization she had to lie facing me on the couch in my office because of her physical distress (the treatment was usually conducted sitting face-to-face). Feelings of not having control over her body led Emily to work on her convictions that she was omnipotent, immortal, and invulnerable. She recalled diving off a chair onto a concrete floor at age three (she imagined she was diving into water) and cutting her chin severely. She talked of magic rituals that, she had been convinced, warded off danger and controlled her world. A nightmare of being stalked by a figure of death led to a discussion in which she became more accepting of her mortality.

To my surprise, having to use the couch was not threatening to Emily; instead it led to moving experiences of feeling good about her body and feeling close to me. She told me of a dream in which I had come to lie on the couch with her. I began to kiss her, but, to her surprise she pushed me away. She talked about a growing sense of propriety as well as the threatening intensity of her feelings. She dreamed she was at a beach party, and a bonfire was burning out of control. A friend was lying in a pose Emily herself sometimes assumed, smoking a cigarette. The friend told Emily she had slept with me, and Emily protested that she didn't believe I would do such a thing. Her associations were to relinquishing pleasures like sex and cigarettes for more integrated ones like the closeness she felt with me. A new and distinctive softness began to replace the familiar flatness of her voice. Her body tingled "like winter" or "like dancing", and she was afraid she might faint. She found the experience orienting but difficult to bear; I felt moved.

When Emily felt good she felt as though she were flying, a sensation she found frightening. Mother's philosophy was that life was misery, and people should be down to earth and learn to live with their feet firmly planted on the ground. I asked Emily what she thought the natural course of these flying feelings might be if they were not "grounded" by misery and suffering. She had difficulty thinking about this and turned her attention to an impending visit from mother, recalling mother feeling her breasts for cancer. She experienced burning anger, had sadistic fantasies about mother's body, and felt an urge to have a climactic, murderous confrontation. She contrasted this with the soft, warm, playful, dizzy, "feel all colours" sensation she felt for me. I remarked that she trusted me. My comment astonished her, and in a spontaneous outburst she quoted Miranda's soliloquy from *The Tempest* about her discovery of a "brave new world" other than her father.

In the last months of our third year, entirely on her own initiative, Emily stopped taking trifluoperazine, joined a group called Smoke Enders and, with surprising ease, relinquished her chronic two- to three-pack-a-day smoking habit; gradually terminated her partial hospital program; and decided to learn to type. She could feel the difference without the trifluoperazine and remarked how she had to talk to herself and will herself to remain in control.

Emily talked with humour about how hard it was to incorporate all the instructions about self-care she had received from her various doctors and the Smoke Enders group and concluded that she guessed we both cared about her and we both cared about me and that was "neat". But she feared she would lose her appeal to mother if she relinquished her vices and took good care of herself, and she feared setting limits regarding her physical privacy, limits based on her new sense of modesty, when mother came to visit lest mother think her crazy! She reasserted her "right" to be self-destructive and in a rage shared fantasies of incinerating me and knifing me to shreds. Finally, she concluded that she was clinging to the valuation of craziness she shared with her mother because it provided romance, privacy in the form of enigmatic withholding, and a sense of triumph and pride. I remarked that we all needed privacy, pride, and romance in our lives but perhaps there were more constructive ways to get these things.

Year Four

At the beginning of our fourth year Emily reported pleasure in her accomplishments, but she cried and said it felt like her mother was dying. She had believed that she would become the messiah of death and destruction and would preach mother's philosophy to the world – indeed, this was the symbolism of the cross carving that had marked my initial Easter meeting with her. As she talked she had to restrain powerful urges to withdraw into a rageful, annihilating hauteur rather than work to prove herself in a forthcoming college interview. She wondered if her messianic fantasies might have been a childish effort to deal with a family full of unverbalized anger and depression, where action was unrestrained and good feeling was not safe because of the absence of boundaries.

Emily began to talk about good feelings as though they were external intrusions. When I pointed this out, she recalled her hypersensitivity to sound and light, which in turn led her to deny perceptions, shut off feelings, cut off thoughts, and tense her lower back and pelvic muscles. This seemed to be a factor in her back spasms. She felt rage as she began to recall bathroom scenes with father, and her fantasies that he would use her for a toilet and kill her. She dreamed of two women, one embracing a man and the other hating men and admonishing the first to end the embrace, and recognised that both were herself. She dreamed of concealing a bandage in a tampon container but having it taken away by a man. Her association was that the penis was a vampire organ that would drain her blood and kill her and that her defense had been to imagine herself with a penis (her arms) and the ability to control the blood flow (by self-mutilation). She experienced new wishes to kiss in lieu of the old urges to smoke cigarettes.

A month before my summer vacation Emily's depressive reaction to the impending separation led her to voice the conviction that she had been breast-fed and abruptly weaned and that she had never accepted a substitute until she encountered me and the verbal presence I represented. She recalled clinging to mother, refusing to learn new things, and embracing the bad feelings that mother so readily responded to. When I reviewed her admission history, I learned that her mother had reported that Emily was weaned at three months because of "colic".

She became excited by her history professor and by her fantasies about his penis but experienced anxiety, gagged hysterically, and felt she didn't want to swallow. She recalled father naked in the bathroom and realized she had transferred her wish for a breast to one for a penis; she recalled imagining being a toilet for father's sperm or excrement, which would get inside and eat away at her. She began to wonder how well she had internalized the soothing functions of our relationship and whether she would need to seek a breast/penis substitute during my absence. She became transiently psychotic and fearful of loss of control, so we made an agreement that she would avoid heterosexual activity while I was gone. In response Emily felt like a ballerina who executes a complex series of steps, lands on her feet, and throws up her arms in joy, triumph and mastery. She dreamed about kissing her history teacher and me while having a comfortable agreement not to go further. She anticipated a positive summer and interesting things to tell me in the fall.

Her prediction proved accurate. When we resumed Emily had successfully begun college. She had a brief flurry of angry oppositionalism to me, during which she recognised that during her adolescence her friends all seemed to hate their mothers, while her mother remained her "best friend". She talked of her fear to move to a place of her own and recalled that her adolescent runaways had always been to YWCAs in other cities, where she would proceed to isolate herself. She became preoccupied with somatic symptoms, imagined she had a fatal disease, and then recognised her wish to use self-destructiveness to terminate her forays into the outside world. This recognition led to a discussion of how she avoided unfamiliar sensations, particularly sensual ones. In two succeeding therapy hours Emily was first convinced that I flaunted an erection in front of her and then that a woman friend was pregnant. This led again to fantasies of being used by father as a toilet and being annihilated, and of her menses as a kind of toilet-flushing. As she recalled father's extensive caressing of her in the guise of a physical examination, she felt a back spasm, and when she moved a bit in my direction on the couch where she sat, her thigh muscles went into spasm. She laughed ruefully, took my footstool, and interposed it between us.

As Emily realised that her self-mutilation had involved efforts to control fear, rage and sexual feelings towards the father she perceived as sadistic, she became more conscious of her own sadism. With laughter at once gleeful and uneasy she revealed fantasies of vengeful intercourse with father involving cutting a "vagina" into his chest and getting in there with her penis-arm-knife to mutilate his insides and dismember him. She wondered how dangerous she might have been to others had she not turned this rage on herself. Fantasies about her relationship with her mother – in which Emily was a princess (mother's name was Victoria) or the Messiah (her mother had used Emily to act out her own protest against prayer in the schools) – were associated with her feelings of omnipotence. She experienced wishes to have her rage contained by a man who would hold her, and she recalled how father would isolate himself elsewhere in the house when she had tantrums as a child.

Emily was behind in her first semester college work, and it was unclear whether she would complete it on time. As tension built she became increasingly rageful and launched attacks on me. She realized that she had always used tantrums to avoid confrontation between her sense of omnipotence and reality. Sexual fantasies about me turned to rageful wishes to pound me into clay. She cursed and came near to attacking me physically. She dreamed of being helpless while a madwoman attacked her. She was so angry she wanted to vomit. With just a small amount of schoolwork remaining to be done, Emily became paralyzed with ambivalence and made the case for becoming psychotic again: she would be able to feel special, and she would not have to face feelings and problems. But she realised it would also mean pushing away the friendship and love of others, and she became sad. She completed her schoolwork on time.

Emily planned a two-week vacation to visit her parents, and then shortened the trip without telling me. When she was told that the therapy hours she had cancelled might now be unavailable, she seemed unable at first to grasp the fact; when she did, she became enraged. Emily returned from the visit in a state of euphoria, bragging that she was everyone's dream girl: she had passively accepted mother's dogmatism and intrusiveness (that is, she was mother's "special shit"), stepfather's thinly veiled sexual embraces (his "playboy bunny"), and the attraction of sister's boyfriend (and victorious in competition with her sister, who experienced herself as Emily's inferior). I did not share her enthusiasm, but responded dryly that she lacked an identity or a dream of her own, and let others use her without limit. I wondered what she might be enacting for me. She angrily retorted that I was "an asshole", and then imagined becoming my perfect cure. But she realised that the price of being a dream girl – suffocation, rage, and self-destruction – was the real "pain in the ass". Emily began to experience a novel sensory-perceptual aliveness, associated with a heightened awareness of her own body and feelings and of others as separate and fascinating beings. She began to generate and act on fantasies of her own. She prepared for a physical examination, which stirred anger and fear related to her father, by planning and acting in such a way as to make the encounter satisfying, and she succeeded. By contrast, she did not anticipate a major scheduled dental procedure, and came in with an enormously swollen jaw and a sordid tale of suffering. She realised, in retrospect, that she had not voiced her doubts when the dentist reviewed the procedure with her and told her he anticipated no problems. She had tried to be his dream girl and not complain, though the procedure was excessively lengthy and painful. As she realised this she experienced biting rage.

As she became more emotional and adventurous Emily felt terrified, out of control, overstimulated, and dizzy. She recalled how hypersensitive and avoidant of stimulation she had been as a child (mother told her she would hide her head in her hands when an airplane flew overhead). After a particularly exciting experience she felt disoriented and developed a fever; she wondered if the new experience was in fact an illness. I called it "growth shock". Emily made many efforts to control these new and exciting feelings by turning them into something dangerous and bad that she could then avoid. For example, she liked ice cream but would tell herself "It's so good it's disgusting!" Then she would literally come to believe that all food was poison. She remembered how wonderful mother said she was when she acted crippled and inept, and she recalled childhood adventures that led to accidents and to painful suturing without anesthesia by her father and without anyone holding her. She realized that making things bad and painful was a form of clinging to her parents and the security of their anhedonic attitudes, that turning unfamiliar sensations of pleasure into badness was a form of self-control and security. We realised that she had gradually worked out an elaborate set of rules and rituals based on the equation that bad equals good, and vice versa, rules and rituals that turned out to be those given her by her hallucinated robed figures.

As she felt more separate from mother, Emily planned an exciting vacation trip with a friend. She had images of flying and dancing. She felt curious about the unknown but insecure as well. Emily wanted to touch and examine my hand. When I allowed her to do this, she seemed to feel more secure about her trip and about her exploration of unfamiliar subjects. She realized in wonderment that I was alive and had feelings like she did but that I was a separate and distinct person.

Year Five

As we began the fifth year of treatment, I observed that Emily's body movements, once wooden and robotic, were becoming more fluid and graceful. When she told me she had not allowed a man she dated to hold her hand because she knew he was involved with another woman, I reminded her that I was involved with another woman. Her requests to hold my hand ceased. Although she wanted to hold my hand again in anticipation of a trip that frightened her, because I represented security, she decided not to act on her wish when she realised that I also represented the most frightening aspect of the unknown world, the penis. This led to more work on her sexual feelings, which were unintegrated and largely experienced as external; for example, in dreams that insects were crawling in and out of her vagina. At this stage awareness of a sexual fantasy or mention of a sexual word could literally make her cringe or jump, or could trigger vaginismus. She dreamed of fleeing from an injured man with a knife and being unable to lock the door of the room she had fled to, of trying to call for help but making no sound, and, finally, of becoming a boy with a woman soothing him. She imagined she had once been a boy and that father had castrated her, but then she realised her sexual disability was an identification with him. She recalled how she had tried to suppress her feelings when father would rub her back at night. Emily dreamed that when she went to a doctor for an internal exam and was told she had an infection, she responded, indignantly, "No I don't; that's me", by which she meant that those were her feelings and they were good. She worried that her attachment to me would cause her mother pain, but at this point she was feeling more estranged from her family, and remarked that her home had been a kind of hospital, with father (a doctor) and mother (nurse by training) both invested in suffering, disability and impotency.

When I returned from a vacation Emily reported that she had finished most of her year's schoolwork and had been able to evoke mental images of our dialogue in situations requiring judgment and self-regulation. Yet she seemed detached, guarded, and fearful. She began to protest about being separate. If she got better she would have to relinquish relationships with her parents and with me, and for what? Even so, she said, she had hung up on mother during one of her depressive litanies in order to finish a school paper and get some sleep for her early morning therapy hour.

Wanting to give me the "cold shoulder", she began to act withdrawn and explosive but responded with amusement when I told her I thought she no longer had to act that way. In fact, Emily's self-image was becoming that of a serious, emotionally intense person who planned for the future and was pleased to receive compliments for her maturity. She made new friends, moved into an apartment of her own, enrolled in a painting class, and decided to transfer to a more challenging university for her junior year.

After the first painting class Emily came to me in a frenzy, which escalated until she shouted, banged her fists on the table, and sobbed. After she had calmed down we talked of her difficulty dealing with stimulation, and she likened the painting class experience to learning to dive into the water headfirst. I recalled her headfirst dive to the basement floor as a child, and the grandiose fantasies that had preceded it. Her next class seemed "dull grey". Mother came to visit, and Emily was able to set some limits, including vetoing mother's wish to sleep in Emily's small studio apartment. She remarked, with asperity, that it was not mother she wanted sleeping next to her. She hungered for real intimacy and had some new experiences, including going to the beach (where she had hitherto feared exposing her body) and participating in a women's rights march.

It was midsummer, and as we anticipated another of my brief vacations and then the fall of Emily's sophomore year, we discovered we had each been thinking about reducing the frequency of our meetings, which enraged the "crazy" part of her and also saddened her for she could foresee an inexorable movement away from me that, she predicted with considerable accuracy, would lead to an end to our work in one or two years.

In the fall of her sophomore year we reduced the frequency of our meetings from four to three per week. Emily's new apartment was robbed, and she felt angry and violated. She was painfully aware of longings to be hugged and loved, but not taken care of. She handled all necessary matters without turning to mother, and our discussions clarified the state of poverty and deprivation in which she had been living, one that seemed so natural to her that she had never talked about it. The apartment had been chosen for its low rent and was in fact in a dangerous neighborhood. Emily's furnishings were meagre. What little clothing she owned was mostly unsuitable. In response to a compelling but foreign inner presence she ate junk food even though she did not like it. Mother called junk food and sweets "poison" but often offered candy to Emily. Mother talked about how Emily deserved the best, but she was very stingy with money and, as I knew from her problem paying Emily's therapy bills on time, was often late or short with Emily's modest allowance. At the same time, mother never encouraged Emily to work and often reiterated her grandiose belief that Emily could do anything she wanted, whenever she made up her mind to do so. In response Emily believed that she could take advanced courses without having had the basic ones and that she could function without adequate food, clothing or sleep. As we talked about Emily's diet of sweets and great expectations, I commented that it was as though she was expected to thrive on a sugar teat rather than the real thing.

As we talked about how Emily might have a lifestyle more compatible with feelings of self-esteem, and more in keeping with the success and affluence of her parents, she felt increasingly angry with her mother. But she feared that if she were to rise above the general level of misery and suffering in her family, she would incur the rage and envy of family members and would leave her mother with nothing. She made several efforts to talk with mother about this. The first one failed when mother "stole her thunder" by claiming she understood completely because she and Emily were just alike. Emily was in high spirits after the second try, however, reporting that mother had called her "crazy" and unable to understand or deal with reality. Mother had never spoken to her like this before, and it felt good. As she concluded her narrative she quoted a passage from A.A.Milne, in which Christopher Robin says "I think I will stay six forever and ever", thus acquainting me with one of the origins of her delusion during the first year of therapy. We shared a laugh.

Emily began to challenge what she called her "fuck up" identity in relation to the males in her family by becoming interested in science and math, hitherto the province of her brother and father. She told me she had "fucked up" a math exam by staying up the night before, but her self-destructiveness seemed to lack its former power; we had to laugh when she subsequently told me she had gotten one of the highest grades in the class. She struggled to complete her university applications in the face of a tendency to deprive herself of food and sleep; she became disorganized, whiny, and self-pitying and then thought of the currently popular song "Vincent", which proclaimed that van Gogh had been too special, brilliant and sensitive to live in this awful world. Emily realised she had been enacting her mother's hatred. She felt an angry, tearing sensation, and she imagined a cornered rat, her psychotic part, clawing and biting her. She began to believe that she had a high potential for achievement, and her resolve to transfer to a top university intensified.

Our attention shifted to the issue of sexuality, which Emily kept avoiding by lashing out whenever she would begin to feel close to me. She realised she could not integrate her sexual and loving feelings, and the awareness that she now had a loving relationship with me encouraged her to work on this. She reviewed numerous memories of having been a passive victim of intrusion and overstimulation by men in her family, experiences that had led to difficulties accepting her sexual feelings as internal. And she realised she had developed a system of self-protection that included inhibition, rejection of her emotions, and projection of rage.

Year Six

As we commenced our sixth and final year, Emily's concerns shifted to fearfulness that mother and her women friends were hostile to her blossoming femininity and her interest in men. She worked on fears and fantasies that she would be neutered and that either she or mother would not survive the changes in her. She recalled with embarrassment and anger how she had carved a cross in her forehead at the hospital while under the delusion that she was the Messiah. She realised she had been sacrificing herself for mother. Now that she was no longer mother's "sidecar shit", to use the symbol of a dream, she imagined mother collapsed, like a broken, lifeless puppet. Emily purchased more feminine clothing, deepened some important relationships with women, and made successful friendship overtures to Mark, a classmate, despite an aversive physical response to his attractiveness – a "no" in her head and a kind of whiny negativism that sounded to me as though she were protesting "I am only a child!" She displaced some of her competitive concerns from mother to Deborah, an accomplished and attractive woman who eventually became Emily's closest female friend.

Emily now felt that she had a personality of her own. She elaborated fantasies about intimacy, pregnancy, childbirth, graduation, career and exhibiting her painting, which was becoming a more central pursuit in her life. Fantasy became a kind of trial thinking preceding action. Seeing me was now experienced as touching home base, as a stepping stone and no longer an end in itself. Emily felt I was now inside her as a benign and supportive presence. For the first time she began to paint on her own, and she reported a constructive inner dialogue between her self-doubts and more encouraging thoughts that incorporated the voice of her painting teacher and my voice, which was less readily identifiable.

Emily cancelled a therapy hour so she could pursue an opportunity that had unexpectedly arisen to get to know Mark better. She was accepted by her first-choice university. She dreamed that she shook mother like a rag doll, heedless of cries from family members that she was heartless, and then called an ambulance to take her away. When her family visited, Emily used humor to make it clear to mother that she now had a life of her own from which mother was excluded. On the other hand, she was indignant when I expressed my doubts about the correctness of her mother's belief that maternal grandmother had Huntington's chorea and that Emily might contract it, then she realised both she and mother had wishes to reinstate the status quo.

With me Emily seemed adolescent and rebellious. She experienced me as an intrusive father in relation to her developing sexuality. The relationship with Mark was developing at a slow and satisfactory pace. Emily had some difficulty distinguishing her consuming interest in him from her relationship with her mother, and distinguishing orgastic from psychotic forms of letting go. And she imagined I would dislike her for completely excluding me from her mind at times of passion with Mark. She marvelled that she had experienced orgasm just from kissing him. They had had their first real fight, which served to bring them closer. But Emily wanted all this to be private. She bridled at my comments and told me, not unkindly, that she could do things herself now and that she had a man of her own.

Emily had some difficulty focusing and finishing her thoughts; she related this to fears of where she might be heading in her life and, specifically, to fears of termination. She was irritable because there was so much she wanted to do and such limited time. In contrast, there were hours when she had little she needed to talk to me about. When my summer vacation approached, Emily acted unaware of the fact and then, at the end of an hour, told me the following dream: She went to purchase an umbrella and selected a beautiful purple one. She brought it to the salesman, who said it was nice, but not waterproof, and perhaps she should not buy it. With this dream she realised she was preparing to grieve our termination.

Emily said she was planning to make love with Mark for the first time (without commenting on the fact that she had chosen a time when I would be away). The backlash occurred when she went walking with him in new shoes that were too tight, denied the pain and got bad blisters. This reminded her of delusionally instigated self-punishments she inflicted for allowing herself to get close to me.

When we resumed her therapy in the fall, Emily felt like an aviator about to take off, not fearfully but with excitement. In contrast, she realised that our relationship had about run its course; we would no longer be struggling to be closer but to say goodbye. Emily thought about the old days at the hospital. Many of her friends she had made there had not been as fortunate as she. She remarked that hers had been a sad story but one with a happy ending. When she brought up a sleep problem, our discussion led nowhere and she realised this was her effort to present herself as crazy and hold on to me.

As Emily began her junior year at the new university, her life did seem to be taking off. She demonstrated an amazing maturity and self-sufficiency, much of it seemingly reflexive, even though we missed a number of appointments (because of difficulties coordinating her new schedule with mine). She dreamed of a disagreement with her mother: mother became a monster who attacked and clawed her face, but Emily fought back.

Emily decided that four months would bring her to the end of her first semester and give her sufficient time to reach an equilibrium with her mother and say goodbye to me. She set a termination date and then concluded a discussion of some problems with Mark by saying, quite oblivious to the significance of her remark "I know we can work it out; after all, neither of us is insane!"

But Emily avoided the termination work. When I eventually commented on this she accused me of devaluing her, as mother did, and lacking confidence that she could meet her commitment. In a rage she began, provocatively, to imagine committing suicide in order to despoil "my" work and destroy me. My crime, she said, was to deprive her of the worry and feeling-free schizophrenic state. Soon she turned the anger on mother for not valuing her accomplishments, but it turned out that Emily had shared few of them with her. I pointed out that she was not assuming responsibility for the work she had done and the person she had chosen to become. After a dream in which she, in the driver's seat, backed up her car but failed to see an obstacle and a murderous mother then tried to take over, Emily decided she should visit her parents and tell them more about herself. In doing so she learned that what she had taken for lack of interest on their part represented mother's concept of how to let her separate and stepfather's belief that she was too fragile to tolerate a response from him. Emily received real emotional responses from both, including learning about mother's longstanding doubts that she would ever get better.

With two months remaining I continued to wait for Emily to begin saying goodbye, while she acted enigmatic and sulky, in a manner reminiscent of the early days of our relationship. Even after we reviewed her wish to assign me responsibility for "seducing" her into the relationship and its consequences, this behaviour continued. I began to worry about whether Emily was ready to terminate, as well as to feel angry, impatient, and devalued. I did not look forward to her therapy hours, and even harbored wishes she were gone, which, I realised, reflected quite an accomplishment on Emily's part considering all we had been through together. In casting around for reasons to avoid intervening and becoming more active in the termination process, I was reassured when Emily told me about a Thanksgiving celebration at her apartment in which she shared preparations and feelings with Mark and an invited group of friends. And it sounded as though she was doing extremely well at school.

Finally, Emily clarified that she had also been waiting for me to do something. If I really believed she could take care of herself and no longer needed to see me, she reasoned, then why didn't I act that way, stop behaving like a therapist with a problem patient, and start acting like a separate person with feelings of my own? Somewhat taken aback, I said I would try, and I moved into this unfamiliar territory by telling her how turned off I had been by her recent behavior. Emily could readily understand this. After some further discussion in which she reviewed some of the changes in herself and reiterated positive feelings about me, she told me she just wanted to be quiet and look at me. But I felt distant and unmoved, like a spectator of her accomplishments and an object of her interest. In accordance with our new understanding I shared my feeling of loss of a sense of "we-ness". Once again Emily interpreted the situation. She said I was acting the way she and her mother had acted, that I was reluctant to let her go, feeling rejected and hurt by her separateness, and that I was looking for problems to keep us together. I had the disorienting sensation that our roles were reversing, but I needed to explore this new direction with her. I thought about the reasons for my reluctance to let her go, ranging from more realistic concerns to various fantasies I entertained about having a nontherapeutic relationship with her. I shared with her the uncertainty I had about terminating with someone as ill as she had been, and I told her I would miss the pleasure of relating to her now that she was her own person. Emily was moved.

The feeling of "we-ness" was briefly restored as we shared the sense of loss of a relationship no-one else could possibly understand. We both felt we had made peace with her leaving. My doubts about her readiness had forced Emily to question herself, and she told me that in all respects the first semester had gone well. Emily remarked on her fearfulness about moving, changing, heading she knew not where. But then she asserted, firmly, that she didn't want to talk about it. She knew that in the future there would be many things she would never again discuss with anyone, for she could carry her own emotional baggage, an accomplishment that left her feeling at once pleased, sad, and alone. When I commented on her freedom I made a slip, and said I wondered what choices "we" would make! Emily intensified her effort to tell me how much our relationship had meant to her. She recalled my gift when she left the hospital and told me of her frustration because she could think of nothing to give me now that would adequately reflect her feelings. With a little more than a week remaining, a sense of calm descended on both of us, a feeling that our work was finished.

In our last hour Emily symbolically relinquished her precious and enigmatic insanity. She gave me journals containing a decade of her psychotic writing, along with her permission to do with them whatever I might wish. She told me how angry she felt toward people who glorify insanity. She said she had learned to lie, without qualms, to people who asked about the scars on her arms, not because she was reluctant to talk about her past, but because her experience had been that the changes in her were so profound that people did not believe her when she would tell them she was once insane. With the notebooks there was a card that read, in part:

Thank you for helping me get on the right path. I think the only way to express adequately how much you mean to me is by living my life as fully as I can.

I have had several letters from Emily in the years since termination, and it appears she is doing just that. She graduated summa cum lauda, the top student in the Fine Arts Department of the university, and she won a major art prize. She played a prominent part in campus life as well. Emily went on to launch a career as artist and art teacher, a career that continues to grow. She and Mark lived together for a few years, and then she decided, as their relationship was not progressing, that it would be better for her to be on her own. Close friendships with women friends have flourished. She has little contact with her parents, but noted in one letter that mother looked better than she had in years: "Clearly our separation has done her good". Emily concluded a recent note as follows: "So that's how things are in my life – pretty good. As far as my psychological growth and development are concerned, I don't think anyone could have hoped for any better, even you!"

CHAPTER 16

VISUALIZATION OF CASE STUDY 1 (DR ROBBINS) USING THE PPCC MODEL: DR STEGGLES

The PPCC model applied to Emily's psychoanalytic therapy (from 'Experiences of Schizophrenia', Michael Robbins)

Stages of Therapy
A Development of the illness

Emily's representational world:
1. Psychoanalyst
   Directs therapeutic activities towards resolving analysand's problems.

2. Experiences
   Born into a depressed, nonverbal family
   Difficult delivery
   Early colic
   Was a baby girl (when her mother wanted a boy)
   Separated temporarily from mother in first year
   Sensitive to loud noises as a child
   Nocturnal phobias, school phobia
   Temper tantrums
   Bullied at school.

3. Dreams/Representations
   Painted well
   Hallucinated advising and admonishing robed figures
   Cut and burnt her body in symbolic patterns
   One teacher called her 'Virginia Woolf' and she secretly began to think of herself as Van Gogh.

4. Observations (non-psychotic thoughts)
   She was naive
   She radiated a charisma

5. Determining Orientation (psychosis and disturbed behaviour)

Schizophrenic Global Perspective 2 (nearly intolerable) 'false self'	Schizophrenic Global Perspective 1 (absolutely intolerable perspective within family)
Having to tolerate surgical assaults by father	Scratched abdomen till it bled
Being forced to reconcile to being attacked by boys	Hallucinated at school and college
Having to miss saluting the flag	Dress and hygiene deteriorated
Being scapegoated by peers	Fits in which she smashed things
She thought she was a possession of her mother's	Several ODs of pills
	Cut and burnt herself
	Wrote incoherently and in a bizarre way of despair and suicide
	Slit her wrists
	Delusional, grandiose and paranoid

(i) 5 Variables of Emily's uncomfortable representational world when initially in therapy (year 1)

VISUALIZATION OF CASE STUDY 1 (DR ROBBINS)

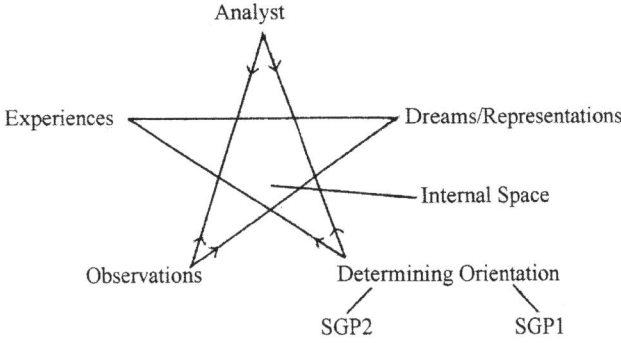

(ii) The PPCC in the paranoid-schizoid position illustrating Emily's representational world and her Schizophrenic Global Perspectives (year 1)

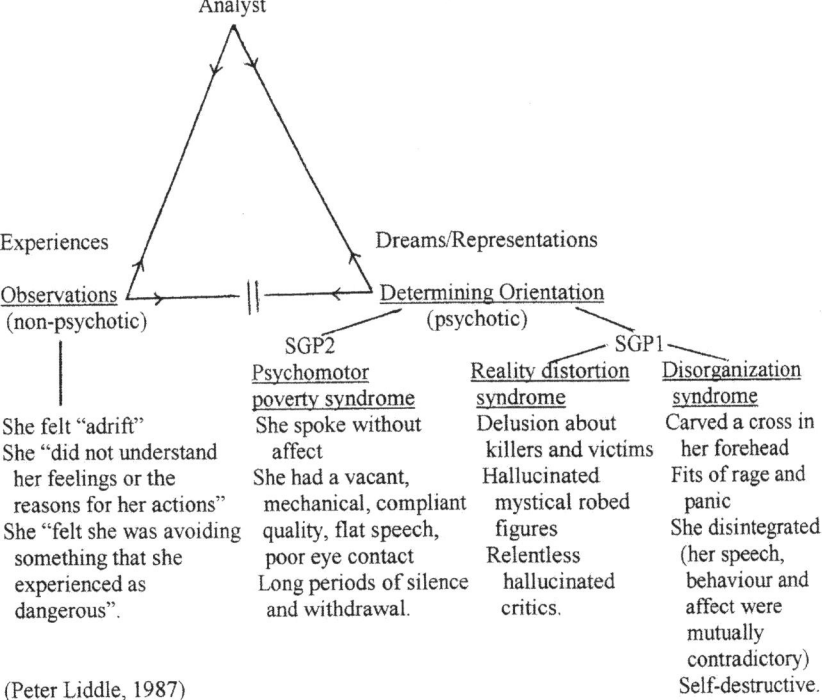

	SGP2 Psychomotor poverty syndrome	SGP1	
		Reality distortion syndrome	Disorganization syndrome
She felt "adrift" She "did not understand her feelings or the reasons for her actions" She "felt she was avoiding something that she experienced as dangerous".	She spoke without affect She had a vacant, mechanical, compliant quality, flat speech, poor eye contact Long periods of silence and withdrawal.	Delusion about killers and victims Hallucinated mystical robed figures Relentless hallucinated critics.	Carved a cross in her forehead Fits of rage and panic She disintegrated (her speech, behaviour and affect were mutually contradictory) Self-destructive.

(Peter Liddle, 1987)

(iii) Emily's limitations interacting with her representational world, leading to block (schizophrenia) (year 1)

B Treatment

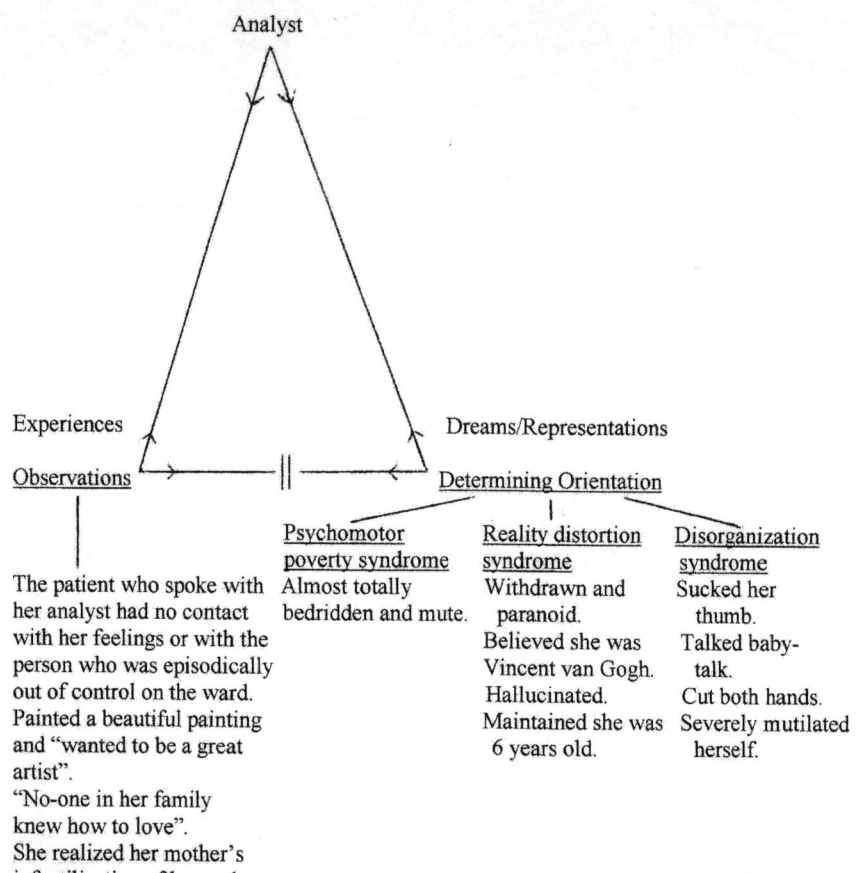

Observations

The patient who spoke with her analyst had no contact with her feelings or with the person who was episodically out of control on the ward. Painted a beautiful painting and "wanted to be a great artist".
"No-one in her family knew how to love".
She realized her mother's infantilization of her and grandiose beliefs about her had prevented her from learning to face and resolve problems.

Psychomotor poverty syndrome
Almost totally bedridden and mute.

Reality distortion syndrome
Withdrawn and paranoid.
Believed she was Vincent van Gogh.
Hallucinated.
Maintained she was 6 years old.

Disorganization syndrome
Sucked her thumb.
Talked baby-talk.
Cut both hands.
Severely mutilated herself.

(Peter Liddle, 1987)

    (iv)   <u>Analysis of Emily's psychosis</u> (years 1-2)

VISUALIZATION OF CASE STUDY 1 (DR ROBBINS)

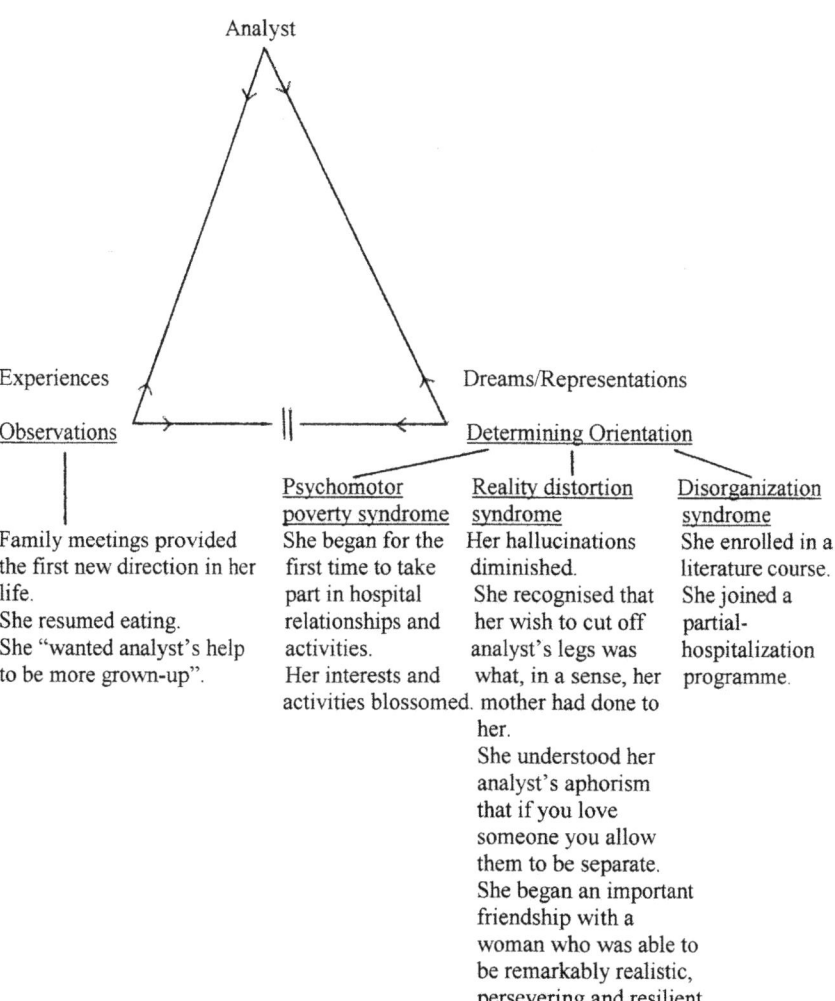

(Peter Liddle, 1987)

(v) Effects of treatment of Emily's psychosis (years 2-3)

C Resolution of the psychosis

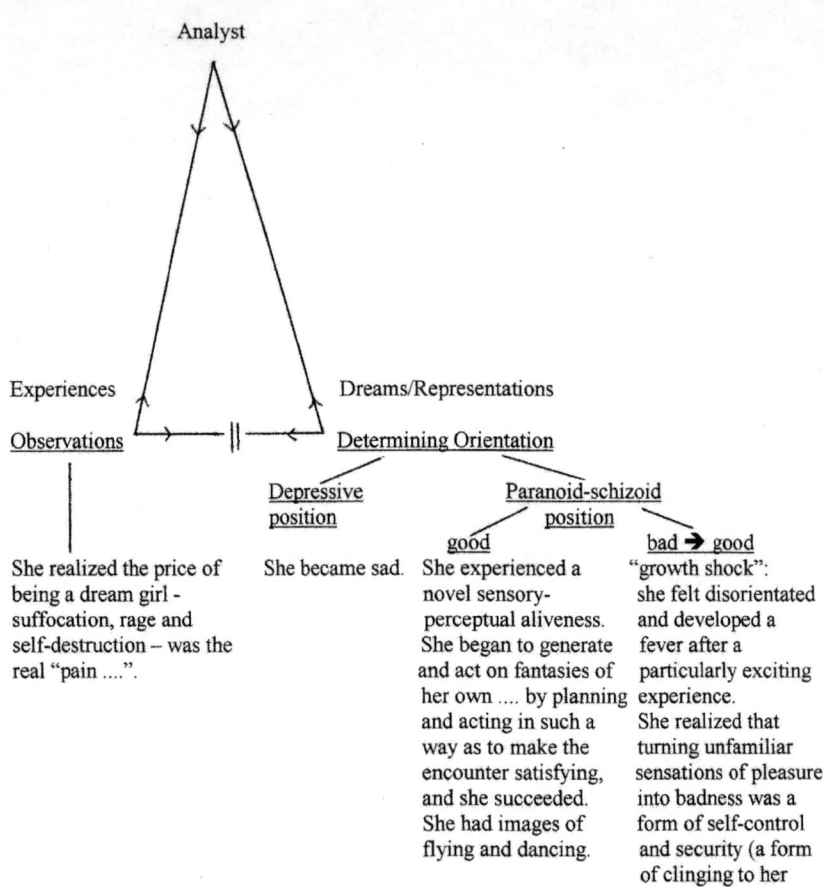

She realized the price of being a dream girl - suffocation, rage and self-destruction – was the real "pain ....".

She became sad.

She experienced a novel sensory-perceptual aliveness. She began to generate and act on fantasies of her own .... by planning and acting in such a way as to make the encounter satisfying, and she succeeded. She had images of flying and dancing.

"growth shock": she felt disorientated and developed a fever after a particularly exciting experience. She realized that turning unfamiliar sensations of pleasure into badness was a form of self-control and security (a form of clinging to her parents).

⇨ She realized becoming psychotic again would mean pushing away the friendship and love of others.

(Melanie Klein, 1935, 1946)

(vi)   Resolution of Emily's psychosis (year 4)

VISUALIZATION OF CASE STUDY 1 (DR ROBBINS)

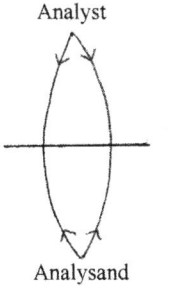 ↔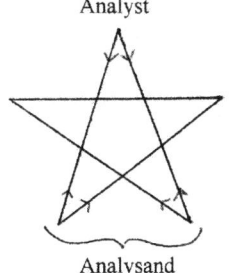

Depressive position   Paranoid-schizoid position

some oscillation
and conflict

Progress.
Emily's self-image was becoming that of a serious, emotionally intense person who planned for the future and was pleased to receive compliments for her maturity.
She made new friends, moved into her own flat, enrolled in a painting class, and transferred to a more challenging university.
She felt increasingly angry with her mother and she successfully challenged her mother's influence over her regarding junk food (an achievement in realism).

Residual self-destructive regress.
Her sexual feelings were unintegrated. Mere mention of a sexual word could literally make her cringe or jump or trigger vaginismus.
She could give her analyst the "cold shoulder", becoming withdrawn and explosive.
She thought she could survive on sweets and junk food.

(Melanie Klein, 1935,1946)

(vii) More therapy, longterm (year 5)

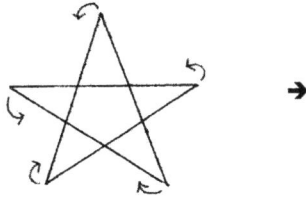 →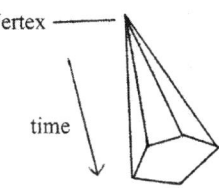

(viii) Closure of the vertex: Orientation and Integration in time, place and person; Establishment of perspective.
"Emily used humour to make it clear to her mother that she now had a life of her own" (year 6).

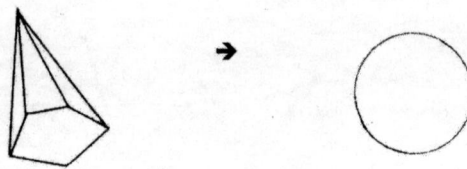

(ix) <u>Rounding of Emily's personality</u> (year 6 and several years later)

"I know we [Emily and boyfriend] can work it out; after all, neither of us is insane!" (Emily was oblivious to the significance of this remark).

.... Emily's experience had been that the changes in her were so profound that people did not believe her when she would tell them she was once insane.

CHAPTER 17

COMMENTARY ON DR ROBBINS' CASE STUDY 1 AND ITS VISUALIZATION:

All views expressed in this chapter are those of Dr Steggles

This chapter discusses the visualization, using the PPCC model, of Case Study 1, a patient called Emily, who was treated with psychoanalytic psychotherapy by Dr Robbins.

The PPCC model visually and graphically describes the process of applying geometric visualization to Case Study 1 (and see also Case Study 2 below), and elucidates conclusively the effectiveness of psychoanalytic psychotherapy for schizophrenia. Emily's therapy with Dr Robbins was "an unusually successful treatment". It represents an ideal outcome for a schizophrenic patient who was stranded in her life without access to means of helping herself out of her lacuna of misery, which is a very common situation among this large population of very ill patients. Half of Dr Robbins' patients had "positive outcomes", and half had "negative outcomes", a very good overall rate of success for his technique. He has described how Elvin Semrad (see Chapter 13) helped him learn to sit with his patients while they struggled with themselves in coming to terms with their substantial difficulties while in his care. But in the final evaluation, it is patient characteristics which determine the use to which a patient is able to put their opportunity of effectively exploring themselves with a view to learning everything they can that might help them live their life more fully than where they have found themselves at the start of treatment. This is why great care is needed in patient selection. Higher than average intelligence is a general requirement, as are personal qualities of patience, determination, courage, the ability to be open and honest with themselves in the acquisition of insight, and a temperament that is essentially well-disposed towards life at core, despite what often emerges as a fundamental rage at their lot in life.

Absolutely excellent, comprehensive clinical reports of a psychoanalysis such as those by Dr Robbins, and reproduced herein, are very rare in the literature. Sensitive, perceptive, academically masterful clinical studies, beautifully written up, these accounts define what can be achieved through psychoanalytic psychotherapy with diagnosed paranoid schizophrenic patients.

They emphasise the ordeal of schizophrenic patients in working through their problems until they find themselves discovering their mind despite their early life experiences. Their rage, despair, pain, terrors, and misery cannot be overstated, endured year after year by the patients. Particularly notable is Dr Robbins' strength in courageously bearing his patients' distress with them as they find their own way through their situations and states of mind, selecting consciously or unconsciously, from among all he says to them, what they can make best use of, at every juncture.

Emily, Case Study 1, was a naturally gifted artist. Her talent and her innate, largely unconscious wish to develop this may have been behind her strength to get well and make something of herself. Originally, she showed signs of being a particularly sensitive baby who responded with difficulty to social and environmental stressors such as loud noises and the dark, and then to her experiences of school. She coped poorly with painful feelings, resorting to self-harm despite succeeding at school with teachers.

These aspects of her life, told to her analyst, Dr Robbins, and in part from other sources as well, reflect how she related to her early world. Collectively, her impressions formed her representational world (see (i) and (ii) of Chapter 16), and can be structured in this way according to the PPCC model (see Part A of Chapter 16: Development of the illness). The Psychodynamic Pentapointed Cognitive Construct (PPCC) sets out the main features of Emily's world, her representational world, as they unconsciously affected her cognition. The main emotional element of her life at the start of her treatment consisted of being overwhelmed and infantilised by her mother. As such, she was quite unable to take responsibility for herself, learn to tackle difficulties, and grow to maturity.

Her Schizophrenic Global Perspectives 1 and 2 (see (i), (ii) and (iii) of Chapter 16) illustrate her conflicted psychological difficulties in terms of Peter Liddle's syndrome form as classical symptoms of schizophrenia (Liddle, 1987). Set out in the PPCC model, the place of these within the sequence of her developing psychology can be clearly seen as part of her schizophrenic mind-set.

Emily's condition at the start of her treatment (Part B of Chapter 16) shows the personal nature of the SGP symptoms as her personally characteristic enactments and psychotic thoughts, and some non-psychotic thoughts that reveal some further detail from the basic schizophrenic symptomatology (see (iv) of Chapter 16). This analysis of Emily's psychosis illustrates very clearly Liddle's syndromes in the context of the PPCC. The PPCC provides a clear framework for Emily's psychology at the start of her psychoanalytic psychotherapeutic treatment.

In (v) some results of Emily's treatment can be seen to have ameliorated her functioning. She became constructive in several different directions, in the hospital, at college, and in her relationships. Most of these developments involved fresh activities with other people, and mark a major change in her focus from worrying internally about herself and self-harming to addressing constructively the world around her.

In Part C, Resolution of the Psychosis (see (vi)), the PPCC illustrates how difficult parts of her psychology, for example the "bad" elements of her paranoid-schizoid position, were beginning to be understood, accepted, and to become more integrated and more like elements of the healthier depressive position. She addressed her difficulties and took initiatives to enjoy her social contacts more, to cease clinging emotionally to her parents, and realistically retracted her desire to live up to a conceptual ideal of herself, recognising the futile pain and ultimate distress this brought her.

At (vii) she still retained some intense difficulties, particularly her physical, personal experiences, with her sexuality, eating, and emotional adjustment. She oscillated, as is usual even with healthy individuals, between the paranoid-schizoid and depressive positions. However, by this time her self-image had progressed into that of "a serious, emotionally intense person", and she was capable of withstanding her physical and emotional difficulties effectively. She was duly able, in line with this, successfully to challenge her mother's influence on her regarding junk food, which illustrates her growing sense of realism.

Subsequently, in (viii), Emily's PPCC vertex closed and she was able to accommodate all aspects of her life with humour and establish distance from her mother. This was reached after six years of work with Dr Robbins, and represents the main stage of success achieved by the therapeutic alliance between them both, in enlightening Emily as to the effects her condition was creating in her thinking, identity, behaviour, and relationships. All of these had developed in her as her response to her mother and to the rest of her environment, perceived unconsciously by her as her representational world, the environment where she had been responding to others as she grew up from birth. But, over time, these responses of hers no longer were sufficient to enable her to manage the new experiences and situations she encountered as her life progressed. By gently pointing out her difficulties and possible realistic reasons for these, Dr Robbins gradually enabled Emily to draw her own conclusions about her present life and make her own choices among possible decisions that would help her mature. When the possibilities of desirable options presented themselves to her, Emily realised good sense and developed her own healthy perspectives and attitudes.

Finally, in (ix), Emily achieved balance with her boyfriend as well, and also with all her other acquaintances, few of whom ever realised how confused and distressed she had once been. This is a measure of the success of this treatment by Dr Robbins on a young woman who had been unable to emerge into her adult life from within the confines of her family. Her experiences, especially those that she assimilated while being cared for by her mother, did not lead to her own mental growth and prosperity. Her overbearing mother stifled Emily's natural responses and prevented Emily from thinking for herself. Dr Robbins' intervention provided an alternative pathway which Emily chose to take, and by doing so helped herself to blossom into the creative artist she had initially shown signs of being, at her school.

The PPCC model thus displays the way Emily's mind changed during the course of her therapy. Initially submerged in the difficulties and pain of her original representational world, signifying as it did the totality of the challenges that conspired to fix her in her bind within her family, she was unable to function normally. Without Dr Robbins' help she would likely have remained there for the duration of her life, debilitated and essentially unhappy: "a schizophrenic patient".

Her contact with the challenging and rectifying influence of Dr Robbins' attitude and encouragement towards her enabled her to see and identify her difficulties as being not only specific and real, but also adjustable and amenable to her own ameliorating efforts. With Dr Robbins constantly supporting her, she was enabled to persevere through her own drive and energy to register and examine her experiences, adjust her attitudes, and take strengthening, progressive decisions for herself.

This is how psychoanalytic psychotherapy brings about fundamental change in the lives of patients who are prepared to put in the work required to evolve up and out of their original life situations, resolve the unhelpfully debilitating and restricting nature of the ways their own mind works, and learn fresh, new, and helpful ways of personally perceiving themselves, life, and others.

Biological psychiatry has a major part to play in the resolution of schizophrenia. Medications can be gratefully received by patients for their efficacious relief of symptoms, despite their sometimes annoying side effects; Dr Robbins commonly prescribed trifluoperazine and occasionally chlorpromazine for his patients when he deemed their influence would be helpful, and has written that taking medication is not a contraindication to talking therapy. But to be enlightened out of a schizophrenic mindset, talking therapies and especially psychoanalytic psychotherapy are the only way known at present that will achieve healthy, reflective mental activity in place of a schizophrenic block, with all its symptoms.

As mentioned above, Dr Robbins has written that he feels one of his most useful strengths as a clinician, which he learnt in his training, was to learn to sit with his patients while they suffered their pain, the pain of recognising how stultified their world has become, and the painful effort of trying to climb out of the mire within which they were bound. These processes take time, which is why long-term psychoanalytic psychotherapy is long-term and, equally, why it is so effective for those patients who can tolerate its own stresses in place of the only alternative, ie. the unpleasantness and stultification of remaining afflicted by their illness; that is, the only alternative apart from more ephemeral or circumstantial therapies which may comfort the patient but not resolve the schizophrenic process in their minds. Dr Robbins' clinical technique requires highly skilled, patient, robust, and alert tending of his patients' minds. Skilled personal supervision is, he is clear, essential during training to be a psychoanalyst who is thereby enabled to deliver psychoanalytic psychotherapy to schizophrenic patients using also his or her psychiatric training in managing psychosis. Good hospital facilities are also essential to take custodial care of patients whose illness renders them unable to live in the community using their own efforts. Episodes of fragmentation repeatedly occur in the analytic treatment of schizophrenia, and robust care systems need to be in place for every such patient.

There can be absolutely no doubt that psychoanalytic psychotherapy is able to save the lives of those psychotic patients who choose to become well, given the chance. In a National Health Schedule for Schizophrenia it would be this opportunity that every suitable patient should be offered. Patient selection would need to be rigorous, discipline strict, and clinicians fully trained. But it is hoped that the methodology described here is clear enough to allow these parameters to be achieved so that some schizophrenic patients, at least, may be alleviated of their distress.

PART V
CASE STUDY 2

· · · · · · · · · · · · · · · · · · · ·

INCLUDED HEREIN BY KIND PERMISSION OF
DR MICHAEL ROBBINS MD
AND OF THE GUILFORD PRESS

CHAPTER 18

CASE STUDY 2: "THE SUCCESSFUL PSYCHOANALYTIC THERAPY OF A SCHIZOPHRENIC WOMAN"

THE WORK OF DR MICHAEL ROBBINS MD

Acknowledgements: This case study is entirely the clinical and literary work of Dr Michael Robbins MD, of Massachusetts, USA, who is a psychiatrist and a psychoanalyst, and a Member of the Boston Psychoanalytical Society. It is reproduced from Psychodynamic Psychiatry, 40(4) 575-608, 2012 with the kind permission of Dr Robbins and of The Guilford Press.

Dr Robbins has, since his clinical work described herein, developed a fascinating new concept of the unconscious mind, described in a number of original works, particularly "The Primordial Mind in Health and Illness: A Cross-Cultural Perspective" (Robbins, 2011).

All aspects of this case study are entirely Dr Robbins' work. None of the case study material is connected in any way with Dr Gillian Steggles, Professor R D Hinshelwood or Dr Miomir Milovanovic. Dr Robbins and his publishers, The Guilford Press, retain all rights and copyright to this case study.

This case study is included herein by permission only to demonstrate how the PPCC model can permit visualization of, and a clear conceptual pathway for, successful treatment of schizophrenia using psychoanalytic psychotherapy, thus conclusively describing the process and illustrating sequentially the efficacy of the treatment.

Disclaimer: Dr Michael Robbins MD is in no way associated with the PPCC Theory, the PPCC structures or the PPCC model.

Abstract

The prevalent sociocultural belief about the psychoses and schizophrenia is that intensive psychoanalytic therapy is ineffective if not destructive and contraindicated, and that the treatment of choice is a combination of psychopharmacology and educational techniques designed to provide symptom relief and rehabilitation. The literature contains few detailed reports of successful intensive psychotherapy that might contradict these beliefs. The psychoanalytic psychotherapy of a woman I shall call Sara, who met DSM criteria for chronic paranoid schizophrenia, is presented in detail. Its success in bringing about a fundamental personality transformation from a seriously self-destructive state in which she was unable to care for herself to one in which she became a mature creative person is confirmed by a follow up two decades after termination. The therapy transpired over an eleven-year period and was conducted for the most part four times per week. It was supported by numerous hospitalizations in the early years as well as pharmacotherapy which she was able to relinquish prior to termination. During treatment Sara separated both physically and psychologically from an undifferentiated destructive relationship with her mother, internalized the capacity to think and represent emotions, and integrated disparate elements of personality to form a cohesive self. She developed psychosexually and formed a mature gender identity. She achieved the capacity for intimacy and motherhood, and had a successful career.

In this era of reductionist neuroscientific thinking the psychoses are believed to be chronic organic conditions like cancer or diabetes whose psychological manifestations are meaningless epiphenomena whose symptoms can be treated and course can be altered but which cannot be cured. Psychiatry has become more or less synonymous with neuroscience and psychopharmacology, in conjunction with brief hospitalizations and educational measures aimed at symptom relief and a modicum of social rehabilitation into the community. It is generally accepted that severely psychotic persons are and will always remain fundamentally different than the rest of us. The concept of psychotherapy if employed at all has become more or less synonymous with such interventions as giving common sense advice and life education and challenging major cognitive and perceptual abnormalities. The idea of working intensively with severely psychotic individuals and exploring in depth their thoughts, feelings, and relationships, with the goal of effecting major personality change has more or less disappeared and in some quarters (for example Torrey, 1983) are considered a destructive regressive practice.

Critics of the efficacy of intensive long term psychoanalytically informed psychotherapy of schizophrenia usually cite the absence of research findings demonstrating statistically significant change on measurable variables in an experimental population in relation to a control group. However, one might argue that a quantitative experimental model is not applicable to complex qualitative systems such as personality and relationship, and that the detailed single clinical case report is a uniquely useful model. Unfortunately, review of the literature reveals a remarkable dearth of detailed reports of entire treatments, start to finish, including follow-up. The reasons for this include, in addition to the aforementioned scepticism about the "scientific" validity of single case reports, issues of confidentiality and the difficulty of making and condensing years of detailed clinical notes into a finite readable credible document.

The need to maintain confidentiality is often invoked as a reason for not presenting detailed reports. While there is danger of identifying people without their permission, I believe it equally true that the issue of confidentiality may be employed as rationalization for not doing the difficult work of condensing and articulating detailed descriptions of what transpires during the course of a prolonged intensive relationship. While I have omitted specific identifying material in the report that follows I have changed very few facts, as I believe one well-intentioned distortion may unwittingly breed others. Protection is afforded by the fact that the work was done several decades ago. The patient had no extra-therapeutic contacts with persons likely to read this report either prior or subsequent to her treatment, and the other mental health personnel involved with her then are mostly gone, one way or another. Sara's permission to publish details of her treatment was obtained around the time her treatment terminated.

Case Report

About a year and a half prior to the preparation of this article I was unexpectedly contacted by Sara, a former patient whose work with me had concluded more than two decades previously. She was passing through the community where I practise and she wanted to say hello and tell me about her subsequent life. Our therapy lasted for more than eleven years. The treatment included intermittent hospitalizations at McLean Hospital where I was at the time a Senior Attending Psychiatrist, as well as intermittent and prolonged periods of time on phenothiazine medications. The report that follows is the condensation of detailed process notes I kept after each of the more than 1100 sessions.

Background

Relevant elements of Sara's history will be presented chronologically as I learned them in the course of our work together so I will only sketch broad outlines here. In addition to what I learned from Sara, history was also obtained from the social worker at the hospital who worked with her mother, and from the records of mother's hospitalization during Sara's prepubertal years which I had the unusual opportunity to peruse with her mother's permission.

Sara was the second of four children. She had two older brothers and a sister five years her junior. Her family was wealthy and aristocratic, and traced its roots back many generations. The family prided itself in equating strength and maturity with masculinity and suppression of emotion. Except for Sara's mother there was no family history of mental illness, but given what you will learn about the family's "ability" to deny blatant problems that information may not be accurate. Sara's mother had no career other than raising her children. She was an angry, depressed woman, intermittently suicidal and prone to fits of rage and bizarre behaviour, examples of which are elaborated in the pages to come. Mother had several brief mental hospitalizations in the years following Sara's birth, some following suicide attempts. Sara's father was senior partner in an international law firm and spent much of his time travelling. By accounts from Sara, and later other family members, he was emotionally unavailable to them and what attention he paid to his children was directed toward doing macho activities with his sons, whereas he left his daughters to fend for themselves. Father's insensitivity was manifest in many ways. For instance, Sara recalls his constructing an outdoor swing for the children hung over a large branch overlooking a steep slope that the neighbors would not permit their children to use because it was dangerous.

As a child Sara did her best to be inconspicuous and hide herself from her mother. She never let mother know when she was hurt or in need. She spent much of her time in the basement of her house, using dangerous tools without instruction or huddling next to the furnace for warmth. When Sara was nine her mother entered McLean hospital for a two-year stay that involved permanent disruption of the nuclear family. There she was diagnosed as a severe borderline personality. Following mother's hospitalization Sara developed magical ritualistic behavior, for example around the number eight, which she eventually told me represented breasts, and she began to hallucinate. Sara's father divorced Sara's mother after her hospitalization, and waged a successful legal battle to gain custody of Sara and her siblings. His attention to his career left him little time to devote to them, and he hired a series of caretakers. He remarried, to a neighbor, when Sara was twelve. When Sara was fourteen he developed a rapidly fatal illness. Sara was sent abruptly and without explanation to France to live with a male business associate, and only informed of his illness when she was summoned home for the funeral. Sara's stepmother was awarded custody, but by that time Sara had begun to run away from home frequently and they had infrequent contact.

Sara regularly ran away from home to skid row areas of cities where she would involve herself with men who abused her sexually in exchange for food and a place to sleep. At age fifteen she was arrested and placed in a youth detention center. From there she was transferred to a public mental hospital where she received phenothiazine medication and unsuccessful psychotherapy for six months until she was expelled for abusing drugs. Despite this chaos Sara managed to complete high school with high grades, and over the course of years punctuated by hospitalizations, to graduate from a good college.

Year One

Sara was twenty-eight when I met her. She was then a patient at a small private hospital in the Boston area, with which I was not affiliated, and to which she had been admitted after having been asked to take a leave of absence from graduate school. She had been told that a condition of her discharge was that she find a therapist. I do not know how she obtained my name, but a friend called to make an appointment for her as Sara was too terrified to call me herself. She was drab, overweight, dressed in baggy clothing and the general impression she conveyed was one of indeterminate gender. Her gaze was vacant, she had a flat whispery voice, made no eye contact, and her discourse was vague. Although she claimed to be nervous she gave little outward evidence. I learned from the hospital psychiatrist that she spent long periods of time huddled in corners, mute and rigid except for bizarre facial expressions, but all Sara told me was that her problem was inability to concentrate and lack of a sense of personal identity. As we talked she reported a sensation that the top of her head was lifting off and she said she was hearing voices that were harassing and frightening her. She said it was difficult to think clearly since thoughts would "short-circuit" and make strange connections so that she could not understand what others were saying or express herself sequentially. After four meetings Sara expressed a wish to work with me. Other than agreeing to my suggestion we meet three times per week we did not discuss much about therapy; in retrospect and in addition to the fact she had difficulty talking with me at all, I had the sense that doing so would be just so many meaningless words. Shortly thereafter she was discharged from the hospital, she stopped taking the medication she had been given there, and she obtained a menial job.

During our appointments Sara would sit near the door with her head averted, often with her coat on and purse clutched to her lap; and she often bolted out the door a few minutes early. Her posture was rigid and her gestures and facial expressions were contorted and contextually inappropriate. She was detached, her voice was flat, whispery, and without affect and she did not make eye contact. There were long silences sometimes punctuated with sotto voce mocking laughter or muttered curses or gibberish about shapes and patterns. She had auditory and visual hallucinations. She believed bombs were planted in the walls and planes and missiles were about to attack and kill her. Our sessions consisted of a curious triadic relationship among Sara, myself, and a Greek chorus of female voices that terrorized her as they instructed her how to cope with the dangerous world she was in and the horrible consequences that would ensue if she disobeyed them. "They" would require that she deprive herself of food and sleep, and undergo various punishments in order to avoid being killed. "They" developed an immediate mistrust and dislike for me and told her they would punish her if she got involved with me because I wanted to kill her. Her thoughts often short-circuited, her sentences fragmented so that they did not make sense. My subjective sense was one of helplessness and defeat, because "they" seemed to control "her" behavior and I was unable to talk to "them" directly. Variants of this behavior recurred, waxed, and waned throughout much of the time I knew her. Occasional astute observations she made and her large vocabulary led me to believe she was unusually intelligent.

Sara was a nocturnal creature. Her voices would not let her sleep. In the middle of the night she often drove her car long distances following big trucks. She frequented bars, pool halls, and gambling casinos and involved herself in the culture of darkness, warmth, drinking, drugs, loud noise, pimps, prostitution and abuse, sexual and otherwise. Remarkably, she never became pregnant. Her goal was to prove that no matter what was done to her it did not upset her emotionally; in that way she could believe she was in control and superior to those around her. Her self-destructiveness included depriving herself of sleep and food, smoking heavily, punishing herself, inducing accidents and injuries and then ignoring the pain and damage. Such activities punctuated our work for many years.

In her previous extensive contacts with psychiatrists she believed she had acted crazy because that was what was expected of her and she was contemptuous because she believed she was successful in fooling them. She soon became frustrated because she felt that unlike others, I gave her little clue about what I wanted from her. However, most of her attention seemed directed toward what "they", her voices, were telling her, and what she was "seeing", about the dangerous world she was in and how to deal with it, in the case of therapy, "telling" her not to relate to me at all.

After a time there appeared transient indications of a wish to relate to me including brief eye contact and flashes of feeling, consisting of deep sadness and insipient tears, and a rage including wishes to "scream bloody murder" and kill everyone. At such times her thoughts short-circuited and she sometimes bolted from the office.

In our fourteenth hour she recounted her first dream: there was a cylindrical eight storey building open inside and resembling a great family dining room, with tables and chairs floating around. One false move and one could take a dangerous fall. Her sister was dying. A clown began to entertain everyone and pushed her sister over the edge. At some point, probably subsequently, I learned that "eight" had longstanding significance representing breasts.

She missed an appointment and I learned that she had gone to Las Vegas and put herself in dangerous situations. She admitted to being angry and wanting to kill me because I had gotten her to like me despite the warning from her voices that I would kill her. Her test for whether she liked someone was whether she thought she could kill them with a gun; she acknowledged she would have trouble shooting me. She was afraid I might die, but if I did it would be a relief, for then she could go to a gambling establishment, lose all her savings, purchase a gun and kill herself. When she violated the commands of her voices that she was not to sleep more than four hours at night, "they" terrified her the following night with the belief that she had jumped from an airplane and her parachute would not open, and "they" regularly arranged punishments for her after any occasion in which she might be more open and communicative with me.

During the twenty-eighth hour I prescribed trifluoperazine. However, it seemed to have no discernable effect. After five months we had our first substantial separation when I took a summer vacation, and despite the fact I gave her a number where she could reach me she decided I was not coming back hence she stopped the medication. She made clear her reluctance to take it and I did not insist she renew the prescription.

There ensued the first of numerous interchanges that challenged my sanity. One day she informed me that she had never really hallucinated and the stories she had been telling me had been manifestations of her ability to fool and manipulate people, including "shrinks" for whom she had great contempt. She described how in the past she had played the roles of a heroin addict in withdrawal, a tough street person, a good girl, and a scholar. She seemed sincere and acted more mature and integrated. After a few sessions in which she was able to talk more directly about her struggle against feelings and dependency and there was no sign that she was hallucinating, I felt both pleased and deeply unsettled. How could I have been so gullible? I consulted informally with two colleagues in an effort to make some sense of what was happening but it did not allay my sense of helplessness and confusion.

She visited her mother, who, according to Sara never made enough food for all her children, and felt jealous of the attentions mother gave to her dog, but added that her mother was planning to have the dog euthanized. Her mother had casually inquired whether Sara had stopped therapy yet, expressing her assumption that, as in the past, Sara would find it valueless. Sara imagined kidnapping Julia Child and forcing her to cook lunch; she went so far as to call her but hung up when Julia answered.

But after eight months of therapy Sara became acutely paranoid. She wondered if the wiring was connected to explosives, if I had a gun in my drawer, and if I was about to strangle her. Between therapy hours she went to a bar, got drunk, and invited attack. In retrospect I believe her false-self state of "normalcy" was also based on paranoid thinking and the change simply made it more obvious. When she became so agitated that she paced my office and said she was going to escape to a distant city I arranged for her admission to McLean Hospital, where she remained on a locked ward for the next one and a half years.

Sara immediately barricaded herself in her hospital room. In terror that staff were trying to kill her she assaulted them, and in order to contain her they had to put her in seclusion and sometimes restraints. In the quiet room she would huddle in corners, grimace and make strange body movements, bang her head against the wall, twist and smash her hands violently, glance around the room apprehensively, and pick at her face. She experienced visual projections of disembodied fragmented floating parts, hallucinated voices either threatening her with terrifying scenarios or "protecting" her by commanding that she act in ways that were self-destructive in order to prevent terrible things from happening to her. When released from seclusion she managed to escape from the hospital several times and place herself in dangerous situations.

CASE STUDY 2

In the hospital Sara was diagnosed according to the then current DSM-III standards as a chronic paranoid schizophrenic. The ward staff consisted of the administrative psychiatrist who "ran" the ward and made decisions about medication, privileges, and restrictions and the like in consultation with myself and other staff; a social worker who met periodically with her mother and occasionally with Sara's siblings; and various staff nurses and occupational and rehabilitative personnel. I met with Sara in an office on the ward when necessary, in my private office in the hospital when possible, and when she needed additional external control and was placed in the quiet room I joined her there for our sessions. I attended ward rounds where staff discussed Sara on at least a weekly basis. And every several months there was a formal review and planning conference about Sara that included a senior consultant from outside the ward.

Shortly after her admission I increased the frequency of our sessions from three to four per week, a frequency we maintained until near the conclusion of our work together. Sara remembered feigning sleep as a child so her father would carry her to bed, as she knew he would not do so if she asked. She told me how she often drove off in her car in the middle of the night and followed big trucks for hundreds of miles, so as not to feel lonely. Despite her paranoid terror of me and the admonitions of her voices she admitted that she was "getting a few crumbs". Between meetings she wrote me a remarkable letter. "I really think I am alive, and if I think about it I get so sad and I get really angry. When I sit in the room with you and I let myself believe you are there I feel so safe I just want to sit there forever. But I can't seem to be able to believe it for very long afterwards. I had no idea what I was getting into by entering therapy and I'm scared and I do hate you, but I also wish I could be with you every minute." Over the ensuing weekend Sara briefly escaped from the hospital in near zero temperature without a coat.

Sara told me that her family refused to believe she had problems that justified her being in the hospital. The social worker who met with her mother and other family members corroborated her impression and told me her mother had almost succeeded in convincing her Sara was only pretending to be ill. As Sara began to show more neediness and emotion on the ward some of the staff began to believe that her therapy was making her sicker. After one of her brothers raised questions about her need for hospitalization Sara wrote to her family:

> I am not dependent on the hospital, in fact I have trouble even asking staff for a towel or for change. I have been operating under

the delusion that I am very confident in taking care of myself and trying to persuade everyone as well as me that this is the case, but it is not. Hanging out on skid row, getting beaten up, putting myself in very dangerous situations wandering around the streets of the big city in the middle of the night totally paranoid, in my apartment all day in what my therapist calls psychotic terror, alone and pretty nuts. My ability to come off as rational, functioning, jobs, school, talk to people, etc. is an integral part of the craziness. When I sit with another person I focus on them entirely, try to figure them out and organize my own self around information I can pick up. It could be described as [S]aran[TM] wrap, weak ego boundaries. The day I arrived in the hospital I thought the staff was going to kill me. I ended up in four-point restraints flat on the mattress with my arms and legs strapped down. I am struggling for my life here because I have gotten crazier as the years go by. I am fighting myself, the part that hates the whole god damn world and doesn't want anything to do with anyone, that part is supported by my saying shit like "I hate Dr Robbins", and I tell myself to get the hell out of the hospital. Part of the treatment is forming a real human relationship with him, telling him I hate him for exposing me to all the rage, sadness, feelings, and that I like him. I have to practice asking for things and saying no to people. I need a safe place to take risks.

This lucid, insightful letter about her capacity to be fraudulent was, of course, another example of the very fraudulence, as subsequent events show how little of what she wrote she really meant.

Year Two

Preceding a short separation Sara became more detached and I commented that she was trying to leave before I did. That night she escaped from the hospital into a cold rainy night. She returned for our final meeting before my absence and I pointed out that she was creating a world of rejection, misery, and abuse and trying to believe that she could control it by not acknowledging how much it disturbed her. On my return she remarked to me sheepishly, "I'm addicted to you; a Robbins addict." It was a cold and wintry day and shortly after telling me of her wish that I would surround her, she said she had an urge to go out into the woods and lie in the snow where she was convinced it would feel warm and secure. I wondered if she was trying to make me feel responsible for the distress she felt when I was gone, and her laughter confirmed the accuracy of my speculation. She told me how as a child she spent much time in the basement of her house, hiding from her mother, snuggling up to the furnace for warmth, and how she taught herself to use dangerous power tools without any sense of fear even though on more than one occasion she had come close to electrocuting herself. Then she remarked that she had been using power tools in the hospital shop and had told the supervisor that she was frightened. She was stunned when he responded that he was glad to hear it, and if she were not afraid he would no longer allow her to use the tools. As she seemed to regain some control she was allowed to visit me in my office in Cambridge. However she immediately became terrified of me and of her voices and said she wanted to split my skull with an axe. She talked of her wish for a womblike world where it would not matter what she thought because I would take care of everything.

We resumed meeting in the hospital where she seemed almost catatonic. I talked with her about how her delusions and hallucinations were reflections of her own mental state of fear and rage but this confused her and made her hate and fear me and wonder if I was driving her crazy. She gave me a self-portrait. In addition to revealing her considerable artistic ability, what was striking was that it looked like an aerial view of a landscape consisting of geometric plots, each filled with busy designs and a large empty space in the middle. She was aware of urges to do violence to me, and her paranoid-determined violent behavior on the ward led to her spending much time in restraints and seclusion. Her trifluoperazine dosage was gradually increased and when there was no discernible improvement chlorpromazine was added. Because she was convinced that the staff had gone crazy and attacked her I asked a staff nurse to join a session. Sara was confused when told that her assaultive, destructive behavior could evoke powerful responses from others, because her family "normally" seemed unaware of her presence. For the first time she felt rage at her family for their failure to appreciate her needs and she began to raise objections when her mother and brother ridiculed psychiatrists and mental hospitals and said she had no need to be in a mental hospital, but she also expressed rage at me for making her know this.

Remarkably, considering her out-of-control states, Sara's capacity to seem rational and logical proved very effective, convincing hospital staff that she was normal and simply feigning illness, and that it was me and my "therapy" that was driving her crazy. Her family was insistent about this to the social worker, who vacillated in her own belief. Over the course of the second year on several occasions the ward psychiatrist and staff raised serious questions about whether therapy was harming her and whether I should stop seeing her. The staff acted out their belief in various ways including waiting for two days after Sara escaped from the hospital before notifying me. At the same time because of her repeated paranoid destructive episodes her medication dosage was increased. There were several formal conferences during these months and fortunately for Sara and our work the outside consultant repeatedly and strongly supported her therapy.

Sara was beginning to note the passage of time in relation to the rhythm of our appointments. She worried about my forthcoming summer vacation. She recalled how her father abruptly sent her to live with an acquaintance in France without explaining that he was dying. She was contemptuous of my "weakness" for continuing to care about her. But she admitted having feelings of caring about me and when I asked her what they were she pointed mutely to her heart. She was able to acknowledge that the hospital was her home for now and decided to keep a diary when I was away.

When I left she escaped and bought a plane ticket to France but she changed her mind and returned to the hospital where she involved herself with a male patient who was known for his violent behaviour. She wrote,

> I am really lost; I am 1,000,000 miles away and I don't know where that is. I have all these fantasies about taking off with him, staying stoned, drunk, getting pimped out, beaten up. I want to cry and scream and hit people and I am so angry. You know I am really smart. I am creative and imaginative. I could've done a hell of a lot with myself, and here I am coming up on thirty and I am sitting in a nut house kissing a fucking psychopath. I am so angry at you. I want to scream, tear the room apart.

When I returned home from my summer vacation Sara said that she was enraged that I had left her but that it had not been safe for her to leave me until I returned. She then lost control and when restrained and placed in the quiet room she giggled, hallucinated, and banged her head against the wall. Yet again I experienced a sense of helplessness and hopelessness similar to what she seemed to feel about relating to another person. I believe that a critical therapeutic element in her treatment was my willingness to experience the kinds of confusion about reality and helplessness and hopelessness she seemed to feel without rejecting her and running away.

The administrative psychiatrist increased her dose of chlorpromazine again. Sara learned that the staff had serious doubts about her therapy and that our relationship might be in jeopardy. She was very distressed and correctly surmised that she was setting others up to enact her hatred and her confusion of sanity and craziness, the part of herself she now associated with the attitudes of her parents. Sara tried to talk to her mother about her feelings of having been neglected, and she told me that in response her mother became enraged, called Sara a bitch, threw an ashtray against the wall, and resisted efforts of staff to calm her. Our responses to her story were curiously congruent; I wondered if Sara had imagined all this (that her mother was actually normal) and Sara herself did not find anything unremarkable about her description of her mother's behavior. Interestingly, her mother's crazy behavior was subsequently confirmed in its particulars by a staff member who had been present. Thus commenced a series of visits between Sara and her mother in the presence of the social worker, after which Sara regularly expected the social worker to conclude that her mother's behavior was unremarkable and was amazed to discover that the social worker was impressed by her mother's caged pacing around the room during their interviews and her threats to leave. This led to Sara's recollection of an incident from early childhood when her mother, in a rage, had literally thrown Sara and her siblings around the room. After telling me this Sara experienced herself fragmented in pieces sitting in several different areas of the room, one part running away from me, and another feeling attached to me and sitting near me as protection against her mother.

We had another review conference in which the nursing staff voiced their near unanimous belief that therapy was not working and that my treatment was making Sara regress, but the consultant supported continued hospitalization and therapy. When Sara escaped from the hospital I was not notified by the staff although it was customary hospital procedure, and first learned about it more than a day later when I found a message from her on my answering machine telling me she had "split" and assuring me she was safe and would return. Sara had gone to Las Vegas but resisted the prompting of her hallucinations to walk the streets late at night. She had also resisted calling me for fear it would make her have feelings and hence "fall apart". On return she talked of her urge to "split" again and we realized that splitting really meant cutting herself off from her feelings. When she observed herself hallucinating she asked the staff to put her in the quiet room where she felt safe. Sara was genuinely confused about whether medication was making her better or as she put it "driving her crazy", and she was aware of a belief that her food was being poisoned. I regularly questioned my own sanity and often I did not know what to believe.

Sadness, anger and related childhood memories began to surface more regularly and Sara looked forward to her hours with me and reported a feeling of security she claimed was entirely novel in her life. Yet she told me she was much more comfortable relating to an assaultive patient on the ward. I responded that while she longed for caring, the only treatment she seemed able to tolerate was a reflection of her own hateful uncaring attitudes. Her condition improved and she was allowed to leave the hospital and come to my private office for therapy appointments. She adopted a motherly role toward an adolescent female patient who repeatedly ran away and got herself into destructive predicaments. It was around this time that her mature sense of identity began to emerge.

But yet again she became paranoid and assaultive, and fought off all efforts to help her. Her privileges to leave the hospital were curtailed, and she required restraint and seclusion in the quiet room. Then she was able to talk about her rageful fantasies of ripping herself apart and blowing up the hospital and me. She felt her head swelling and occupying all corners of the room.

I was impressed that she did not seem to be attending to anything I said but she laughed and tried to convince me that my perceptions were not accurate. I suggested she might tape-record her sessions to help her determine who is accurate (Robbins, 1988) and she agreed to do so. Sara was responsible for the taping and the tapes were in her possession to use as she chose. Once again I had to deal with my helplessness and uncertainty about what use she might make of the recordings. However she soon informed me that she was learning how little she actually listened to me. She told me this was the first experience in her life of a caring relationship with another person in which her needs were satisfied and the realization made her depressed and enraged. Caring was a chink in her armor and a threat to her "independence". She remembered an incident in which her mother had taken her and her siblings sailing and threw them in the ocean in order to teach them not to be frightened and prove to herself that she could rescue them if need be. Soon afterward Sara again escaped from the hospital, went to a bar, got drunk, and had casual sex. When she literally tried to tear her face off she was put back in restraints. There she told me "you can only destroy what you have".

Year Three

Sara was again confined to the quiet room because she had begun to tear at the skin on her face in an admitted effort to tear her face off. I shared with her my feelings of helplessness and distress and we both marvelled at the power of her hatred. She regained some self-control and became very sad as she realized her drive to destroy what was important to her. She realized that she was trying to drive me crazy. Paranoid terrors that her mother would kill her, and episodes when she shouted at the ward staff and had urges to blow up the world, were followed by memories of having been attacked by her mother as a child.

Sara gradually regained more consistent self-control and discharge planning began. She began to drive to her therapy appointments at my office which was now in my home some distance from the hospital grounds. When her car would not start after an appointment she frantically pushed it away from my house and down a nearby hill and almost into a main street full of rush-hour traffic, so terrified was she that I might notice her predicament and she might have to ask for help.

After twenty-six months and 355 hours of therapy and one and a half years of hospitalization Sara moved to a halfway house. She realized the hospital had become a kind of home and family to her. In the new setting she felt her mother was omnipresent in other women, and she sensed there was a lion outside her bedroom at night and a presence hiding behind my office plants.

She anticipated my summer vacation with terror and articulated her fear that I was abandoning her to the clutches of a crazy woman. We agreed that the woman was no longer her mother but part of herself. She realized how unaware she tended to be of injury, illness, fatigue, hunger, and sexual feelings and for the first time was frighteningly aware that her self-protective instincts were deficient and that the things that upset most people did not bother her. I added that the feelings that signified home to most people, such as intimacy, terrified her. Finally Sara concluded that she might need to return to the hospital while I was gone, and immediately she felt better. She said she loved me and she gave me a gift of a lovely ceramic car she had made, which she called her "getaway" car. She remembered having swum much too far out in the ocean until she was no longer certain she could get back, only to realize that the prospect of trying to return was so terrifying she did not want to try. Turning off her feelings was a form of triumph; it meant no-one could hurt her. Episodes of caring, work, and insight were small oases in a desert of paranoid detachment and lengthy silence and I found myself responding with sleepiness and boredom to the rhythmic alternation. When she noticed this, Sara articulated wishes to tease and torture me and put me in a dark place so that I would feel trapped and alone, give up hope as she had done, detach myself from my body and feelings and go crazy. She was relieved next hour to find I was still intact.

These ideas alternated with memories of having such things done to her, first by mother, then brother, and ultimately some of the sadistic men she had apprenticed herself to.

When we separated for my month-long vacation Sara re-entered the hospital as planned, but she quickly realized she no longer knew anyone there. She escaped and went to London where in fact she knew no-one, but she called to reassure me that she was well and taking care of herself, and she sent me a card from Freud's house.

She was pleased to see me on my return and seemed positive about our relationship and aware of her problems with self-care but her characteristic paranoid withdrawal and muteness followed, with regular interpretation of my countertransference drowsiness and detachment in terms of her wishes to drive me crazy as had been done to her. When a destructive act was committed at the halfway house, although the perpetrator was known, Sara was almost convinced she had done it. It seemed that we were immobilized in the throes of a mutual struggle between on the one hand gaining sanity in her case and retaining it in mine, and on the other hand a powerful pull toward a state of hopelessness and resignation to losing our minds. I told her I was thinking about recommending re-hospitalization and to my surprise she cried, felt closer to me. She construed my setting limits on her as the actions of a good parent. She felt pleasure when a policeman stopped her for speeding. She dreamed chickens had escaped the coop and a racoon was about to kill them. She recalled unsuccessfully concealing from her mother the fact that she had cut her finger rather badly. When they arrived at the hospital the doctor wanted to suture the wound but her mother objected and would not permit it. She told me that her mother never made enough food for her and forced her to eat things she did not want, and associated to how she performed fellatio on abusive men in the belief that she was controlling them.

In the fall Sara began constructive planning and returned to graduate school. But once again she pulled the rug of sanity and reality out from under me. She said, very convincingly, that she was upset because she had been untruthful with me and that she really did not hallucinate, and the stories of abuse and skid row were fabrications. She said when she was in London and had wanted attention and sympathy she went to a restaurant and convinced the waiter that she was a bereaved widow revisiting the scene of her marriage. I felt shocked and a bit sick to my stomach and I wondered aloud whether I could trust my senses about what was real. Sara tried to convince me that she was telling me these "truths" because our relationship was deepening and she cared, but I felt suspicious, a bit paranoid as I struggled with what was real. Fortunately I observed and I pointed out that she was sitting in the farthest corner of the room and showing no emotion. In response she reported that the room was becoming animated in sinister and threatening ways and she feared that I was going crazy.

She told me life was becoming meaningful to her, that she was taking better care of herself and she expressed gratitude. She had felt pain immediately when she jabbed her hand on a nail head. For the first time in her life she took a stuffed animal to bed with her. She attended a family dinner and recounted that her mother had called her granddaughter hysterical when she fell downstairs and cried, and called her daughter-in-law overprotective for comforting her.

She asked her mother for permission to see her mother's hospital records and to talk with her former therapist so she might find out what had really happened to her as a child. To her surprise her mother agreed. But her mother did not follow through. After dreaming she was in a world of seductive vampires and had to decide whether to swallow a concoction and become like them Sara again asked her mother. This time her mother got angry and accused Sara of trying to persecute her. Sara began to express rage at her mother and a wish to kill or drive her crazy but her talk was punctuated by disruptions, self-derision, and the sensation of choking and suffocating. She wrote me a letter that included: "I hate the whole fucking world. Not only does my head get splintered up but the room goes to pieces and words get blasted into meaningless letters. So the four walls of the room no longer join and I don't feel safe here. Everything gets unglued. I get so angry I just want to blow up the world. Where the hell are you?" She seemed more aware of how identical her own attitudes and behaviors were to those of her mother and how unreliable and inconsistent both of them were.

Sara then revealed that she did not believe her mother had been in a mental hospital or had been mentally ill and she subscribed to the family belief that her mother had been hospitalized for a physical problem. Nonetheless I received detailed records of her mother's hospitalization along with her permission to share what I thought appropriate. Sara wondered whether they contained information about whether her mother cared about her. After reading the notes I responded that there was little concern about her marriage or her children. Sara told me she was chopping up her thoughts and physically choking back massive rage and that she might kill me. When Sara reported delusions of a terrifying woman in the doorway of her room at night I read her a nursing report that mentioned her mother's abusiveness, threats of violence and suicide, running away, periods of disorientation and immobility lasting for hours, and her mother's terrifying hallucinations of a persecutory old woman. We realized how similar she and her mother were and how much she had been invested in her efforts to control mother's behavior by invisibility and compliance.

Year Four

For the first time she shared fantasies of having a home and a husband of her own but then she withdrew, told me that she was crazy and that there was a bomb bursting in her head. Around the time of Sara's birthday Sara struggled with feelings of homelessness and wishes to be my little child on the one hand, and terror of me because I looked crazy, associated with the urge to speed, get picked up by the police, attack them and get killed. Eventually, she sought help from the staff at the halfway house and was briefly and constructively re-hospitalized. She said "if I'm going to feel all this stuff then I want to have people around all the time to share it with".

After a conversation in which her mother told her how hard she had tried to select a birthday gift for her that Sara would not interpret as a rejection, Sara came away with a more balanced view of a mother who was making an effort. She went to a family gathering at her mother's house and told one of her brothers how important he was to her and how angry she was at some of the ways he treated her. He became angry, withdrew, and uttered a mocking laugh she was very familiar with. To Sara's surprise her mother empathized with her and attempted to stop the quarrel.

When she talked about how the barroom atmosphere of darkness, drunkenness, and abuse was a "home" of deadness where she felt no-one could touch her I asked her to agree not to go to a bar again. She did so reluctantly and was overwhelmed with feelings of homelessness and rage. Sara moved out of the halfway house and into a house she rented jointly with several women. At night when she began to be terrified and paranoid she hugged her stuffed animal.

My summer vacation approached. After another episode of rage and fantasies of bombing and destroying the entire East Coast Sara laughed and told me that she had fooled me yet again, this time into believing that we were getting closer. When she observed my drowsiness in response to her detached silence she vehemently asserted that it was because she didn't want me near her. Seemingly oblivious to what she was doing she tracked mud over my office rug with dirty sneakers. She wished to go to a foreign country where she did not speak the language so there could be no communication. I commented that that country was called the land of backward schizophrenia.

Nonetheless she managed our separation well, obtained a job as a preschool teacher's aide and undertook more course work. Her teaching experience exposed her to scenarios of infants crying for their mothers and mothers claiming them. She felt overwhelming sadness and rage, associated her feelings to my vacation and voiced confusion about whether she was a small child and I had in fact abandoned her. She reported that at the end of the previous hour she had stood outside the office door wanting to knock and tell me she needed a hug for security. Instead she went to a bar and got drunk. The theme was that of an abandoned child who feels so overwhelmed with pain that eventually she no longer wants anyone to come and make her aware of it.

After another period of paranoid detachment she remarked that going crazy was a terrible price to pay for not being able to say no to her mother, and the nature of the current conflict emerged. Her mother had recently had surgery, and Sara had been driving her mother to the hospital for her treatments. She recalled a childhood incident where she had hidden from her mother but her mother had found her, hit her, and told her that if she saw her again she would cook her in the oven and eat her for dinner. She was able to tell her mother that she could not see her in the foreseeable future and her mother was surprisingly accepting, This too enraged Sara, for she felt that it came much too late and she had no forgiveness in her heart, only hatred.

She began to keep a diary between sessions in the form of letters to me. She wrote:

> *I would like to kill a lot of people and they don't know it but really I don't want to kill you. I wish I could give you a big hug and tell you how I feel, that I am so lonely and tired and so scared and I can't sleep. I know it won't be you that kills me, it is my feelings that I think will kill me; feeling good, safe, loving you, wanting to hug you and never leave. I think of you sitting in your chair and I feel warm inside and safe and so sad I can hardly bear it, like I could cry forever.*

She told me about the summer that she was sent abroad when her father was dying and she remembered visiting an old baker to whom she became very attached. He had an endearing pet name for her and she recalled wishing that he would adopt her. I had a familiar sense of surprise and disorientation learning of this hitherto unmentioned oasis of caring in her life. But the very next hour Sara informed me that she had listened to her tape-recording and realized that what she told me was what she had wanted to believe whereas in fact she had only run errands for the baker. She described her terrifying mother, tall and wiry, "wired up" all the time. I recalled some of her delusional preoccupations with electricity and some of the near serious mishaps she had experienced when she did electrical wiring; she laughed and related this to her wish and fear to hold on, adding "if the voltage is high and you hold on with both hands the current will go through your heart and kill you".

She learned mother was planning to move to another state. Sara rapidly oscillated between pleasure in seeing me and wishes to hug me and wishes to hit me which were associated with reflexive fist clenching and demonstrations of her right cross. She said "The biggest mistake I ever made was to start seeing you." She literally made fists at me, which meant "touch me emotionally and I'll clobber you". She started to pick up a small statue and throw it at me and when I moved it away from her she became confused; for a time she could not "locate" her anger.

When her mother moved, Sara felt sad and alone. She had derived a perverse sense of security and predictability from being able to anticipate and cope with her mother's disturbances by being invisible, elusive, and inconsistent, and now she felt exposed and vulnerable and did not know how to be in a situation that required direct emotional expression and assertion.

She decided she needed to talk to me about sex since she wanted to have children of her own, and she was beginning to show some interest in men. She remembered the experiences she had when she performed fellatio, and how she transformed her feelings of helplessness and the wish to vomit, to hit, and to bite off the penis, into a sense of mastery and control in which she felt superior, in control, and belittling of the man for being so insanely excited. I suggested that real control was based in consistency, knowledge of her emotions, and selective action based on that knowledge. She responded that for the first time in her life she felt listened to and attended to, and she realized that the more she accepted her upset feelings the less she hallucinated, and she was sleeping better at night.

Year Five

Another birthday approached. Sara imagined that I came over to her and removed a tiny baby from within her and nurtured it. She recalled that her mother was unable to remember any of the children's birthdays. I gave her a birthday card and wrote "We all deserve the opportunity to be special to someone. I hope you won't let the misfortunes of your past imprison you so that you won't have yours." Her response was a fragmented combination of tense laughter, sadness, anger, and flat words of thanks. I had upset her expectation that I would not remember.

She began to envision a future and for the first time feel hopeful. She was doing very well at school and would become a full-fledged teacher the following year. But she fought with me over everything, remained withdrawn, and would allow a bit of contact only just before the end of an hour. We began to wonder whether the best she could do was to be like a squirrel that gets its nut and then runs. She reported a nightmare in which she was with a former patient who was wheelchair bound, her hands and feet amputated, and Sara was hugging her and trying to estimate just how much she was capable of learning to do. We talked about her chronically hunched over position in the office which was an effort to deny the existence of her body and sexuality. She was literally unable to sit back. When she tried she felt dizzy and nauseated with powerful sensation of terror that she would be attacked, ripped apart, and annihilated. She told me this is why she had never felt safe enough to wear a skirt.

She received her master's degree and at graduation fellow students and teachers expressed caring for her and described her as gifted and creative. She told me that for the first time in her life she felt optimistic and excited and had even purchased a dress to wear to a job interview. She was certain she now had enough control so that she would not become psychotic during the upcoming summer separation. At the conclusion of the last hour she shook my hand, expressed her gratitude to me for having "put up" with her and said she would miss me. I remarked that she had had to put up with me as well and that it hadn't been easy and with a brief burst of sadistic laughter she departed.

When we resumed she had begun a full-time teaching position. She dreamed she was observing a person of indeterminate gender who was wearing a plastic raincoat and who set her or himself on fire. No-one paid attention. The victim was amazed to find out that he or she had not died but the coat had melted into the person's body. After this she recalled a childhood incident when her mother's sailboat tipped over, throwing her into the water with the sail on top of her. Because she had followed her mother's instructions and had worn a life preserver she was trapped beneath the sail and could not get out.

Sara was less rigid physically and emotionally, and more spontaneous. She was more sensitive to temperature and pain. She sat a bit closer to me in the room, spontaneously clapped her hands when she said something, and wanted to examine an object of interest in my office. At times she sat back and relaxed, and once yelled in an angry voice, "fuck you". These gestures and expressions of emotion terrified her. She feared she would be attacked but she realized it was she who had been attacking everything both of us did or said.

For the first time she began to worry about real problems in her life like finding a caring husband rather than about her hallucinations and delusions. She realized that she wanted to have children and that there were now men she liked and she would be forced to talk to me about sex if she wanted a man in her life. We concluded that this idea was a concrete reflection of her belief that in order to get any semblance of attention or affection she was forced to perform oral sex. She perceived me as a crazy man, out of control of my sexuality and sadism, and she concluded I had been trying to disrupt our relationship by prematurely forcing the subject of sex on her. Nonetheless she took the unprecedented step of telling her oldest and perhaps only male friend that she cared about him. He responded that he did not reciprocate her feelings. She fled to a pool hall where she proceeded to take out her pool stick and defeat every man who would play with her.

Despite her concern that I would not want her to do it, Sara planned a holiday trip abroad with a friend. She gave me a small gift before leaving and shook my hand, demonstrating a violent oscillation I now associated with alternating holding on and breaking off. At the beginning of our separation Sara had the first dream that she could recall in which I figured, which she told me on her return. She was in my office and there was a big window against which lay a monstrous dead whale. It seemed normal to her that it be there, until my teenage daughter came along and Sara asked her what the whale looked like from outside the window. Sara saw me approach from another building and feared I would get angry at my daughter for talking to her. She related the dream to her deadness identity and to a childhood memory of seeing people pick apart a dead whale that washed up on the beach. "Dead whale" became an important therapy metaphor for the state of being she continued to strive to achieve.

Year Six

Sara uncharacteristically showed emotional upset at a family dinner and when she tried to leave, one of her brothers followed her. She burst into tears as they shared their mutual mistrust of others and the belief that the ability to be detached and unfeeling represented control, and her brother hugged her. Sara angrily blamed me for this. Soon thereafter she reported a nightmare in which she had entrusted the care of her students to someone else and went off and forgot their existence. When she remembered and returned it was evident that something terrible had happened to one of the students. I told Sara that I knew what had happened, that it had been unbearable for the student to be left alone so she had gotten herself beaten into unconsciousness. I commented that Sara had to make a choice between the mother of caring and attention to thoughts and feelings and the mother of rage, destruction of her mind, and deadness.

When her first teaching year ended, students, their parents, and faculty expressed praise and gratitude to her. Once again our relationship seemed stalemated and when our summer vacation separation approached she wrote me a letter:

You shouldn't bother with me and should take a painkiller and sleep. You know I do hear you and I feel I am being attacked because it is not too pleasant what you're saying. I just want to tell you to go to hell and take your damn caring with you because I want to blast everyone to hell especially someone who cares. It is becoming clear what I want and what I don't want and I didn't get and that clarity makes me so angry it scares the hell out of me.

She then dreamed that someone killed her brother, cooked his appendix and gave it to her to eat as though this were normal. In the dream she was terribly upset, screamed, and then awoke. It turned out that the brother image represented things she liked and valued in her life, whereas her cannibalism represented the killing of caring. As my summer vacation approached Sara reproached me for leaving, saying "look who you're leaving me with!"

When we met in the fall Sara told me how constructive her month had been. She had purchased a house of her own in a safe neighborhood, was being assertive and creative at work, and had maintained a sense of me within her that helped her make good decisions. As usual there was another side. She began to miss appointments and then reported a dream in which she had spilled coffee on the lovely dining table she had purchased for her home, and in order to avoid awareness of the contrast between the marred area and the rest of the tabletop she had hacked it to pieces.

Sara told me she was afraid she might wear two mismatched shoes to a forthcoming parents' meeting, and she realized this represented how little dialogue there was between the caring and hating parts of herself. I suggested that she try to find names for each one and that she sit in different chairs in the office when talking from each position. She called the two parts "black" and "red" and over the next five weeks we elaborated the characteristics of each. Ms Black turned away from me and muttered curses. When expressing Ms Red she told me that Ms Black was thoughtless, ignorant, rigid, hateful and destructive, and possessed a vocabulary limited to name-calling. She began to panic and said that I did not understand that she would punish herself for this conversation once she got herself alone.

She reported a nightmare: her house was burning down, she walked down a dark, empty street with burns on her feet, but she did not seem to care. She told me how she had burned some food and burned her hands removing it from the oven and she twisted her fingers violently. At the same time she began to express horror at the Ms Black part of herself, calling it mean and "Neanderthal". But she felt frightened and told me that her mind was exploding and her thoughts were flying apart, and she was barely able to speak.

When Sara told me how she had cared for two children at school who had been injured I contrasted her capacity to care with her refusal to take care of herself. She responded by telling me how she was walking around with a hole in her shoe, that she habitually drove without a seatbelt, that she allowed her house to remain a mess, did not allow herself sleep, and physically tortured her hands so badly when expressing her caring for me that she worried that she might break her fingers. After sharing her impulse to travel to a nearby city where the news media reported a mass murderer had been killing women Sara reported a nightmare. She had cancer and was being her own doctor. She took slices of herself and put them in the oven to incubate, and they grew to be monstrous, black, gross, and disgusting. She said "if I lock up this Neanderthal part then I will have lost the only part that has ever taken care of me and I will feel intolerably alone".

We began to talk about her broken heart and she remembered sitting immobilized after her mother was hospitalized. In our last hour before a separation she admonished me to take care of myself so that nothing would happen to me and she would not be heartbroken. I responded that she needed to take care of herself which meant bearing her feelings. She struggled against the urge to cry. She imagined having me sit next to her and put my arm around her so that she would feel secure and might be able to fall asleep. But she panicked until she realized that it was because her image of me had changed into that of her mother, with long fingernails, ready to strangle her.

Year Seven

After reiterating her belief that she had to perform oral sex in order to have a relationship, Sara realized that it was after her mother's hospitalization that she began to run away and got men to abuse her and force her to do that even though it made her choke and want to vomit. She began to cry. She knew she had been breast fed and began to wonder what it had been like. She became terrified of me.

On Sara's birthday, our 998th hour, I gave her another card on which I wrote: "I am sorry I can't be the loving mother you never had. And I can't take away your memories and feelings about never having had one. But I would like to help you put these things where they belong so that you can get some love in the future." Sara clutched it for the entire hour, interrupted at times by the feeling that her mother was about to take it from her, and at other times by her own wish to get away. She told me that she had kept on her person for half a year the other card I had given her. At the conclusion of this hour she said, quite unaware, "I'm going to take care of myself even if it kills me!"

After another deadening stalemate I remarked somewhat facetiously that I needed a consultation from her. Little did I know I was mobilizing her ability to write, think, reflect, and be artistically creative, presaging some of her later accomplishments. In response she began to bring me a series of documents, beautifully illustrated as though they were children's stories, with the theme that holding onto her mother was a barrier between us and that she needed to face her rage and tears over having had no mother. She wrote about how she had been destroying her life and our relationship, adding: "I don't want to spend my life doing a Woody Allen impersonation. The pendulum has been swinging for thirty-five years, without any joy, love, sadness, company. I want more with you and I want the rest of my life also. I want lots of things but the minute you show up I don't want anything but to drive you nuts and run." There followed a section written in red ink to indicate the thoughts of Ms Red which concluded with: "so I waste my time getting revenge on you who has never hurt me in any way and in reality getting revenge on myself, carrying out my mother's misdirected revenge on me". After a sentence in black starting with "this is a bunch of bullshit" she concluded in red that she was taking courses with me, "feelings 101" and "elementary language".

Year Eight

Preceding my summer vacation the stalemate between the two sides of Sara intensified along with her anger at me no matter what I did, and I struggled during her hours with the urge to lose consciousness and fall asleep. Sara commented that she wanted me to experience what had been forced on her: a terrified state of helplessness, hopelessness, futility and paralysis. Then she spontaneously decided to tell me a story. It was about a little donkey and his caring mother. The mother was shot by a bad boy, leaving the little donkey all alone, staring into the mud and rain. I commented that this was a story about heartbreak and the end of the world. There ensued more self-destructive behaviors and grisly fantasies and we realized that the "crazy" part of herself not only did not think but had no words. She began to use words more to describe this part and I felt relief, and told her that when she put it into words and talked about it I felt less crazy because her words made sense in relation to my experience of her.

During our summer separation she enrolled in a program abroad and when we resumed in the fall she was tanned, well dressed, and had lost weight. She talked enthusiastically about her adventures, new relationships, and the future.

She was distressed that she had a dream in which I appeared because it indicated my importance. We were sleeping in separate sleeping bags, entirely zipped up, on a beach on the northern coast. We had been there a long time, there was water and a line of seaweed over much of us, and she was half awake. This clear illustration of our relationship was most troubling to Sara; our disengagement, the deadness, and endlessness. She admitted that she missed me and had pretended the teddy bear she now used for comfort represented me, but then she called herself a "stupid jerk".

She said with regret that despite her love of children she would probably never be able to have any of her own because she was now in her mid-thirties. I likened the way she led her life to how she customarily waited until the end of therapy hours to get anything from our relationship and wondered if she might be inventing a new form of self-punishment by making herself wait until it was too late in life to get what she wanted. As she struggled over her heartbroken childlike longing to cry, be comforted and fall asleep, she tried to cover herself with the blanket on my couch but her striking motor inability to hold it enacted her difficulty holding onto caring feelings. Sara told me she had gotten drunk and had slept with a "loser" who lived in her neighborhood for some time. She began to hallucinate cursing commentary on her relationship with me; she told me that over the holiday she had felt rejected and excluded from my family. I suggested and she agreed that she resume trifluoperazine. For perhaps the first time she allowed medication to help her and to think and talk about what was happening. Almost immediately her hallucinations diminished and she became calmer and better able to sleep, to focus attention and concentrate and organize her life. She recalled her struggles in the hospital to fight off the effects of medication and felt terrified that she was allowing someone to get into her mouth and influence her. She tried to sit closer to me and had a fantasy of being dragged back into the corner by her hair. I encouraged her to identify the parts of herself by moving from one chair to another again. In the "black" chair she talked about her contempt for human beings, relationships, and her own wellbeing. In the "red" chair she told me she had made a new female friend, had joined a health club, and was expressing anger more appropriately when people mistreated her. At the end of this hour she reported "a splitting headache".

Disturbing memories of performing fellatio made her consider whether this had been a repetition of her breast-feeding experiences. She talked about being force fed and having to pretend that she enjoyed it while experiencing sensations of suffocation, gagging, and wishes to bite. She remembered it was after her mother was hospitalized that she began to run away and engage in the enslavement relationships that involved sucking the penis to ejaculation. She had a sudden urge to suck her thumb. She dreamed she and her brother were attempting to escape from her home of origin through an underground garage but their mother came along in the car and flattened them. In another dream she came to my house for an appointment but there was a party and she could find no place to park. She dreamed of travelling down a jungle river with a guide. On the last part of the journey they went over rapids and she fell overboard, swallowed water, and drowned. She felt certain that the dream and memory of almost drowning under the sail when her mother's boat capsized related to her breast-feeding experience. She recalled her mother in the kitchen, cursing, threatening, throwing things, baking a cake and making the children sit in a circle on the floor and one by one lick the remains of the batter from her finger.

She recalled her terror at watching her mother shaving her legs, and watching her newborn sister lose a piece of umbilical cord. Perhaps her mother had done something to her. She had the urge to sleep with a man and I wondered if this was her way of assuaging doubts about her gender. To my surprise Sara agreed and began to talk about the feeling that she had been "ripped off" and forced to be a girl in a world where boys got everything. She recalled childhood activities using a blow-torch in her basement which we now believed were efforts to construct a penis. She was apprehensive that I might want "a blow job" from her. She wrote me a letter in which she described a dream:

I was searching for something but there was this demon following me around in the shadows killing people. It was like some robot that ripped the tops of people's heads off and ate their brains and hands. It killed everyone that I saw or talked to. What a vivid picture of what I am doing! The monster is obviously me and I can't kill it and you can't kill it because all it does is constantly try to kill you. I don't think you really understand what a monster I am. I get you where it hurts. I get you to care about me and try to help and then kick you in the head over and over.

We returned to the subject of castration and discovered that she believed all children are essentially male. Males have power and control but they are "pricks, have brains in their crotch". Some children get "ripped off" and become eunuchs. In my notes subsequent to this session I subsequently realized I had written "it is like pulling teeth to get her to continue to think about this". She realized that getting beaten up and "ripped off" and trying to control the penis and get it inside her was re-enacting her struggle to get a penis as well as the feeding struggle with her mother. She realized that she tried to control me by withholding her thoughts and feelings, withdrawing and "ripping me off".

Year Nine

She reported a "splitting headache" as she contemplated the part of her that wanted to be close to people and the part that was enraged at human beings. She missed hours and made the tape recorder malfunction. She picked fights with me over everything and wanted to "kick my balls". She resumed sleeping with an old boyfriend and hallucinating. She insisted on stopping the trifluoperazine because it made her feel drunk. I suggested it was helping her wake up but she was adamant and I decided she needed to bear the consequences of her decisions. The thoughtful work that had characterized recent sessions stopped as well. She walked in front of her car after parking it on a hill without setting the brake and nearly succeeded in running herself over. When she said that I looked like I felt helpless I readily assented. She felt as though we were saying goodbye and she were attending her own funeral. After a long silence she said that it was pointless, that she was not going to change and that although she would miss me, tomorrow would be our last hour. Perhaps she was right, I thought, and in any case I felt I needed to accept her right to control her life, so I shared my concern for her and my sadness.

Sara called me soon thereafter to say she had reconsidered and she told me her fantasy had been to quit therapy, stop caring, quit her job, and drive off. We agreed that she wanted to take a trip from the city of caring and loving to one of hatred, insanity, and perhaps suicide. She talked about how little it would disturb her family if this were to happen and I responded that I cared and it would distress me deeply. She was touched and cried. When she left the session she discovered that she had locked herself out of her car and had to return to the office for help. The next hour, after preliminary curses, she said she had been relieved to find herself locked out of her car because she was certain that had been her unconscious effort to keep herself from driving off and quitting, and this was the first instance she could recall in which her unconscious motivation had been constructive!

Unlike other positive moments in our work this incident heralded a permanent change. Sara no longer seemed psychotic. She told me that to her surprise she had never been this depressed before without having delusions and hallucinations. She decided to cut back to once-weekly therapy. We met for another year and a half prior to terminating and although our relationship remained stalemated there was no recurrence of hallucinations or delusions. Sara reported progressive expansion in the areas of close friendships and work. She began to develop an identity as an educational crusader as evidenced by meteoric career advancement and the high esteem in which she was held by other educators, parents, and most of all the children she taught. It became clear that the extent of her professional ambition and effort would be the only limiting factor in the success of her career.

About seven months after we decreased the frequency of her appointments Sara gave me another one of her illustrated letters as a kind of Christmas gift. After summarizing her accomplishments she concluded:

> *From the quiet room to this. That is saying a lot. For a huge chunk of each day I am happy, enjoying myself, challenged. You stuck by me. Thank you for your amazing patience and caring. I did everything I could to drive you away, and I continue to keep you at a distance with all the ways I have worked out over the years. But at the same time I take little pieces of our friendship and use them to patch my broken heart. You have given me a good life with friends and a satisfying job. You have also, like you said a long time ago, given me choices. My happiness with what I have now fuels my rage and urge to destroy you and my feelings, destroy myself. But much of me wants more and thinks that I can go further.*

Although she realized it was unlikely that she could attain her goal of intimacy with a man without further intensive work with me, each gesture in that direction was regularly followed by some form of destructiveness. She seemed to be saying "I won't" to the prospect of more intensive emotional involvement with me. Finally I suggested that she was saying by her angry negative behavior what she was unable to say in words, namely that she did not wish to go further in therapy. Then it turned out that Sara did not want to experience the intense sadness of termination, either. She seemed to want to continue our ambivalent contact endlessly without movement. She seemed no more capable of saying goodbye than she was of continuing our work. We agreed to her wish to visit and report to me every half year or so, in the hope that eventually she might be able to reach a more definitive decision of one kind or another. During one such interval she wrote me:

> *There are nights when I get so depressed and feel helpless and angry and want to die, but I can survive them, I have control and know more clearly that the feelings will not kill me. I do not take drastic action anymore. Often I don't pay attention to my feelings and it is only when I get very close to being psychotic that I force myself to figure out what is going on. You helped me to do this many, many times. I can do it myself now. Thank you for your patience and caring. Thank you for giving me choices. You sat there for years waiting for me to show up. You ran the risk of holding out your caring and being rejected over and over and over. I know that I didn't entirely arrive, but I am happy. I know that it is not ideal that I carry you around in my head as a watchdog. Ideally it should be me that does this but the part of me that wants to destroy all caring and all life is very powerful and I need you there in my mind as a third party.*

After another hiatus in our sessions Sara returned and informed me that she had made a very satisfying relationship with a man she described as kind and intelligent. She shared the surprising news that they had a good sexual relationship because she realized that in order to retain her sanity during sex she had to reserve the right to ask him to stop lovemaking at any time; a condition he was willing to honour. He lived in a distant city and they had concluded that in order to decide whether they wanted to make a commitment to one another they would first need to live together. This awareness coincided fortuitously with Sara's conclusion that in order to advance her career she needed to change jobs and get a Ph.D. and this might just as well be done in the city where he lived. She knew I would be pleased and she had come to say goodbye. She expressed moving tears of farewell and gratitude.

Epilogue

More than twenty years elapsed before Sara unexpectedly contacted me and came to visit. I felt I was in the presence of an impressively mature woman with a solid sense of self who made direct eye and emotional contact with me, had a sense of values and purpose, and was highly intelligent and articulate. She described a very satisfying marriage to the man she had told me about in that final session. She and her husband had adopted a very disturbed adolescent boy and raised him to a constructive and mature manhood. In her career as teacher and educational innovator she was greatly valued by colleagues and by the community. She had resigned her position some years previously after a dispute with authorities in which she had the backing of her colleagues and the community, and obtained a Masters degree in creative writing. She had written and illustrated a coming-of-age novel for nine to twelve year olds, which had been published and very favourably reviewed. She had never again sought or required therapy or medication. Remarkably what she recalled most about our work was not things I had said to her, but my unwavering patience and caring during her long periods of silence and disengagement.

Discussion and Conclusion

I believe Sara met the criteria for chronic paranoid schizophrenia, whether according to the version of DSM that was in use when I treated her or the current version. Space does not permit exploration of whether there is a distinction between psychoses like Sara's, in which there is a major history of childhood trauma at the hands of parental figures, and ones in which there may be a lesser component of trauma alongside evidence suggestive of constitutional predisposition.

The treatment I described was based on fundamental psychoanalytic principles: uncovering of unconscious meaning and analysis of transference and dreams. It was not a conventional psychoanalysis, however, because Sara never used the couch except to sit on, and for the most part she was not encouraged to free associate, in so far as this promoted disintegration and undermined her reflective and integrative capabilities. Instead, I tried to establish eye contact as an essential element of relationship, and meaning was uncovered by dialectic interchanges in which I tried to hold in mind what I thought she was communicating to me by her behaviour, gestures and facial expressions, speech peculiarities and prosody, as well as her actual words; to mirror my impressions back to her as speculations; and to encourage her to confirm or deny their accuracy. Particularly in the early years the work required creation of a holding environment where her destructiveness might be contained and she might be encouraged to think, a capacity that can usually be assumed to exist at or near the beginning of an ordinary psychoanalysis. The availability of a supportive long-term environment was essential in this regard and it was sorely tested by Sara's destructiveness not only to herself, but toward both myself and ward staff by undermining our sense of reality and pressuring us to enact toward one another the unintegrated rage and suspiciousness that she was unable to represent, bear, and think about. The role of medication in her treatment was unclear; there were times it clearly helped, and others in which it exacerbated her paranoia as she fought its effects or did not take it as prescribed.

I have chosen to present the work as it unfolded and for the most part not to interject my theoretical thinking and hypotheses along the way. Our work might readily be formulated in terms of Klein's (1935, 1946) theories of the paranoid-schizoid position with splitting, projective identification, and phantasy; Bion's (1957, 1959) theory of failure of alpha functioning and dreaming that ordinarily metabolizes beta elements of raw experience and creates a gradient between conscious thought and unconscious process, an evacuation of raw beta elements in the form of delusion and hallucination; Matte-Blanco's (1988) model of symmetrical logic; and even Kohut's (1971) theory of failure of self cohesion and presence of an archaic bipolar self. I prefer my own theory of primordial mental activity (Robbins, 2011, 2012), a mental process distinctive from thought that is related to Freud's (1900) primary process and dreaming, and Klein's paranoid-schizoid position. Sara's development seemed to be fixated at a dissociated oral sadistic/ masochistic level. Confusing as our relationship seemed during much of the treatment, in retrospect the transference and my reciprocal countertransference were simple in outline. They involved Sara's undifferentiated relationship with her mother and with me, and included efforts, at first unconscious and gradually made conscious in the course of our work, to make me the object of the kind of annihilating rage, mindbending distortions of reality, and disruptions of continuity and trust to which she had been subject by her mother that she could not hold in thoughtful representational mind and memory. In so doing she induced in me reciprocal feelings of confusion about reality as well as hopelessness, helplessness, and at times anger, and she pushed me toward a mind-numbing paranoid psychosis such as she experienced. It was my task to demonstrate to her that one could not only survive such assaults, but learn to deal with them in a more constructive effective way by thinking, representing her emotions, and remembering. Another element of the dissociated oral transference was Sara's masochistic drive toward an annihilating relationship such as she had with her mother. The related fantasies toward me that seriously impeded our work involved threats of oral invasion not only by my penis but by medication and by the very words that were the means of my communicating with her. Sara compensated for her fears by a subtle grandiosity that was manifest as a conviction that she knew how to take care of herself better than anyone else and that she was superior because no matter what was done to her she experienced no emotional pain or distress. She was full of rage and had a deep contempt for men, whom she believed she was manipulating and controlling by what seemed from an objective perspective her manifestly masochistic behavior. Her malignant rage led her to the brink of ending our relationship on many occasions, at first through her unconscious enactments but later when she had come to realize more consciously her sadistic determination to destroy my efforts and make me suffer no matter what I did, as well as her oral masochistic terror that I would destroy her.

What was mutative in my work with Sara? The relative stability of my own sense of self and my sometimes shaky faith in my own sanity and reality sense was essential. Of most importance, I believe, was my capacity to sit with Sara through not only the vicissitudes of her own suffering but her unconscious efforts to drive me insane by making me experience the kinds of reality bending experiences and overwhelmingly painful affects of helplessness, hopelessness, confusion and inchoate rage, and to remain thoughtful and help her metabolize these into thoughtful language and emotional representation. In my psychiatric training many decades ago at the Massachusetts Mental Health Center I was taught to learn not by reading theory but by sitting with my patient and bearing and helping her bear her hitherto unbearable pain. I believe my knowledge of psychosis and what ability I have to work with deeply disturbed persons came from this intensive interpersonal immersion in a way it could never have come from didactic cookbook instruction.

The fact that I could fall back on a theory of mind (Robbins, 1993, 2002, 2011, in press) was critical to my ability to comprehend what was going on with her when she was doing her unconscious best to destroy my capacity for sane thought. There are those who believe that theory is unnecessary, that it is used by the therapist as a defensive barrier to relating to the patient, and that all that is necessary is a benevolent, kind, caring attitude along with patience and common sense. Sara's follow-up comment that what she recalled most about our work was not things I had said to her, but my unwavering patience and caring, might be taken as support for such a belief. But I think such an a-theoretical attitude is responsible for the long-term stalemates and ultimate disillusionments that so often accompany efforts to work with severely psychotic persons. The fact that Sara did not immediately recall the details of our work says more about memory than about therapeutic efficacy. Consider child development. While many adults do recall specific kinds of teaching from their parents, the fundamentals of teaching a child to walk, to talk, to become socialized, to think and use his or her mind, are never remembered in their specifics. They have become internalized as a part of the adult personality. What adults do remember is parental caring (or, in pathological instances, lack thereof). In the course of our work Sara informed me how she gradually transformed the things I tried to "teach" her about her mind from an alien threatening presence she wanted to destroy, to a third party in her mind, and eventually to a valued part of herself that helped her to face painful feelings and not run away into psychosis. At that point "I" had become a part of her more than a set of specific memories.

In the course of our work Sara underwent a fundamental personality transformation. Recall that her chief complaint was inability to concentrate and lack of a sense of personal identity with her psychotic sadistic mother who distorted reality, attacked Sara's efforts to care and to develop an integrated continuous sense of herself. She developed the capacity to care, internalized the capacity to represent emotions, integrated the disparate elements in her personality to form a coherent cohesive sense of self, and became capable of experiencing and resolving intrapsychic conflict. She underwent significant psychosexual development from a dissociated sadistic/masochistic oral relationship with her mother and the belief that she was a castrated male, to establishment of a mature gender role identity, and she achieved the capacity for intimacy, motherhood, and a successful career.

References

Arieti, S (1955). *Interpretation of schizophrenia*. New York: Basic Books.
Bion, W (1957). Differentiation of the psychotic from the non-psychotic personalities. *International Journal of Psycho-Analysis*, **38**, 266-275.
Bion, W (1959). Attacks on linking. *International Journal of Psycho-Analysis*, **40**, 308-315.
Freud, S (1900). The interpretation of dreams. In J.Strachey (Ed. & Trans.) *The standard edition of the complete psychological works of Sigmund Freud* (Vols. 4-5). London: Hogarth Press.

Klein, M (1935). A contribution to the psychogenesis of manic-depressive states. In M.Klein, *Love, guilt and reparation and other works, 1921-1945* (pp.262-289). London: Hogarth Press.

Klein, M (1946). Notes on some schizoid mechanisms. In M.Klein, *Envy and gratitude and other works, 1946-1963* (pp.1-24). London: Hogarth Press.

Kohut, H (1971). *The analysis of the self*. New York: International Universities Press.

Matte-Blanco, I (1988). *Thinking, feeling and being: Clinical reflections on the fundamental antinomy of human beings and world*. London: Routledge.

Robbins, M (1988). Use of audiotape recording in impasses with severely disturbed personalities. *Journal of the American Psychoanalytic Association*, **36**, 61-75.

Robbins, M (1993). *Experiences of schizophrenia*. New York: Guilford.

Robbins, M (2002). The language of schizophrenia and the world of delusion. *International Journal of Psycho-Analysis*, **83**, 383-405.

Robbins, M (2011). *The primordial mind in health and illness: A cross-cultural perspective*. London & New York: Routledge.

Robbins, M (2012). The primordial mind and the psychoses. *Psychosis*, **4**, 258-268.

Robbins, M (in press). Affect and psychosis. In A.Gumley, A.Gillham, K.Taylor & M.Schwannauer (Eds), *Psychosis and emotion: The role of emotions in understanding psychosis, therapy and recovery*. London & New York: Routledge.

Searles, H (1965). *Collected papers on schizophrenia and related subjects*. New York: International Universities Press.

Sullivan, H (1953). *Schizophrenia as a human process*. New York: Norton.

Torrey, E (1983). *Surviving schizophrenia*. New York: Harper.

CHAPTER 19

VISUALIZATION OF CASE STUDY 2 (DR ROBBINS) USING THE PPCC MODEL: DR STEGGLES

VISUALIZATION OF CASE STUDY 2 (DR ROBBINS)

M Robbins: "The successful psychoanalytic therapy of a schizophrenic woman" (2012):
An academic process analysis according to the Psychodynamic Pentapointed Cognitive
Construct (PPCC) Theory (2012)   Gillian R M Steggles

A combined academic and clinical study of the successful 11-year psychoanalytic therapy of a 28 year old chronic paranoid schizophrenic woman.

Stages of Therapy
A Development of the illness
  (i) 5 Variables of the patient's impoverished representational world when initially in therapy (years 1-2):
1. Psychoanalyst
   Directs therapeutic activities towards resolving analysand's problems.

2. Experiences
   Childhood trauma
   Neglect by mother
   Inadequate nourishment
   Exposure to danger by mother and by self
   Insensitivity and emotional unavailability of father
   Exposure to severe isolation abroad when only a child
   Family pride in equating strength and maturity with masculinity
      and expectation of suppression of emotion.

3. Dreams/Representations
   Mentally unstable mother
   Emotionally absent father
   'Macho' brothers, one of whom she was fond of, but one who queried her need for hospitalization
   Conveyed impression of self as a person of indeterminate gender, and believed that she, like all girls, was a castrated male.
   Dream: of a great family dining-room in a cylindrical 8-storey building containing dangerously floating tables and chairs which could be injurious. A clown caused the death of her sister.

4. Observations (non-psychotic thoughts)
   Patient was "getting a few crumbs".
   "I really think I am alive, and if I think about it I get so sad and I get really angry".

5. Determining Orientation (psychosis and disturbed behaviour)

Schizophrenic Global Perspective 2	Schizophrenic Global Perspective 1
(nearly intolerable)	(absolutely intolerable
'false self'	perspective within family)
Tried to be inconspicuous and hide herself from her mother. Concealed badly cut finger from her mother.	Tried to run away from home to skid row areas of cities; where Her low self-esteem allowed men to abuse her sexually in exchange for food and a place to sleep.

223

The PPCC:

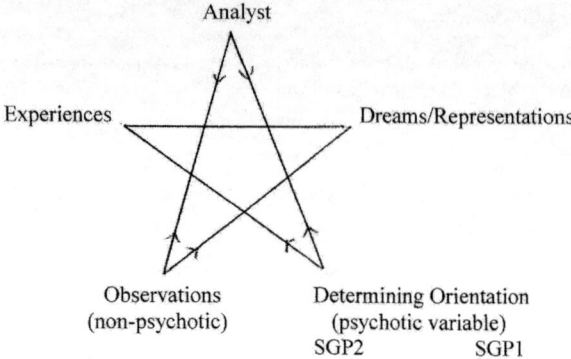

(ii) Patient's limitations interacting with representational world, leading to block (schizophrenia) (year 1):

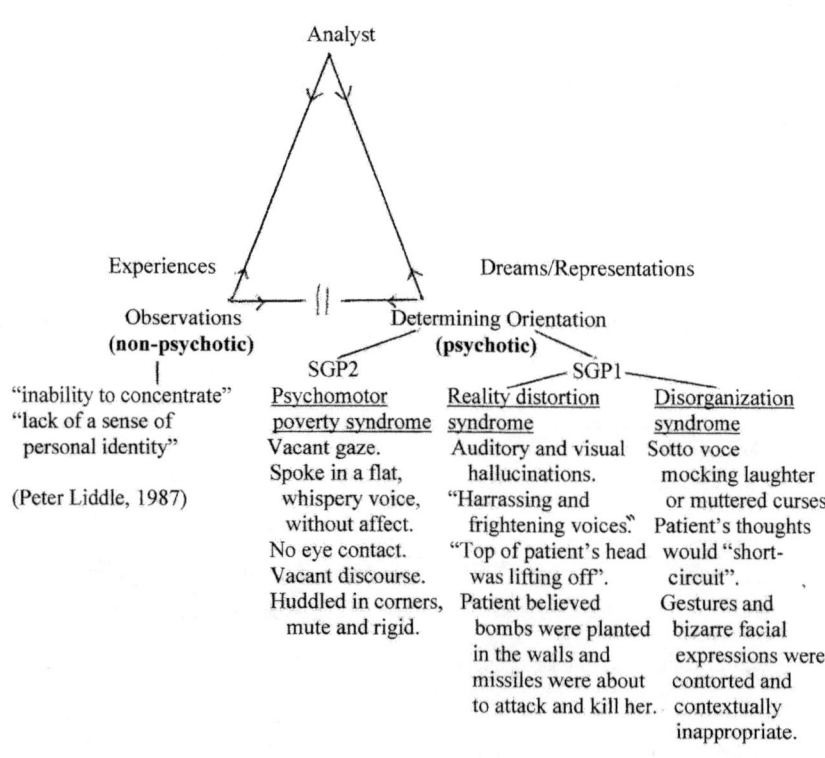

VISUALIZATION OF CASE STUDY 2 (DR ROBBINS)

B Treatment
  (iii) Analysis of the psychosis (year 3):

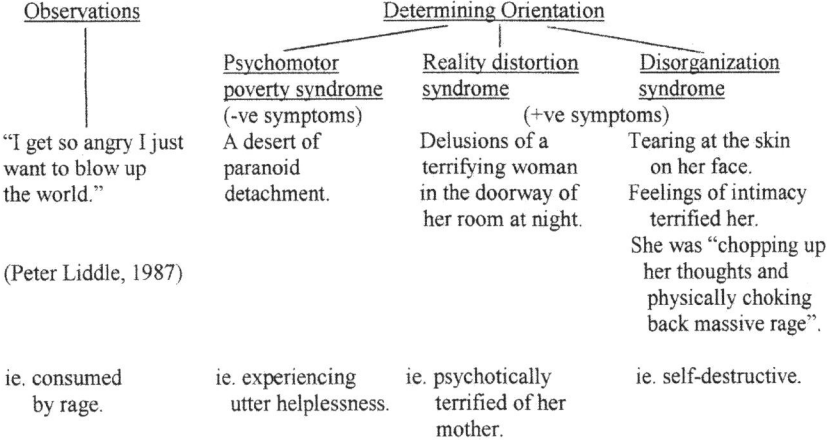

Observations	Determining Orientation		
	Psychomotor poverty syndrome (-ve symptoms)	Reality distortion syndrome (+ve symptoms)	Disorganization syndrome
"I get so angry I just want to blow up the world."	A desert of paranoid detachment.	Delusions of a terrifying woman in the doorway of her room at night.	Tearing at the skin on her face. Feelings of intimacy terrified her. She was "chopping up her thoughts and physically choking back massive rage".
(Peter Liddle, 1987)			
ie. consumed by rage.	ie. experiencing utter helplessness.	ie. psychotically terrified of her mother.	ie. self-destructive.

  (iv) Effects of treatment of the psychosis (years 1-11):
       Psychoanalytic therapy

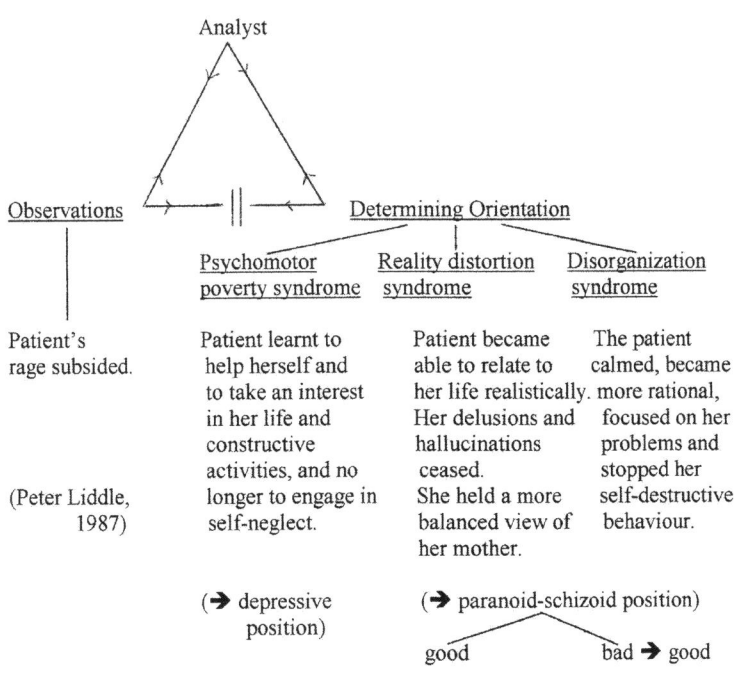

Observations	Determining Orientation		
	Psychomotor poverty syndrome	Reality distortion syndrome	Disorganization syndrome
Patient's rage subsided.	Patient learnt to help herself and to take an interest in her life and constructive activities, and no longer to engage in self-neglect.	Patient became able to relate to her life realistically. Her delusions and hallucinations ceased. She held a more balanced view of her mother.	The patient calmed, became more rational, focused on her problems and stopped her self-destructive behaviour.
(Peter Liddle, 1987)			
	(→ depressive position)	(→ paranoid-schizoid position) good bad → good	

225

C Resolution of the psychosis

(v) Resolution of the psychosis (years 1-7): (a long process)

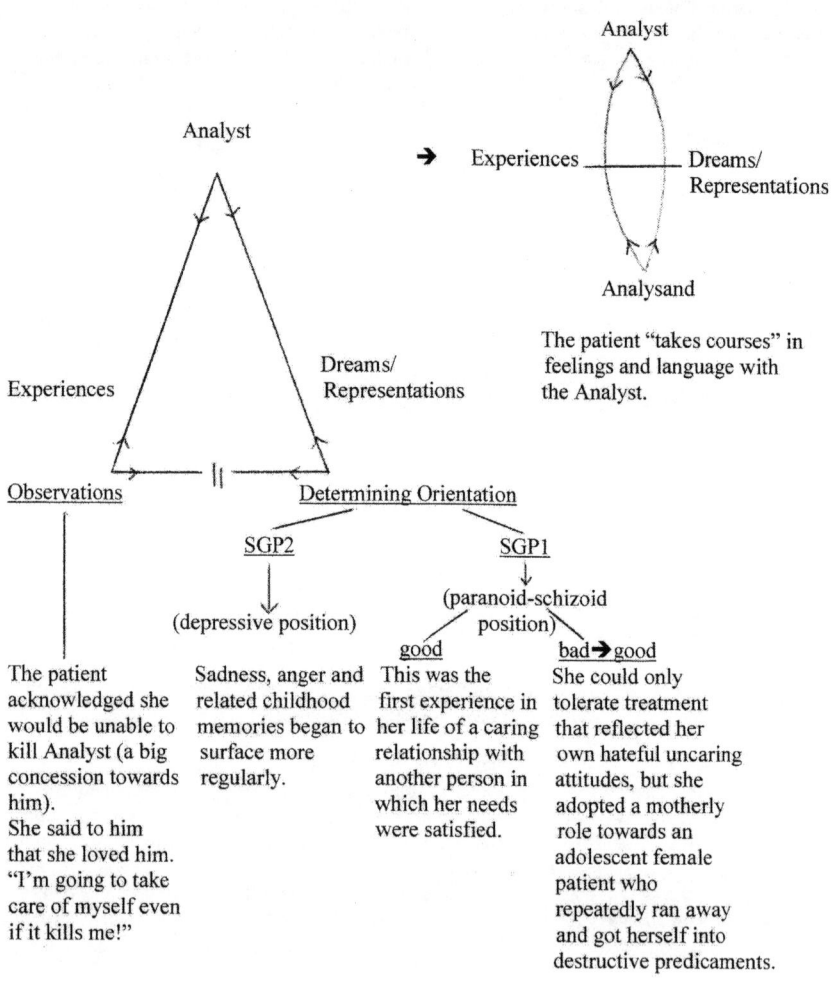

VISUALIZATION OF CASE STUDY 2 (DR ROBBINS)

(vi) More therapy, longterm:

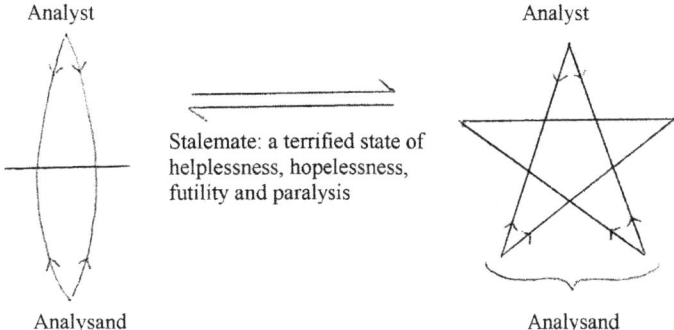

The PPCC: depressive position	The PPCC: paranoid-schizoid position
"Ms Red"	"Ms Black"
The patient was "taking courses" with the Analyst, in feelings and language. She made a new female friend, joined a health club and expressed appropriate anger when mistreated by people.	The patient turned away from the Analyst and muttered curses. She was thoughtless, ignorant, rigid, hateful and destructive. She had a "name-calling vocabulary". She had contempt for human beings, relationships and her own well-being. In this black chair she described herself as mean and "Neanderthal".

(vii) Closure of the vertex (years 7-8):
(Establishment of perspective)

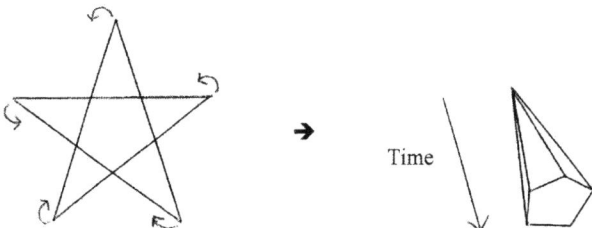

"The pendulum has been swinging for 35 years, without any joy, love, sadness, company. I want more with you [the Analyst] and I want the rest of my life also".

She talked enthusiastically about her adventures, new relationships, and the future.

(viii) <u>Rounding of the personality</u> (11 years of treatment + 20 year interval):

<u>Closed vertex:</u>
Integration in time, place and person.

<u>A healthy psyche</u>

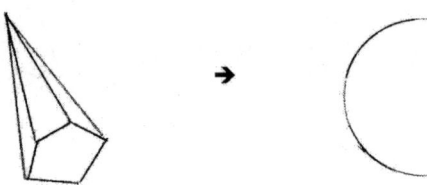

<u>Time</u>: 35 years of oscillation in many dimensions, now actively and happily rooted in the present.
<u>Place</u>: The patient no longer escapes on self-destructive visits to skid-row parts of town or to desolate pubs which were 'a "home" of deadness where she felt no-one could touch her' but has instead a home with her husband and son.
<u>Person</u>: She became an impressively mature woman with a solid sense of self who made direct eye contact with the Analyst, had a sense of values and purpose, and was highly intelligent and articulate.

She formed a mature gender identity.
She achieved progressive expansion in the areas of close friendships and work.
She formed a very satisfying marriage to a kind and intelligent man.
She adopted a very disturbed adolescent boy and raised him to a constructive and mature manhood.
She became a teacher and educational innovator.
She achieved a Masters degree in creative writing.
She wrote and illustrated a novel for children.

CHAPTER 20

COMMENTARY ON DR ROBBINS' CASE STUDY 2 AND ITS VISUALIZATION

All views expressed in this chapter are those of Dr Steggles

The subject of Dr Robbins' Case Study 2, Sara, showed every sign of suffering typically among those patients with a diagnosis of paranoid schizophrenia. At the start of her therapy she had a thoroughly destructive relationship with her mother and was quite unable to care for herself. She engaged in dangerous activities on the streets of large cities, and for some time experienced near-destitution but for the constant support of Dr Robbins. At the end of her therapy she pronounced that the feature of it which was most profoundly helpful to her was Dr Robbins' steadfast, steady presence during the long silences while she sat with him, saying nothing, in her confused and miserable states while she was trying to make sense of what she was experiencing in his consulting room.

This experience, of blank confusion, appears to be common among untreated schizophrenic patients. Dr Robbins describes in the Abstract to his paper the prevalent belief that "intensive psychoanalytic therapy is ineffective if not destructive and contraindicated, and that the treatment of choice is a combination of psychopharmacology and educational techniques designed to provide symptom relief and rehabilitation". His work with Sara demonstrates beyond doubt that psychoanalytic therapy in skilled hands can resolve schizophrenia. Sara went on to complete a Masters degree, marry, mother a needy young man, and have a successful career. The challenge for clinicians, I believe, is to identify how to conduct an effective psychoanalytic psychotherapy treatment; how to determine beforehand that a patient is likely to respond to all the demands that this treatment makes on its subjects; and, in mastering these, to identify all those schizophrenic patients whose illness could be resolved or greatly alleviated by this treatment. Sara may not have appeared to be a likely candidate, but Dr Robbins had noticed early in his relationship with her that she was unusually intelligent, for example from her wide vocabulary and occasional astute observations that she made, and so he persevered with faith that this aspect of her would carry her through her treatment.

The PPCC model initially describes Sara's Representational World. This summarises aspects of Sara's early environments up to the time of commencement of her therapy, the representational world being Joseph Sandler and Bernard Rosenblatt's conception (Sandler and Rosenblatt, 1962) that in a young child it forms a preconscious, or unconscious, collection of the most notable aspects, to the child, of all the environments it has so far encountered; it is adjustable, gradually changing, as the child develops, in its role as a guide for the child's future experiences. The contents of Sara's representational world are enumerated in (i) at the beginning of Chapter 19, and then displayed visually as "The PPCC". Sara's representational world clearly illustrates within the range of elements of Sara's mind, thus Experiences, Dreams/Representations, Observations and the psychotic Determining Orientation, how deficient were Sara's early experiences, her early life, her early relationships, and how deeply unhappy she had consequently become. She appeared not to feel this deep unhappiness to start with, due to her numbing of her feelings in accordance with her family's attitudes to independence and "macho" assertiveness against the world. The PPCC's pentapointed construct, shown in part (i) of the visualization of Case 2, shows how all parts of Sara's mind were caught up in her utterly dismal perspective on the world in general and within her immediate relationships in particular. This is the presentation in Sara accepted by Dr Robbins for treatment with psychoanalytic psychotherapy which, as he says, would be generally rejected by many psychiatrists as "ineffective if not destructive and contraindicated"; he clearly demonstrates that it is highly effective, even for a chronic schizophrenic patient like the intelligent Sara who was, however, learning to trust him and who continued to sit with Dr Robbins for hour after hour trying to understand and make sense of her issues, attitudes, decisions, and her efforts to find herself within herself. The pentapointed construct sets out these issues, attitudes, and potential decisions in a structured way so that the relation between their elements may be appreciated. Sara's psychoanalyst, Dr Robbins, held all the elements of Sara's mind, known and unknown, in his mind while he sat with Sara, putting into practice what he describes as his having learned from Elvin Semrad about how to bear with the schizophrenic patient their pain, distress, confusion, and despair. This situation is precisely what some psychiatrists claim is "ineffective". Talking treatments are all based upon the human elements of contact, communication, identification, empathy, sensitivity, sharing, compassion, generosity of spirit, and the human social instinct. Schizophrenic patients have commonly spent most if not all of their lives so far, like Sara before her treatment, in environments where they have simply not experienced any opportunity to reflect within themselves about their own value or potential. They have become cowed, withdrawn, submissive, easily manipulated, frequently bullied, and hopeless. They have not identified their own chances to show initiative, to be creative, or to flourish in any way. This can clearly be seen in Sara's earlier life before therapy, from observing her representational world. Once recovered after her therapy, as noted by Dr Robbins, she had achieved her Masters degree, had married, and with her husband was successfully bringing up a needful young man.

    At the start of treatment, Sara's illness involved a constant state of psychosis where she remained largely out of touch with Dr Robbins, with a few isolated indications of connection such as when she could acknowledge to him that she was being subjected to "harassing and frightening voices". This block in her mental functioning is displayed visually in section (ii) of Chapter 19, in the PPCC model's triangular form. Here it may be seen that her non-psychotic self, as Observations, was completely out of contact at this time with her psychotic elements, which are displayed as her Determining Orientation, ie. her Schizophrenic Global Perspectives 1 and 2, consisting as they do of the three main symptomatic syndromes identified by Peter Liddle in 1987 (Liddle, 1987): the Psychomotor Poverty Syndrome, the Reality Distortion Syndrome and the Disorganization Syndrome. This diagram clarifies the relations of Sara's psychotic elements to the non-psychotic Observations part of her mind, which was accessible to Dr Robbins to reason with her and suggest ideas that she might find helpful as she progressed on her long path towards health. The scale of her confused distress may be appreciated from looking at this diagram. Sometimes psychoanalysts are able to calm imminent psychosis by talking to their patient so that the patient does not consciously accept or reject the analyst's interpretations, but rather assimilates the tone of his or her voice, their calm body language, and the kindness of their facial expression. Section (ii) describes the early phase of hard work being tackled by the therapeutic dyad: the arrows represent the mechanism of resolution of the difficulties, ie. dialogue between the analyst, both with Sara's accessible, non-psychotic mind making Observations, and with her blocked off clinical syndromes that constituted her Schizophrenic Global Perspectives.

The effect of Sara's treatment on her psychosis can be seen to begin in Section B (iii). Initially she seemed to face even worse problems than her denial and adopted toughness; relinquishing these exposed her raw self to the treatment process. Here she was beginning to experience and face her emotional difficulties more squarely and specifically. Her symptoms have become more concentrated into features of her life, eg. being overcome by rage, feeling utterly helpless, realising she was overwhelmingly terrified of her mother, and becoming overtly self-destructive. This was, of all the suffering she underwent during her ordeals, one of the most painful times for her when she felt completely helpless and out of her own control. She sat mute in her chair in Dr Robbins' consulting room, silently stuck and fixed in her predicament. All that could be done was for Dr Robbins to make sure she knew he was there with her and for her, despite her aggression towards him that resulted from her despair, confusion, and fears, for example, of her mother. During this time her mind will have been moving among her very unpleasant experiences and trying to relate them to her present situation, and particularly to Dr Robbins. It took time for her injured mind to be able to think, reflect, reason within herself, and come to itself as the person she was, and to begin to be able to conduct a reasoned conversation as speaking truly from herself and not within the persona she used with her mother and her family, ie. denying pain, and being macho and unthinking. This activity, this skilled process of enabling a schizophrenic patient to learn gradually to speak as themselves, is the material that evidences the justification of rejecting some psychiatrists' belief that trying to bring schizophrenic patients' minds into mental health is "ineffective if not destructive and contraindicated". Psychiatrists may validly be very cautious about this new therapeutic application of psychoanalytic psychotherapy. It certainly carries risks, and any other approach would be cavalier. But when very carefully supervised, as demonstrated in Case Studies 1 and 2, it can be remedial. The PPCC model elucidates visually the process of the psychoanalytic psychotherapeutic dialogue and its effects on the schizophrenic patient. This potentially efficacious nature of the process of psychoanalytic psychotherapy on schizophrenic illness in carefully selected patients, very carefully observed and managed, has thus been demonstrated, with a view to replicating it equally carefully, initially in a small and carefully selected cohort of patients suffering from paranoid schizophrenia or schizoaffective disorder.

Section (iv) shows how the PPCC illustrates further effects of therapy on Sara's mind. Having addressed her emotional rawness she began to be able to address nicer aspects of her environments than her family circle had afforded her, as her developmental representational world. Her rage subsided. In place of her self-neglect and self-destructive behaviour she learned to help herself and to take constructive initiatives. Her hallucinatory and delusional symptoms ceased. This was not due to medication change. It was due to her mind's stresses and fears and miseries being replaced by enlightened conversation with Dr Robbins. It was no temporal coincidence, coinciding with her therapy. This is an example of how psychological influences can have power over mental function. Such influences may have a different time frame from medications, but their power is at least as strong because the person's thinking itself has become changed. That person can still remember her previous attitudes but is beginning to build new experiences and new memories. Sara oscillated quite frequently, during the middle years of her therapy, between her family-induced thinking and the enlightened thinking that at times she exchanged with Dr Robbins; but here she was finding herself unable to choose between them, as an interim phase of her treatment. When she finally did choose, she consciously chose sanity with Dr Robbins. She no longer required medication and her treatment was complete, an effect of psychological management.

The Resolution of Sara's psychosis, a long process, is described in Section C (v). Her Schizophrenic Global Perspectives here illustrate adaptive resolution of her mind's schizophrenic characteristics. She was now able to adopt Klein's depressive position, for example her wild, unfocused rage about the world and "wanting to blow it up" subsided, and she now felt specific sadness and anger about her childhood. She felt for the first time in her life that, with Dr Robbins, she was experiencing a caring relationship with another person in which her needs were satisfied. This experience grew into her adopting a motherly relationship with another female patient who repeatedly ran away and got herself into destructive predicaments, just as she herself had previously done.

In Section (vi) Sara's oscillations may be seen between adopting security, peace, and warm feelings as "Ms Red" in her "red chair", and her contrasted sitting as "Ms Black" in her "black chair" (an idea of Dr Robbins to help her distinguish her self-identified darker side, "Ms Black", from her nicer self, "Ms Red"). As Ms Black, her aggressive, rejecting, hateful, and destructive states of mind predominated and made her feel "Neanderthal". As she oscillated, she felt herself to be in a terrified state of helplessness, hopelessness, futility, and paralysis. Some psychiatrists may have some difficulty in evaluating or understanding these psychoanalytic psychological states. But psychoanalysis makes it possible to follow patients' minds, and "psychiatry" means "medical management of the soul (or psyche)".

Following how patients' minds may be healed is what psychiatrists try to do when they treat patients with serious mental illnesses, hoping to make them well, or at least better and suffering less. By this stage, Dr Robbins had worked with Sara for long enough to enable her both to understand how deficient her early life had been of nourishment, kindness, and loving care on the one hand, and also actively to experience some of the benefits of rationality, openness to the world and to emotions, and of self-care, on the other. So Dr Robbins knew that Sara had this knowledge and experience, and that what she chose to do now with her life, after her oscillations, was down to her. A biological psychiatrist in possession of Dr Robbins' knowledge would probably be of a similar view. All that is needed for this knowledge's value and potential benefit for schizophrenic patients to be realised by all psychiatrists is for it to be shared and understood, and used for patients, with the help of medications.

In years seven to eight of her treatment, as shown in stage (vii), Sara was able to "close her vertex", ie. acknowledge and assimilate all her life's previous experiences in such a way that she no longer felt threatened or upset by them. This was a tremendous step for her to achieve at last, after all this time in treatment with Dr Robbins. She had developed maturity and had built on her rationality and academic abilities. She felt that "the pendulum has been swinging for thirty-five years, without any joy, love, sadness, company", and she wanted to do something about it and live fully the rest of her life. Finally, in stage (viii), Sara's personality rounded, and, as Dr Robbins saw when she came to see him some twenty years after completion of her therapy, she had flourished as a wife, mother, and teacher. She had a Masters degree, and a flourishing career working with children and their parents and other staff, all of whom like her own family thoroughly appreciated her. So Dr Robbins' psychoanalytic psychotherapeutic technique and work with her saved Sara's life, and from his detailed report of his excellent work he presents its undeniable evidence, together with the evidence he also presents (see Part IV) of his patient Emily.

PART VI

A PROPOSED NATIONAL HEALTH SCHEDULE FOR SCHIZOPHRENIA

....

DR GILLIAN STEGGLES

CHAPTER 21

PRINCIPAL AVAILABLE TREATMENTS FOR SCHIZOPHRENIA AND SCHIZOAFFECTIVE DISORDER

Treatment interventions and maintenance for patients suffering from schizophrenia and schizoaffective disorder are expensive, but so are the financial, not to mention humanitarian, costs of not applying them. The suffering of schizophrenic and schizoaffective patients more than justifies the application of the most suitable treatment, from among the different modes of treatment available, for each individual patient. The Schizophrenia Commission Report (Andrews et al, 2012) outlines current practice generally available to schizophrenia sufferers.

Schizophrenic patients vary considerably in their functioning capacities. Schizoaffective patients are generally more able than those suffering from schizophrenia, which is thought to be associated with the greater affective component of their illness. Treatments for these patients are carefully selected and tailored for the individual, and changed or added to as required as the patient develops in recovery. Psychoanalytic psychotherapy, the most intensive and long-term therapy, which is under discussion in this volume, is the most expensive treatment, but also the most effective, when provided to suitable patients.

Early Intervention Services

Early intervention services (EIS) are effective at rescuing as much as possible of the personality and nature of a young person in their first acute crisis. Sometimes they can detect prodromal symptoms in a young person following early referral, before psychosis has become established. The duration of untreated psychosis is directly relevant to the overall prognosis (Marshall et al, 2005), so early interventions can be instrumental in securing a young person's future mental health.

Antipsychotic medications

Antipsychotic medications have been the mainstay of treatment, and very helpful in the management, of schizophrenic and schizoaffective patients since the 1960s (see Chapter 4). Since then, a broad range of antipsychotic effects have been observed with both the first and second generations of these medications, which act on D2 dopamine receptors in the mesolimbic tract in the brain to suppress the symptoms of psychosis. Almost all psychotic patients are prescribed these medications, which are found to be almost universally helpful, although side effects have to be monitored, and treated with anticholinergic drugs if necessary. Taking antipsychotic medication is not a contraindication to the use of psychological therapy for a patient.

Electroconvulsive Therapy

Electroconvulsive Therapy (ECT) is used to treat extremely depressed patients. It is rarely used to treat schizophrenic patients, but schizoaffectively disordered patients may be helped by it if they become severely depressed.

Individual Placement and Support

Individual placement and support (IPS) schemes offer supported employment to schizophrenic patients who wish to engage in paid competitive work alongside unaffected colleagues. IPS schemes firstly place schizophrenic patients, even severely affected ones, in a competitive work role, and then offer training and support. This differs from standard vocational schemes, where a long apprenticeship is considered a necessary prerequisite to working. IPS schemes are, today, quite effective in obtaining competitive, salaried positions appropriate to individual schizophrenic patients' specific abilities.

Family Therapy

Family therapy (FT) offers help of many kinds to families and patients affected by schizophrenia. It provides information about the illness, and supports patients and carers by providing practical solutions to problems where possible. Expressed emotion is identified as a recognised trigger factor for precipitating immediate problems for the patient, commonly including relapse, so families can be helped to avoid this. The family is well-placed to give support to their affected member and, given the opportunity to learn how they can best do this, most relatives are keen to make what contribution they can towards easing the life they all, collectively, have to address when one of them is taken ill.

Social Skills Therapy

Social skills therapy improves patients' ability to function in relation to other people. It gives the patients specific skills such as being able to hold a conversation without feeling unduly anxious, or being able to cook a meal and serve it to friends. Practice at skills such as these allows patients to progress better in relationships with more confidence, and can make a very helpful contribution towards patients' recovery from schizophrenic illness.

Criminal Justice System Diversion

Schizophrenic patients and others with severe mental illness are over-represented in the prison population (10% compared with 1-3% in the general population), and are not helped there as they should be. Even short prison sentences do not allow support in the way that suspended sentences or mental healthcare in the community through Community Orders do. Criminal Justice System Diversion (CJSD) seeks to ensure that people with mental health problems who come into contact with the criminal justice system are identified and directed towards appropriate mental healthcare, particularly as an alternative to imprisonment. Community Orders result in greatly reduced re-offending rates. The Mental Health Treatment Requirement (MHTR) can be placed by magistrates and judges on those who receive a Community Order or a Suspended Sentence Order, although the MHTR is not much used due to practical difficulties in its implementation (Khanom et al. 2009; Seymour and Rutherford, 2008). Nonetheless, where possible, it is still much more effective, more cost-effective, and evidently more humane as well, to divert people with schizophrenia out of prison and into the community.

Treatment of substance misuse

Substance misuse, including that of alcohol and cigarettes, is much higher in schizophrenic patients than among non-psychotically ill individuals. As described above in Chapter 4, a high proportion of schizophrenic patients smoke (61%) compared with the normal population (33%), as reported in the clinical records of 1.7 million people by the Schizophrenia Commission in 2012. The same source found that 26.1% of schizophrenic patients misused alcohol compared with 11.9% of healthy people, and 17.8% of schizophrenic patients abused other substances compared with only 7.0%

of the general population. Psychological treatments such as Cognitive Behavioural Therapy and Motivational Interviewing (see below) are used to help patients with a dual diagnosis of substance misuse or addiction and schizophrenia. These interventions have been found in a number of studies to be cost-effective and gave favourable clinical results, but the size of the samples was small and so the studies' results should be considered with caution.

Maintenance of physical health

The physical health of schizophrenic patients as a group has only recently been addressed seriously by clinical health staff. Some of the drugs used to treat schizophrenia, particularly olanzapine, can cause weight gain, and patients can also be at risk for cardiovascular disease and diabetes. There has been limited study of obesity and its treatment in schizophrenia. The risks from smoking are nearly doubled in schizophrenic patients compared with the normal population but, again, there is little positive evidence for the reducibility of this risk; bupropion, nicotine replacement therapy, and group therapy are the main physical treatments that have been applied, without marked success.

Critical Time Interventions

Homelessness among schizophrenic patients is addressed by Critical Time Interventions (CTI) workers, who apply the interventions over a period of nine months. The interventions consist of three phases: the transition phase, the try-out phase, and the transfer of care phase. The CTI worker gives home visits, co-ordinates care-givers, and develops long-term plans and goals (Herman et al. 2007). One study estimated that the CTI service led to a five-fold decrease in the risk of homelessness in New York City (Herman et al, 2011).

Assertive Community Treatment

Assertive community treatment (ACT) delivers clinical outpatient care to schizophrenic patients in the community. It has led to an improvement in symptoms and satisfaction among users of the service, and may be a cost-effective intervention for homeless people with severe mental illness. A large study has questioned ACT's efficacy in reducing homelessness among schizophrenic people, and also its economic efficacy (Slade et al, 2012), but many different community services now embody the principles of assertive outreach.

Outreach programmes

Outreach programmes aim to improve outcomes for homeless people with mental illness by engaging with homeless people who are unwilling to find help on their own, and providing help to these groups. Such a scheme was implemented in New York City, and like other similar schemes was found to increase costs. These schemes very often bring people into contact with services who otherwise would not have been in contact, thus causing the increased costs. Their value depends on society's evaluation of the benefits they bring to homeless people. Supported housing has rarely been studied in the literature, but seems to provide superior efficacy at a greater cost.

Crisis Resolution Home Treatment

Crisis resolution home treatment (CRHT) teams provide intensive care in the community to individuals who require immediate treatment and support. CRHT teams can reduce bed occupancy both by acting as a "gatekeeper" in decreasing the likelihood of an admission, and in permitting earlier discharge. The extent to which this applies in practice is, however, put somewhat in doubt by other factors influencing bed occupancy, and by the CRHT teams apparently not being utilised to their full potential. But considerable financial savings are implied if the teams were to be fully utilised; and even now, many young lives are preserved more intact by the work of CRHT teams than if the disruption of a psychiatric hospital admission were to be encountered.

Peer-support workers

Peer-support workers are those who have experienced mental illness and who then help and support similar individuals while they in turn work through their own experiences of illness, treatment, and recovery. "Recovery" is a concept dating from the 1970s which describes "overall wellbeing beyond symptom management", and furthermore "with the expectation that patients can lead normal lives, and secure employment, further education and training, and independent housing". Peer-support workers have progressed further along their path to recovery (Deegan, 1996; Repper and Carter, 2011; Davidson et al, 2006). They have gained in experience and learnt perceptions, beliefs, and knowledge of mental illness which in turn, when shared with current patients, can pass on confidence, drive for autonomy and independence, and hope and encouragement at every stage in the process of healing.

Advanced Treatment Directives

Advanced Treatment Directives (ATDs) are summaries of patients' wishes, written while they are contemplating future illness episodes and deciding how they would best like to be managed at such a time. The ATDs can be overridden under the Mental Health Act, but they are nonetheless popular at personal, existential, and ethical levels, as they give the schizophrenic patient influence over their own future situations when this might otherwise not be possible. It was found in one study (Henderson et al, 2004) that, using ATDs, compulsory admissions were reduced by more than one half.

Cognitive Behavioural Therapy

Cognitive behavioural therapy (CBT) sessions comprise discussions with the therapist about negative beliefs and behavioural patterns in which beliefs are tested through behavioural changes. It is a highly structured therapy that focuses on practical issues in the here-and-now. It may help schizophrenia sufferers by helping them to cope with difficult thoughts and behaviours. In this way it may help the patient to avoid relapse and thereby decrease service usage. The guidelines learnt in CBT sessions could also help the patient to continue in their employment, by enabling them to deal effectively with everyday occurrences, using their recent CBT experiences in practice.

Psychoanalytic Psychotherapy

Psychoanalytic psychotherapy may be used to resolve the schizophrenic or schizoaffective psychological disease process. Total commitment to the therapy is required, as is usually the case also with other therapies for them to be effective, and the treatment is reserved for those patients who can tolerate its painful self-scrutiny, loneliness, stresses, distress, and anxieties. The financial burden can be around £13,800 pa, and the treatment may continue for four to eight years or so, or sometimes slightly longer. But psychoanalytic psychotherapy has the potential successfully to resolve schizophrenic illness psychologically, thereby permitting the patient to understand themselves and so forestalling future episodes of illness. Once insight into the self is gained, the patient's resilience is robustly strengthened and this protects the patient from further illness.

Group Psychodynamic Psychotherapy

It can be quite difficult to persuade schizophrenic patients to attend group therapy, particularly those who tend to be peripatetic in character. But group therapy can provide much-needed social contact for the isolated schizophrenic individual, and may be a stepping-stone towards accepting help with housing, finance, and avoiding destitution. Groups are a helpful influence when the schizophrenic patient tries to stop smoking, providing moral support among contacts who the patient can see have similarities to themselves. There is scope in group psychodynamic psychotherapy for the schizophrenic patient to learn about themselves, and to find acceptance, which may be welcome if they have reached a point in their life when they are ready to accept help. More stabilised schizophrenic patients may likewise benefit from the regularity of familiar contacts and the opportunity to consolidate what they have already learned about themselves during their illness, with a new chance to apply their social skills with others. Groups such as these provide much-needed continuity in the lives of those who are in need of stabilisation and reassurance but without being troubled by loss of independence. For these patients commitment may be difficult, but through it they may learn to commit themselves to their own actual needs, which is a step in the right direction in assisting those trying to help them out of what are often quite dire circumstances.

Avatar Therapy

Avatar therapy is a novel psychological therapy devised by Professor Julian Leff (Leff et al, 2013) which was developed to alleviate schizophrenic patients of auditory hallucinations when these intrude as a symptom. In fact, avatar therapy has been known to banish auditory hallucinations and to cause a patient to be able to thank his psychiatrist "for giving him his life back". The avatar is a moving cartoon image on a video recorder, selected by the patient, so that, together with the patient's choice of voice type, it most closely "fits" the patient's imagined image and voice of his hallucinations. The psychiatrist speaks through the avatar, which moves its facial expressions and mouth appropriately as the psychiatrist speaks. Initially, in the first few sessions, the avatar is (the psychiatrist pretends to be) hostile, but gradually becomes benign and even complimentary. The patient believes the avatar is his or her voice speaking, and gradually the voice merges into normality and the patient's hallucinations are resolved. Avatar therapy has shown very promising early results (in 2018) and is being used to treat patients at the Maudsley Hospital in South London.

Anticipatory Pleasure Skills Training

Anhedonia, or lack of experiencing pleasure, is a challenging symptom of schizophrenia. The prevalence among schizophrenic patients of high levels of anxiety may be related to this finding. The intrinsic motivation of schizophrenic patients, ie. motivation which does not depend upon external rewards, appears to be generally similar to that of non-schizophrenic individuals. However, their extrinsic motivation, that which is aroused by the prospect of future, often unseen, rewards, seems to be inhibited. It is not known why this should be the case, but it appears to hinder schizophrenic patients in their self-mobilisation and effort towards future goals. Anticipatory pleasure skills training aims to incentivise schizophrenic patients in this direction by encouraging them to imagine future rewards and goals which appeal to them, and then towards extra effort in attaining these rewards and goals. Contemplating the nature of the rewards and goals, different aspects of them, and how the patient would enjoy them is the focus of the treatment, as is holding them in mind while the endeavour proceeds. It is hoped that anticipatory pleasure skills training may have a generally favourable effect upon schizophrenic patients' level of anhedonia and their daily experience and functioning.

Motivational Interviewing

This is an approach to motivating the patient where the decisions are taken only by themselves. The interviewer helps the patient review all possible options relating to a specific problem or difficulty that the patient is addressing. The interviewer can help with suggestions, but does not offer their views; only the patient's views on the suggestions are considered, and the interviewer's task is to confirm and approve the patient's opinions and decisions. In this way, the patient's mind is made up only of his or her own chosen perspectives. The interviewer understands and accepts this, and encourages the patient in their continuing progress as they work through their problems.

Dental care

Schizophrenic and schizoaffective patients can spend long intervals of time on their own, unsupervised and unattended by health staff. The condition of their mouths and teeth can degenerate to a serious extent, and dental care should be provided at centres where their antipsychotic medication and physical condition is monitored. Dental hygiene is not a priority of these patients, and responsibility for this aspect of their health should be accepted by health centres along with care of their general physical wellbeing.

In a National Health Schedule for Schizophrenia the most suitable treatments for every patient suffering from schizophrenic illness would be selected for them. This includes treatment for the most intelligent and able patients. For these patients, palliative care and supportive management alone is simply not enough, and they deserve enlightenment as best they are capable of reaching it. Psychoanalytic psychotherapy may contradict some of their beliefs and assumptions; but unless these mistaken attitudes of mind are corrected at root, these patients will never be well, like all their contemporary schizophrenia sufferers.

Reaching a state of mind where the patient will be receptive to thinking differently in this way is only possible in psychoanalytic psychotherapy, where support is afforded in the analyst's consulting room and in the therapeutic ward environment where the patient is being accommodated. Here, with all this necessary support, the patient is given the opportunity for correcting their views in a positive direction that will strengthen them in their search for autonomy and independence, for example, learning that not all grown men are predictably threatening towards them, or that sometimes complete strangers can be very kind.

Intelligent and diligent and determined patients suffering from schizophrenic illnesses actually require this opportunity to rethink their experience of life while under psychiatric care. Only psychoanalytic psychotherapy can access the deepest levels of their psyche in order for this relearning to take place, and psychiatrists need to be aware of its processes and potential to give their schizophrenic and schizoaffective patients their deserved opportunity of recovery.

CHAPTER 22

PATIENT SAFETY DURING THE PSYCHOANALYTIC PSYCHOTHERAPEUTIC TREATMENT OF SCHIZOPHRENIC AND SCHIZOAFFECTIVE PATIENTS

Patient safety is held to be the single most important aspect of all clinical care. Raanan Gillon's four ethical principles (Gillon, 1994) include non-malfeasance alongside beneficence; and the phrase "First do no harm" – primum non nocere – is believed to date from as far back as the seventeenth century as a part of apprentice doctors' ethical principles.

In psychological medicine, as in all other medical specialties, it is imperative to learn from past mistakes. This is especially true in the psychoanalytic psychotherapy of schizophrenic and schizoaffective patients, as this is a recent application of a treatment in depth to a highly complex illness. Patient related factors, staff related factors, and the role of leaders in the teams overseeing the treatment, ie. hospital consultants, senior managers, and the therapists themselves, all need to interrelate closely with each other to retain flexible and sensitive care for every patient's needs. Vigilance and applied forward thinking by staff, thus putting themselves into the patient's shoes and anticipating difficulty or danger in likely situations, must be attended to in order to install preparatory protections and ensure the patient's safety in that future situation.

Patient related factors may be those common to all schizophrenic or schizoaffective patients undergoing psychoanalytic psychotherapy, or they may be factors that relate specifically to an individual patient. If there are unusual and unique aspects to a patient then their clinicians need to be aware of these and appropriate support provided. Sometimes a patient may be particularly vulnerable physically, eg. nearly blind, which affects their ability to travel to and from analytic sessions. Or they may have been exposed to very strange ideas as they grew up, which have considerably distorted their perspective before their mind has been adjusted in treatment. Strange ideas may be very dangerous regarding patient safety because unusual assumptions can easily place the patient or others at risk. The responsible clinician may be wrong-footed by an unusual patient with unusual needs, through no fault of the patient or the clinician, and due only to a highly improbable set of factors which have been their mutual misfortune to encounter. For example, the patient may have been subject to unusually forceful parental pressure, with psychotically grandiose ambitions for the patient, who has been initially unable to stand up to them and develop normally. The regular safety measures must nonetheless be applied to the patient, and safeguarding borne in mind, to be ready if required.

Many safety factors apply to all schizophrenic and schizoaffective patients receiving psychoanalytic psychotherapy. Good staff relationships with the patients, and a will towards maintaining and constantly improving these, are one of the best ways to ensure that healthy self-care is practised by patients when on their own away from the ward and its staff. Good relationships between staff in different capacities, with effective and early sharing of new information among themselves, will ensure that new needs are not overlooked by anyone when the patient's circumstances or characteristics change. Consistency of management helps considerably in maintaining equanimity and calm, both in individual patients and within the ward's ambience. Continuity as far as possible of the psychological environment, including both the ward and the analyst's consulting-room, helps to frame the patient's mind in a non-disturbing setting, so that any changes in the patient's mind tend to be either therapeutically-derived or surfacing effects of the patient's illness and not, therefore, irrelevant and an interference in the treatment. Relationships between staff members and the patient's relatives can also prove to be helpful if they are actively cultivated rather than ignored or dismissed. Staff may learn useful details about their patient from a mother or supportive friend, as well as this potentially leading to much better-constructed care arrangements if staff are aware of the family's viewpoints when the patient is discharged home from hospital.

Harm is less likely to befall a patient if they have previously been able to rebuff harmful difficulty. If they have shown resilience to strain and to increased demands upon their robustness, and shown initiative or resourcefulness, then new dangers or challenges may reasonably be expected to present only quite a manageable situation for the patient to deal with. When a patient has a sense of themselves as an individual, they naturally and instinctively will be active in their own self-defence. Early in treatment, this may not be the case, particularly in schizophrenic illness, and the vulnerability of these patients new to treatment really requires vigilant thought and consideration as to exactly what their needs might be. They will be inexperienced in caring for themselves in a thoughtful way, and not at all used to troubleshooting for themselves. So, being nearly wholly dependent on the staff for their care, they will trust and hope for a safe passage through their treatment.

The reliability of patients is an individual characteristic which must be taken into account for their successful management. Reliability builds up over a lifetime, and its relevant periodicity is the recent past. It can be affected by, among other factors, mood, stability, attitude that is dependent upon the present environment and relationships, current preoccupations, and motivation. Good relationships with staff, as described above, can prove seminal in cultivating reliability in a patient, which of course, in turn, makes the staff's tasks much easier.

The reliability of the psychotherapy unit's clinical systems and processes is equally relevant to developing safety and security for the psychotherapy treatment's progress. It is widely held that aspects of therapy, interactions, clinical expertise, and experience are the drivers of therapeutic change, and that systems and processes take very much a back seat in mental healthcare. But applied policy regarding ward numbers, locked or unlocked ward door decisions, ward psychotherapy group routines, care over occupational therapy and other off-ward arrangements, visiting hours, and constant checking over patient whereabouts all greatly contribute to patient safety when routines that are reliable are established. If the patient becomes quite used to what they can expect as a patient on that ward, they do tend to settle and think as normally and healthily as their condition will allow.

When the ward feels safe in its predictability to the patient, their sensitivity to cooperation with the staff becomes gentler and their attitudes more biddable. Life as a mental hospital patient can seem very daunting to them, but if they feel safe the staff will be able to gain best access to their psychological core in order to be able to treat them psychologically. When feeling safe, patients are able to access much deeper parts of themselves in ward psychotherapy groups than when anxious about their situation.

And when they are feeling their care is safe today, they are much more likely to demonstrate preparedness for the future in coming days and weeks, and for any as yet unforeseen challenges or difficulties that they may in due course encounter.

Patients' views of harm generally coincide with each other's views regarding obviously undesirable events but, due to the broad differences in their self-defence abilities, they may differ considerably in both their ability to take decisions and their needs for safety measures taken on their behalf. For example, a locked ward door in position to prevent absconding from the ward may make one patient feel safe while another feels claustrophobic and angry because of it. Generally, mental health patients, including schizophrenic and schizoaffective patients, are generous and forgiving about incidents that have gone wrong, and are more concerned about the coordination of their care than about isolated incidents, even though these can be extremely serious. Schizophrenic and schizoaffective patients can learn to trust their staff in practical terms as well as psychological ones, so great care really should be taken over a patient's likely interpretation and psychological processes in an anticipated situation when the consequences of these going wrong could be quite disastrous.

Mental health staff, like many others, often work within restrictions of time, energy, specific and general responsibilities, academic rigour, maintenance of harmonious interactions among themselves, and often the strictures visited upon them at work by their institution's state of finance. Up-to-date training and professional development needs to be constantly maintained by the staff's hospital or academic centre, and within this remit attending to safety becomes an ongoing business and everyone's job. The academic institution or hospital has to maintain the full picture as taught to the staff, from the absence of harm to the presence of safety. It needs to create a culture of staff happiness, which tends to lead to successful staff practice. Maintaining staff happiness affects their behaviour, engagement, empowerment, and wellbeing, leading to a positive ambience for patients on the ward and to patient safety because of the absence of likely harm. The mental health of the patients remains within an ambit of perceived safety when their perception does not dwell on matters likely to be dangerous or harmful to them. But if they are likely to be exposed to very real danger then the psychological processes they will need to undergo to handle the danger must be rehearsed in relation to their likely illness-derived mental deficits like thought block or loss of memory, such as a simple but clear warning, which will confer guidance in dangerously confusing situations. Unusual patients may already be afflicted by unusual attitudes or concerns from their earlier lives, which staff may discover from their artwork or writing. A patient may have suffered considerable interference from within their family and, if this can be detected by the staff, the patient's safety could be greatly enhanced by keeping the family at a distance from him or her, and reassuring them. Failure to clarify the patient's psychological characteristics may lead to imprecise communication with them which, as already argued, is a critical ingredient in patient safety.

Clinical staff, from trainee psychiatric nurses to senior consultant psychiatrists, try to promote an environment where both knowledge and kindness for mentally ill patients abound. Each staff member will have joined their profession through inspiration for alleviating suffering, and is usually highly motivated to work with their colleagues in this direction. The more senior staff may hold seminars for the others in their team, and go themselves to lectures and conferences on relevant topics. The professional literature contains many instances of cases where a patient has responded unusually well to treatment, demonstrating therapeutic truths hitherto only referred to in theory and not widely known about; these transformational cases tend to strengthen resolve among the staff for their work. Accurate knowledge of their fields, and a kind, tolerant approach allow mental health staff to get the best results for their patients after their earlier states of total disorder, confusion and fear which brought them to hospital.

Clinical supervision is recognised as being very helpful to staff working in mental health. Working clinically in a mental health capacity can create considerable strain on the clinician's capacity to live a normal, healthy life, and to perform safely at work. Clinical supervision of their work is regarded by many as being absolutely essential for good working practice. It provides valuable and necessary opportunities for the clinical worker to share their experiences, test ideas and often to offload anxieties so that these may be scrutinised, analysed and resolved, and no longer interfere within the staff member's daily working life.

Undergoing their own psychoanalysis is a sound way of securely managing staff's personal resilience to events in their own life and their ability to retain their innate robustness whatever they have to address. This can also strengthen their reactions to their work, and is adopted by many workers in mental health. Mindfulness and reflective practice enable staff to reach appropriate conclusions about episodes or encounters with patients and others during working practice. Simple reactions to these can be painful or even create inappropriate responses in staff which they need a chance to address and resolve. Mindfulness stills the mind, bringing it back to the present moment. While calm, the mind can observe aspects of a recent troubling situation that had previously not been noticed. The mind can sometimes utilise this review to answer questions which had previously only given rise to worry. Reflective practice may calm anxieties by placing troubling factors or observations in context. Specific difficulties may be seen within a broader framework, where different parts of this can provide answers or explanations for the original problems.

One's own role in a team may be seen as leadership within one's own work's requirements; and safety is every team member's business, both their own safety and that of the patients, so each staff member can lead with suggestions and any good ideas for safety plans. If a staff member is responsible for output according to a patient's requirements, leadership can be shown in producing that output. Success is due to the whole team's efforts, with each worker enacting leadership where appropriate according to their own role, and co-ordinating their work with other team members and the overall aims of the team within its guidelines. Safety is promoted by the absence of bullying, racism, and discrimination. As well as adopting responsibilities in keeping with leadership, a staff member can be a good team player, promoting teamwork, accountability, and forward thinking, all of which contribute to the safety of a therapeutic environment. By keeping their own words, behaviour, habits, values, and hopes open and positive, staff can enhance the destiny of the patients on the wards who pick up, in their plight in hospital in the staff's care, all of the psychological legacy that the staff endow to them. Staff have to develop resilience, always remain polite, and learn from any mistakes so as to improve the quality of their work. Openness, honesty and transparency are needed to facilitate this learning and ensure the developmental process of establishing and enhancing the new psychoanalytic psychotherapeutic treatment of schizophrenic illness. This treatment of schizophrenia and schizoaffective disorder is still only infrequently practised, so everything that can be should be learned from all current and recent instances of its practice. We should be thinking ahead towards a time when the common pitfalls associated with it are well enough known to ensure safety for the large majority of patients who are given the treatment.

Open and clear communication is conducive to patient safety, especially regarding known hazard points. Schizophrenic and schizoaffective patients often can only think slowly or inaccurately; their memories may be adversely affected by their illness, and sometimes they experience clouding of consciousness. IQs can fall by ten to twelve points due to a schizophrenic illness. If they are likely to face actual danger, it makes sense to place them in sheltered accommodation until their minds are capable of protecting themselves as they deserve to be protected. The objective of ensuring patient safety is to prevent harm. The risks and benefits of the treatment to be undertaken should be explained, together with the consequences of doing nothing as contrasted with receiving the treatment. But if all the parties, ie. the patient, their relatives, the intended therapist, and the hospital consultant, all agree to undertake the treatment, then thought must be given to the most likely hazards and effective psychological management put in place.

Risks may be embraced, managed, or avoided. Clinical supervision, reflective practice and staff's own psychoanalyses embrace existing risk for themselves and for their patients, and are an effective means whereby risk can be embraced. Managing psychological risk is a substantial arm of clinical psychiatric training. Profound knowledge of psychiatric disorders is required to achieve good psychological management of patients on a psychiatric ward, and to sustain effective safety measures. Managing risk needs to be practised for physical as well as psychological risk. Supervision of patients' physical health has recently been greatly intensified nationally, which is certainly needed because schizophrenic patients' life spans have in the past trailed by fifteen to twenty years behind the life expectancy of psychologically healthy people. In addition, psychiatric patients are also at physical risk, especially early in their treatment, of becoming lost during their journeys between hospital and their analyst's consulting room and back to hospital if several transport systems have to be used. This possibility could be lessened by providing clear details of the bus routes or railway stations to be used. If the analyst is worried about the patient's mental state they can be sent back to the hospital in a taxi. Registering what time they leave the ward or the analyst's consulting room is another way of being sure that they remain safe until they arrive at the due time at the other end of their journey. If they are late, steps may be taken to find them. Knowing the patient's location always, clinical vigilance, and good staff training are all ways of managing risk.

Ways of avoiding risk would be regular fire drills, checking discretely, and, if necessary, for the absence of weapons, and ensuring generous funding for the hospital unit. But being risk averse in a psychologically therapeutic environment can invite harm because, in working with the mind, trying to eliminate risk can engage its presence as a possibility, and it may then become a reality in some form in people's minds, either the staff's minds or in the patients' minds. So the presence of possible risk should be borne in the staff's minds and managed, with steps taken to render its actualisation very unlikely. Where possible risk is likely, and particularly where the potential danger is great or very serious, the patient must be protected from harm. Careful forethought and planning by the team working with the patient can usually forestall dangers such as these.

CHAPTER 23

FUNDING, ON A PAR WITH PHYSICAL TREATMENTS: CONCEPTUAL BLOCKS

The treatment and management of mental illnesses have been underfunded for many decades compared with the treatment and management of physical illnesses. It is true that most advances in psychiatry during this time have been in the production and use of new medications. Some new psychological therapies have also been developed, such as Avatar Therapy, and also Cognitive Behaviour Therapy (CBT), Cognitive Analytic Therapy (CAT), and motivational interviewing techniques, for which treatments patients are referred to psychologists by psychiatrists. Psychoanalysis is continually evolving, so today's psychoanalysts tend to develop Freud's original tenets even if from outside they appear to manifest internal disagreement within this profession.

But these innovative new understandings usually indicate progress in grasping patients' psychological functioning, and should not be regarded from outside the profession as mere internal wranglings. Gradually, psychoanalysis is establishing universally observed unconscious phenomena, and some of these, which every analyst would espouse, include transference effects, repetition of mental behaviour in an individual patient, internalisation of aspects of their surrounding environments, and projection of parts of themselves into other people. Freud was not aware of many of the recently identified phenomena, but adherence to their existence by successive generations of psychoanalysts does not necessarily represent a departure on their part from much of the foundation he established for psychoanalysis.

With clinicians working in this way, the general public nonetheless cry out for psychological or "talking therapies", and these may be very effective once any basic requirement for medication by a patient has been met. Psychological treatments, together with skilful prescribing of the best medications available, are capable of resolving the problems of many of today's individual patients who seek help from psychiatry; sometimes the remedy only lasts in the short-term, however, which tends to be the case with CBT. Deeper psychological exploration such as that provided by psychoanalytic psychotherapy may be needed to access fundamental rifts in mental construction. The question that has to be asked is: is it worth plumbing these depths in individual patients? If they are plumbed safely, the patient is likely to be able to go on to a thoroughly flourishing and fruitful life, like any other patient who has had a heart transplant and is greeted back at work with enthusiasm when they return, recovered. As yet there are only a few of these joyful psychologically restored patients outside the psychoanalytic profession who come to notice. This may be partly because they are encouraged to get on with their lives and not look backwards. But there is a bedrock of people who have enormously benefited from a psychoanalysis. Why should this work not be examined closely, its necessities of protection, defence, and care of its patients, the facilities needed, and the most successful clinical techniques, evaluated, and the process learned from start to finish the way Christiaan Barnard developed heart transplants?

This author thinks the reason is that psychological treatments are invisible, intangible and difficult to conceptualise, whereas physical treatments are visible, tangible, and easy to understand. This, the author thinks, is the reason for a general block among most groups of people except in the psychological professions in accepting that psychological issues, including curative techniques that potentially resolve illnesses, are as real as physical objects like artificial limbs or mobility chairs, or cochlear implants that people can look at before being hidden inside their head and enabling them to hear. The value of implanting a helpful idea inside their own head is not so easy to perceive. The cost of a cochlear implant in 2017 is £21,158.82 (Department of Health, 2017) which would pay for nearly two years of psychoanalytic psychotherapy, ie. approximately one third of an average duration of an analytic treatment's sessions for a schizophrenic patient. And enabling a schizophrenic patient to think differently could save their life. Highly intelligent, determined, patient and forgiving schizophrenic patients are capable of responding to clinical initiatives. And once they understand how far they are misguided, equivalent to the clinical state prior to insertion of a cochlear implant, what they make of their opportunities then is up to them, like the use the cochlear implant patient will make of their new hearing ability; and all clinicians hope that the schizophrenic patient will accept the analyst's presentation of reality and reject their own mistaken presumptions, attitudes, and beliefs. Their cognitive functioning may have been damaged meanwhile, however, and although cognitive exercises may be helpful, full restoration is not generally found to be the likely outcome. Nonetheless, their improvements in insight, broad-based comprehension, emotional stability, peace of mind, and access to their own innate initiative do offer scope for a fresh approach to the world for the recovering patient, who may, one way or another, find alternative ways and means of compensating for their partial loss of their original cognitive abilities.

Lack of personnel is another probable reason why funding tends to be scarce in psychiatry compared with cardiology or orthopaedics. Without adequate staffing, funding cannot be used for patient benefit. Training a psychoanalyst is very expensive. And to treat schizophrenic patients it is necessary first to train in psychiatry in order to be able to recognise and then handle clinically any psychotic episode the patient may manifest during her analytic therapy. The expensive training, and its length, may deter all but the most dedicated clinicians from pursuing their ambitions to alleviate schizophrenic patients from their illnesses.

So trained staff are needed to implement psychologically resolving cures that have been developed to treat psychologically suffering patients as much as delivering artificial limbs, new hearts, cochlear implants or mobility chairs to treat amputees, heart failure, deafness or immobility. A fresh, new mind is as useful to a needy patient as being able to get about, hear, or exercise. Training psychiatric and psychoanalytic staff is as important to Medicine as manufacturing artificial limbs, mobility chairs, heart valves, and cochlear implants. Showing psychiatric and psychoanalytic trainees what is possible in their professions is money very well spent. One of the PPCC model's uses is that it presents the reality of psychoanalytic psychotherapeutic treatment in a clear and undeniably practical form which is justifiably applicable to suitable cases of schizophrenic illness. This could be very useful in helping physicians and surgeons and non-psychologists to understand the treatment during discussions about funding.

People experiencing their first psychotic breakdown are extremely fortunate if they are contacted by an Early Intervention Service (EIS). These EIS services are recorded in the recent Schizophrenia Commission report, "Effective interventions in schizophrenia, the economic case: A report prepared for the Schizophrenia Commission" of November 2012 (Andrews et al, 2012), as saving £5,493 to the NHS per service user in the first year of psychosis, mainly due to saved costs of bed occupancy. The same report identifies this cost as being that a night in a mental health inpatient bed costs £321. Thus this saving is explained by avoiding a two and a half week long admission, which would save not only money but also avoid the considerable trauma of admission to a psychiatric ward. So, already, psychological treatment is seen to promote a basically sound approach to saving the NHS money.

The cost of a psychoanalytic psychotherapy treatment with a psychoanalyst is usually approximately £60 per day. With five sessions per week and allowing for six weeks holiday for the analyst per year, this amounts to an annual cost of £13,800; and for a whole eight year treatment, which is a generous allowance, this cost would be £110,400. With bed occupancy at £321 per night, accommodation costs in hospital as an inpatient for one year would be £117,165, and for, typically, five years during an individual treatment, the sum would be £586,000. Thus the treatment and accommodation costs would amount to £696,400.

This compares not unfavourably with the cost in British £s sterling of a heart transplant in the USA in 2011 of £799,631, and of a double lung transplant of £639,000 (UNOS, 2011). A heart-lung transplant in 2011 would have cost £920,413, a kidney transplant £210,707, and an intestine transplant £967,219. All these costs are very expensive indeed, but with careful patient selection, where these operations are seriously needed they do save the life of the patient. And the accommodation costs in hospital, as well as hostels, of untreated schizophrenic patients over their lifetime can be very high, and often at least the £586,000 spent on a schizophrenic patient in treatment.

The British newspaper *The Times* on 22 December 2016 carried an article headed "First patients to get bionic eyes on NHS". It read, in part, "[Professor Paulo Stanga, of the Manchester Royal Eye Hospital] was confident that the £150,000 US-made system would be routine within five years". A mind capable of fresh insight endows at least as much clarity of vision as a bionic eye. The bionic eye is visible, tangible, and its function easily understood. Psychoanalytic psychotherapy is invisible, intangible, and challenging to understand. But psychoanalytic psychotherapy can be practised, has been practised, and will be again, and in skilled hands does restore personal clarity of vision to patients feeling as desperate as those without an eye. A new mind is no less influential in a patient's life than a new eye; the cost of a new eye happens to be only 0.25 that of a new mind, but the benefits to the patient are remarkably similar.

The ongoing costs in a recovered schizophrenic patient include medications, outpatient appointments, GP appointments, and possibly Community psychiatric nurse visits initially, while confidence builds. But in a successful treatment there will be major savings in NHS and community care resource usage over the considerable use by untreated or minimally treated schizophrenic patients. These considerably used resources include increased hospital bed occupancy, ie. over the lifetime minus that during treated patients' treatment; hostel staff salaries and all accommodation costs; Accident and Emergency Department visits; police vigilance in safety management, ie. sleeping rough recovery and collection from destitution on the streets, alcoholic behaviour, and any social misbehaviour; day care centre community services costs, eg. staff salaries, heating, lighting, overheads, meals, occupational therapy, transport; social care arrangements, eg. social worker support, clothing, nutrition, hygiene; and benefits payments. There will also be the ongoing costs as in recovered schizophrenic patients of medication; outpatient appointments at times until return to GP care; and increased CPN care. A hospital outpatient appointment cost £114 in 2015, and an Accident and Emergency Department attendance £132 (Department of Health, 2015). A recovered schizophrenic patient may need an occasional GP or other appointment, but because they have recovered their mind they will on increasingly frequent occasions be resourceful enough to find their own solutions rather than present in a vacuous, helpless state yet again to doctors and clinical staff.

Just as kidney transplants subsidise all other types of organ transplantation because of obviating the high costs of dialysis, so it is anticipated that those intelligent, determined, patient, forgiving patients who really want to be well are likely to provide returns in different ways to society in gratitude to the systems that provided their care. Patients' own initiatives are the key to the success of this process and of their own destinies. They need protection during their treatment of a kind that the professions will learn with the experience of treating successive cases. If this care is provided when needed then the patients' own initiative may begin to flourish and thereby lead them into their lives without needing further help beyond occasional check-ups with their GP.

The average amount potentially earned by a healthy recovered schizophrenic patient aged thirty-five to sixty-five years might be, for example, £25,000 pa. If they then worked for thirty years their amassed total earnings would be £750,000. Even for a single recovered patient this would supersede the costs of their analytic treatment of £110,400 and hospital accommodation of £586,000, amounting to £696,400. Given that the annual cost to society of schizophrenia is £60,000 per patient (Andrews et al, 2012), over a restricted lifetime of, say, fifty years (schizophrenic patients tend to die fifteen to twenty years earlier than healthy others), a patient diagnosed aged twenty would cost society £1,800,000, and more if they lived longer. These are all large sums of money, but the costs have to be spent because the patients will not go away. The only way to see the patients "go away" is to make them well so they want to "go away". Then, with their initiative flourishing – and most schizophrenic patients show some element of initiative, for example in occupational therapy – with help and the clear understanding that only they can help themselves long-term, they may remove themselves from major elements of NHS care.

This argument is not very different from the rationale of the transplant system. In February 2009 the UK transplant programme realised annual gross savings of £316m per annum to the NHS compared with the cost of alternative medical treatment such as kidney dialysis (NHS Blood and Transplant, 2009). Increasing organ transplantation rates by 50% could achieve a further cost saving of £200m per annum to NHS commissioners. Transplanting kidneys saves life-long dialysis, and renal transplantation subsidises all other types of organ transplantation. The more of it that is done, therefore, the better, benefiting not just grateful patients but also the NHS.

The Report of the Schizophrenia Commission in November 2012 (not The Economic Case) described schizophrenia as "The Abandoned Illness" (The Schizophrenia Commission, 2012). There is no need for it to be abandoned. Intensive psychoanalytic work with it is increasingly being conducted in America (Robbins, 1993), Sweden (Cullberg, 1991), (Cullberg and Levander, 1991), the UK (Jackson and Williams, 1994), (Williams,1999) and in Denmark (Rosenbaum et al, 2005), with results that are clarifying how schizophrenic illness may be treated and sometimes resolved. Susan Hingley writes about the contribution of psychodynamic theory and practice to the treatment of psychosis (Hingley, 2006, p. 211): "......research reports, case studies, and reviews published over the past ten years have pointed towards a small sub-group of sufferers fulfilling DSM-III-R criteria for schizophrenia who can respond to intensive, often long-term, psychodynamically-oriented psychotherapy". And the second generation of antipsychotic medications certainly have their uses in contributing to the efficacy of long-term psychological treatments, even if they have to be prescribed with care due to unwanted side-effects. The results of recent psychoanalytic work into schizophrenia have generally agreed on a number of consensus points, eg. that addressing schizophrenic patients directly and with enough latitude can help them to engage effectively with themselves as a focus which they can then change and adapt; that through intensive work a degree of self-reliance can develop, thus decreasing needfulness of care by supportive agencies; that learning to tolerate unpleasant affects at some times can lead to appreciation of better affects at other times, and improve sociability; and that an improved sense of reality may develop, enabling the patient to fend better for themselves in the real world they are living in.

The number of schizophrenic patients receiving psychoanalytic psychotherapy who have been studied is not great, and exploration in this direction is in its very early stages, but addressing this previously "abandoned illness" psychologically is well underway; for example ISPS, the International Society for the Psychological and Social Treatment of Schizophrenia and Other Psychoses, and its publications, has led to a great and increasingly active expansion in psychological understanding of schizophrenia. Common denominators are observed, as described above, in those aspects of the illness which may be more easily alleviated. Generalisations should be made cautiously so that false hopes are not raised. The numbers treated with deeply reaching treatments such as psychoanalytic psychotherapy should initially be kept small and patients carefully selected so that accurate results may be carefully obtained and learned from, so that scarce financial resources remain well spent, and so that good care can be taken of the patients. Schizophrenia will only be abandoned if those involved in managing patients with it abandon it, and there is every sign in today's psychiatry that there is enthusiasm for engaging deeply with schizophrenic patients. Analytic treatments are rigorous, and a high level of clinical skill is required for good results. But the extension of clinical skills from those experienced in them to their successors, before psychiatric psychoanalytic skills become lost to the patient population's access to them, may yet be possible. There still are working psychiatrically trained psychoanalysts who have this knowledge and could be invited to share it before it disappears.

PART VII

PSYCHIATRY AND RELATED PHILOSOPHICAL CONCEPTS OF HEALING

....

DR GILLIAN STEGGLES

CHAPTER 24

MEDICAL ETHICS: THE ETHICS OF TRANSFORMATIVE MENTAL HEALTH TREATMENTS

Medical ethics as a discipline may be traced back at least to the time of Hippocrates in ancient Greece, in the fifth century BC. Hippocrates himself did not aver "First do no harm", although this is often attributed to him (Sokol, 2013). But his Hippocratic Oath did contain the seeds of ethical responsibility that all of today's doctors address when they graduate in Medicine and take up clinical duties.

Raanan Gillon was at the forefront of British medical ethics when he published in 1986 his book "Philosophical medical ethics", based on a twenty-six part series in the British Medical Journal (Gillon, 1994). He introduced to BMJ readers an approach to medical ethics developed by the Americans Beauchamp and Childress (Beauchamp and Childress, 1989), which adheres to four prima facie moral principles and attention to these principles' scope of application. This "four principles plus scope" approach has become a cornerstone since the 1980s of the medical ethics taught in medical schools, and is also respected in the USA.

The four principles plus scope approach claims that all of us, from a wide range of cultural, political, religious, racial, and moral backgrounds and beliefs, will be able to adhere to these four principles, and also fundamentally understand and effect their scope of application. The four prima facie principles are: respect for autonomy, beneficence, non-maleficence, and justice. "Scope" indicates how the principles are applied. "Prima facie" means that the principle is binding unless it conflicts with another moral principle – if it does we have to choose between them (Gillon, 1994). Gillon is at pains to point out that this four principles plus scope approach does not provide answers to problems in any way automatically, but rather provides "a common set of moral commitments, a common moral language, and a common set of moral issues". Gillon insists

"We should consider these in each case, before coming to our own answer using our preferred moral theory or other approach, to choose between these principles when they conflict."

Respect for autonomy is the moral obligation to respect the deliberated self-rule (autonomy) of others in so far as such respect is compatible with equal respect for the autonomy of all potentially affected. In Immanuel Kant's terms, respect for autonomy is also described as treating others as ends in themselves and never merely as means (Gillon, 1994).

Medical ethics requires us to respect patients' autonomy with many implicit prima facie obligations. Thus, as Gillon says, we have to obtain informed consent from patients before subjecting them to any procedure to try to help them. Healthcare workers explicitly or implicitly promise their patients and clients that they will keep confidential the information confided to them. Keeping promises is a way of respecting people's autonomy, in the same way as we rely on the promises made to us by others. Equally, we must not deceive each other, for example about patients' diagnosed illnesses, unless they clearly wish to be deceived. Being on time for appointments respects the other's autonomy, as the appointment amounts to a kind of mutual promise; if we do not keep an appointment we break the promise (Gillon, 1994).

Good communication skills permit respect for patients' autonomy to be exercised; the clinician is able to regulate how much or how little information is provided to the patient about, for example, a proposed intervention. In doing so, the patient's autonomy is liberated into its own decision-making capacity, and the ethical principle of respect for autonomy is fulfilled. Gillon emphasises the importance of listening as well as telling during clinical consultations such as these, in order to uphold their ethical probity.

Respect for autonomy remains valid in psychiatric care even when illnesses as serious as schizophrenia are considered. Indeed, working with the patient's autonomy, as contrasted with their expostulations resulting from exasperation with the illness, is one of the surest ways to obtain cooperation for unpleasant aspects of care. Most psychiatric patients are subject to distasteful experiences such as taking medication, whether tablets or injections, exeat restrictions on sorties outside the locked ward, or even simply having to attend sessions and appointments when they would rather not. Consistency, firmness, and good humour are the best techniques for dissolving resistance, especially when directed specifically towards the patient's autonomy, and sometimes an oblique approach can also be successful.

Relatives' and carers' needs and wishes must be taken into account when working with matters of a patient's autonomy, but great care is needed to retain the patient's personal perspective independently from theirs, as sometimes he or she needs a certain space in which to "try to be well as themselves" without interference. Here their sense of themselves may be nursed slowly and carefully so that it can begin to grow alongside their self-helping autonomy and alongside the family's wishes being kept at arms' length from the safety of the ward. Where the patient is being treated as an outpatient, their autonomy tends to be more assertive due to the experienced stressors and stresses of life in the community. Their autonomy needs to be respected and worked with, to help the patient make the best use of what care and support is available to them at this stage in their illness' management. A patient who feels empowered by their autonomy being respected is likely to make much better progress than one who senses that what they have to say makes no difference to their own management.

Gillon's summary (Gillon, 1994) of the four principles plus scope approach to medical ethics considers beneficence and non-maleficence, like his review of autonomy, in a similarly helpful context that indicates their respective importance. He shows that they need to be considered together, because whenever we try to help others we inevitably risk harming them; healthcare workers always aim at producing net benefit over harm. And even if we have or recognise no obligation of beneficence to others we still have an obligation not to harm them. So the ethical objective is to achieve beneficence with non-maleficence, a task that involves taking great care concerning very many aspects of the patient's treatment. Assessments of harm and benefit require accuracy in evaluating risk and probability, which in psychiatric care is at least as difficult as in physical medicine. Gillon says that empowerment is relevant when considering beneficence, even perhaps as a new moral obligation: "On reflection I think that empowerment is however, essentially an action that combines the two moral obligations of beneficence and respect for autonomy to help patients in ways that not only respect but also enhance their autonomy."

In psychiatric illness the patient's autonomy is commonly particularly compromised by the illness preventing the patient having access to it within themselves. Sometimes the interference is due to compromised mental functions such as cognition or memory. Alternatively, the patient's mind may not yet be able to grasp aspects of their life which later they may wish to adopt in their own way. Protection by clinicians of the patient's options is thus critically important for the psychiatric patient's future, at a time when they are unable to protect themselves.

The fourth prima facie moral principle, justice, is often regarded as being synonymous with fairness, as Gillon describes. He divides justice into three categories: fair distribution of scarce resources (distribution justice), respect for people's rights (rights based justice), and respect for morally acceptable laws (legal justice) (Gillon, 1994). It can be argued that at times it is as important to treat unequals unequally as to treat equals equally. Giving priority in healthcare to those who most need it, or who most deserve it, balanced against those who most want it requires a form of justice that can rarely be fully answered in all its aspects simultaneously.

It could thus be argued in isolation that every patient suffering from perhaps the most severe and serious mental illness of all, schizophrenia, who has the potential to emerge out of it, given the resources, should justly be given the opportunity to learn about themselves and their illness in psychoanalytic psychotherapy. The relative costs of this, as has been argued in Chapter 23, compare favourably with equivalent major physical procedures, with no less risk but with potentially equivalent benefit in QALYs, quality adjusted life years. Schizophrenia causes as much individual debility as heart disease, and the human suffering involved is at least as intense. The alleviation of this suffering arrives much more slowly in psychiatric treatment than through a heart transplant operation, but is as effective in a successful treatment. Careful patient selection is key to identifying those who do have the potential to use psychoanalytic psychotherapy effectively, and to applying the treatment successfully within psychiatry's armamentarium. Previous evident application to a discipline or effort during their earlier life, and attributes of insight, patience, tolerance, determination, and courage are among the characteristics that augur well for a particular patient's intention to undergo and complete the treatment.

Scope of application of the four prima facie principles, ie. respect for autonomy, beneficence and non-maleficence, and justice, may be a source of radical disagreement, however much we agree upon our moral commitments and moral obligations to others, as Gillon describes (Gillon, 1994). And as he writes, the rights of agencies that should morally be taken into account may be disputed if these agencies include the environment, works of art, and live animals or plants; should some, or any, of these agencies be considered as having rights? But by far the most usual scope that is discussed in medical ethics is that available to a particular patient with a particular combination of factors contributing to their ill health.

Psychiatric patients fall within the scope of application by psychiatric mental healthcare staff in their work. And here the need for justice, autonomy, and the moral scope for application could not be stronger. Being trapped within schizophrenia is surely one of the most terrifying situations known to humankind. It is very important not to let malfeasance occur, as this can ruin a patient's life. The beneficence of alleviating schizophrenic illness using psychoanalytic psychotherapy is a clinical ambition that has grounds for optimism because it can be done. The traps and pitfalls of the procedure are still being identified because it is such a novel treatment for schizophrenic illness. But the more it is carried out, the better will be the results if lessons are learned each time something does go wrong. The suffering of untreated schizophrenic patients is so terrible that clinicians do feel driven to try the best possible therapeutic solutions where these might be effective. And there are always environmental factors that may need special attention regarding patient safety, when a careful appraisal of the patient's anticipated vulnerabilities must be conducted.

The question of justice in distributing healthcare has been discussed by Norman Daniels (Daniels, 1985). This was followed by his later book describing justice as it spans all socially controllable factors of health (Daniels, 2008). He asserts that his theory of justice for health is integrated, practical, and global in scope. But perhaps he does not consider how deeply intertwined health is with social justice? Should these not be considered separately? Also, relative inequality can have an impact on health no matter where the baseline is set. And would his liberal views be supported globally? (Rid and Biller-Andorno, 2009).

These questions apply to justice in distributing general healthcare. They form one of the arguments that have been, largely unconsciously, used against psychiatric care in Medicine. Healthcare is seen widely as care of the health of the community; that is, "seen" as needing to be supplied. What is not seen is not focused on. A vagrant in the community needs a home, food, fresh clothes. But the quality of his mind is "him", the person who he or she is, what he or she says; it is his or her present state, invisible to many medical people as much as to the community. Isn't it something best left alone or dealt with as an intrinsic part of the person who is rehoused, fed, and re-clothed?

The truth is, he or she almost certainly actually needs psychiatric management if they are distractible, talking to themselves or behaving oddly. And their young counterparts receiving Outreach and Early Intervention services require definitive treatment after the intensive first year of support, to prevent them reaching this state after sliding down a long, slippery slope of despair and decline. These young acutely ill schizophrenic patients should be reclaimed from schizophrenia whenever possible. The disease process, starting psychologically in pathological experiences that progress destructively within their early environments, needs to be terminated in treatment, and clear thinking stimulated to replace it so that the patient becomes able to help themselves. This is perfectly possible with psychoanalytic psychotherapy in skilled, experienced hands.

Morally and ethically it is fair and equitable that a young, energetic person full of potential should be given the chance to use their mind for the rest of their life as much as a middle-aged person with responsibilities should be given the opportunities consequent upon receiving a new heart for the rest of their life. No doubt symposia will need to be held to develop checks and balances in funding healthcare, such as building on NICE's experience and advice. What needs to be made absolutely clear is that remedial treatment of schizophrenia is possible; clinicians need to be adequately trained; patients must be cautiously and expertly assessed and selected; and the treatments must be carried out very carefully with every due regard for the safety of the patients. Heart transplants no longer raise eyebrows. Recovery from schizophrenia should similarly be expected as a genuine possibility from a treatment that is known to be potentially remedial, in suitable patients. For success, the treatment should be based securely in suitable accommodation, everyone in the team must be fully informed and knowledgeable, the ward base adequately funded for long enough, the patients should have access to sufficient ancillary services such as occupational therapy and clinical psychologists who can administer specific ancillary treatments where needs arise, and every provision should be made for the safety of the patients, whose mental functioning is so badly compromised. They have been selected for their personal characteristics rendering them suitable for the treatment; they know they are expected to work hard at it. But until mental agility returns to them, often several years hence, their cognitive functioning may be poor and beyond their own efforts to restore. Close observation of the patients should be maintained so as to understand exactly the issues that they are addressing. Oversight is very difficult to avoid, but can cause serious problems if something important is missed. If all the team and the patient have developed trust, however, the patient may still recover and the mistakes made may be learned. If a clear ethical stance has been maintained throughout, good and strong decisions are much more likely to be made than if any woolliness of thinking at all is tolerated; and good, strong decisions tend to lead to good patient outcomes. Some early heart transplant patients did lose their lives but, as well as exercising their own free choice, also acted in the cause of future successes so that more patients could be helped to live.

CHAPTER 25

THE PHILOSOPHY AND VALUES OF THE NHS IN RELATION TO PSYCHIATRIC PATIENTS

When Aneurin Bevan created the National Health Service to provide healthcare for the people of Britain on 5 July 1948 he shared with the British people his vision of protecting their health "from the cradle to the grave" based on three central principles:

1. That it should meet the needs of everyone
2. That it should be free at the point of delivery
3. That it should be based on clinical need, not ability to pay.

Since 1948, and with very few exceptions, these principles have governed how the NHS is run, in most people's minds and understanding of it as an organisation. It could be stated that the NHS is virtually the most loved institution in Britain, with only one or two others equally loved by its population, and whenever there is a financial crisis or turbulence, the NHS is regularly "ring-fenced" to preserve its functioning as normal. The NHS's influence is ubiquitous within the British population's life, affecting the lives of every one of us without exception, and usually multiples of times for each individual. It is a great luxury to be able to depend upon it when we really need it, and we are aware that we are the envy of the world for this. Its three central principles endear it to our sense of fairness, community, generosity, security, and, to a large extent, our cohesion as a nation. Feelings run very strong among the population and the NHS's workforce alike that its ethos and values should be preserved come what may to our nation or politics, and loyalty to it is intensely felt and acted upon whenever it or its running comes under threat; some of its workforce have been known to strike, including quite recently, when a sector feels its safety or another aspect has been singled out for change that is contested.

Psychological aspects of people's health have tended, in modern Britain as in other developed parts of the world, but not so much in India and the East, to be thought of in terms of the Cartesian division between mind and body. In India and many other parts of Asia psychological wellbeing is conceptualised as being wholly integrated with bodily health, and commonly in these regions a person will say they are feeling pain in some part of their body when actually, upon careful overall observation, it may become apparent that they are depressed. Equally, with severe physical pain, they may express spiritual anxieties about their future. Physical and psychological distress are much more integrated as an aspect of their lives, relating to wellbeing or not being well at all. But in Britain, in the last hundred years or so, advances in physical medicine have raced ahead of understanding of psychological medicine, which has been considered a quite different field of study. Modern day genetics, tissue operations such as heart transplants, electronic prostheses like limb extensions, and exoskeletons that enable ambulation in otherwise wheelchair-bound individuals have all reached advanced stages of sophistication while psychological medicine science has somewhat lagged behind.

But this is changing. By 2017 the British population is aware how strained our services for psychological welfare maintenance have become. This strain is due, mainly, to lack of knowledge and understanding about psychological medicine, what it can achieve, how effective it can be, and strains of many kinds on clinicians. Heart transplants, electronic prostheses, mobility chairs, and genetic manipulations can all transform appropriate patients' lives. Exactly the same process is possible for psychologically afflicted patients when the treatment chosen is the right one, when the patient is prepared to persevere with the treatment, when a clinician with the right skills is available to deliver it, and when suitable facilities are available near enough to the patient's home community.

It is probably because psychological treatments are invisible, difficult to conceptualise, and cannot be physically touched or handled, that the public find both them, the illnesses they have the ability to resolve, and patients suffering from mental illnesses, subjects to be avoided and sometimes disdained. This is a phenomenon not to be simply criticised, however, because its basis amounts to ignorance, fear, perplexity, some horror, and so much compassion that the public generally have difficulty in overcoming these obstacles to be able to engage with mental illness calmly and constructively. Education is key to helping the treatment of mental illness to find a similar level of understanding as physical illness among the public, the government, and patients and their families, in the same way as psychiatrists are, or really should be, regarded with the same parity of esteem as physicians and surgeons. And among psychiatrists, psychological psychiatrists really should be held in the same regard as biological psychiatrists. But why the schism within psychiatry? Psychiatry needs to reconcile itself to integration of the mind at its deepest, unconscious level, with the evident, conscious mind. Neuropsychoanalysis offers many good bridges between the unconscious mind and brain functioning. The unconscious and neuropsychoanalysis should be embraced to facilitate interrelationship between patients' minds and disorders of neuronal chemical transmitters. If that were done by all psychiatrists, psychiatry might unite and be a very strong branch of Medicine. And as such, it could oversee clinically all the independent psychological branches of mental science that at the moment are disparate, and weak as a whole therefore. Good psychological science needs to be done as well as physiological sciences, neuroscience, pharmaceutical research, and research in psychosomatic Medicine. With good psychological science, this gap within psychiatry could be closed, and psychiatrists could justifiably claim a third, or equivalently costed proportion, of the healthcare budget together with physicians and surgeons.

When we have really good psychological science that in these ways integrates fully with the physical sciences, and when all medical clinicians including within psychiatry work together, it will be much less difficult to find justification for arguing for funded mental health treatments. All medical clinicians will agree, certainly, that psychological wellbeing permits much less physical deterioration in, for example, schizophrenic patients. A good proportion of psychologically afflicted patients, even schizophrenic patients suitably treated, will recover and go back to work, and the costs of welfare benefits and allowances will shrink as the minds of previously ill patients begin to work normally again, allowing them to emerge as the individuals they have been trying to become. Very good science and clinical practice are needed to be able to allocate the best treatments for each patient, with all the expense that that entails. Finance on its own is not the answer. Application of expertise is key, backed up by finance and facilities. Careful management of finances also is important. But if changes of these kinds are co-ordinated, then psychological sciences could earn mental healthcare its place in the philosophy of the NHS, in practice.

Meeting the psychological needs of everyone, one of Aneurin Bevan's adapted key principles, is clearly a tall order. In practice in the NHS, this would have to be restricted to psychological illnesses, which is within the gift of psychiatrists, rather than simply conceding to wishful thinking or desires or personal demands among the public. Such requests for psychological help as these are increasingly being successfully met by IAPT, encouragement towards self-help, and themed community groups; this enables psychiatrists to concentrate on the clinically ill public. At the moment, in 2018, not all patients with mental illnesses are being treated, but fresh impetus is being put into addressing this gap in provision. Psychiatrists are working very hard to make provision for patients' needs with inadequate resources of workforce, inadequate places of refuge such as psychiatric hospital wards in which to attend their patients, and inadequate time at their disposal. Ideas that are the modern-day equivalent of the drastic step taken in the twentieth century of closing all the very large long-stay mental hospitals are, to some extent, in flux at the moment while the best ways of administering psychiatric care are worked out. The public's views change, but are also needed because it is they whom psychiatry serves.

The great majority of psychiatric care is now practised in the community, in day centres rather than generally in hospital wards. Maintenance of schizophrenic patients is currently aimed at, once they have received their treatment selection and have learned their own ways of managing themselves as well as they can. This is generally the goal of psychiatry; but as is, also, to open up possibilities of better mental health to those patients who want to work harder on themselves. Opportunities such as these are what are likely to shape the future of psychiatry. Even schizophrenia may be better understood today by those who study it, although there is a long way to go before its full comprehension; and alleviating it in suitable patients will return individuals to the wide pool of society, to contribute to it as healthy people. Already it is recognised that if a threshold of psychotherapeutic care can be provided, patients sometimes are delighted to pick up their lives again and progress further. Care in patient selection for stressful treatments is mandatory, but so is providing those treatments to each patient of which they could make their best personal use. In these ways the psychological needs of patients not to be mentally ill, or to be as fit as they could become, could be met, in the skilled hands of psychiatrists.

Schizophrenic patients generally have very little money of their own, but deserve their treatments, and not necessarily the most stressful or the most expensive, on the same basis as other British people. A difficulty for many medical people is the contrast between the complete lack of financial resources of schizophrenic people, especially long-standing, chronically ill schizophrenic people, and the extent of their need. It must seem like a bottomless pit to those doctors who do not understand schizophrenia. But it is equally important to remember that schizophrenia is an illness that, as far as can be known at present, affects in its proportion of around 1% as wide a range of people as there are in the normal community. There is therefore a wide range of schizophrenic patients. Some are very intelligent, despite the damage to intellect and cognition that is usually wrought by the illness. Many originally have ordinary intelligence, and some are below averagely intelligent. Some are artistic, while some are practical in orientation; Case Study 1 and Case Study 2, herein, describe the different personalities of two of Dr Robbins' schizophrenic patients. But for the very intelligent schizophrenic patients, like others, the NHS principles state that they should be treated according to their need. They need to be enabled to apply their intelligence to the communal good of society, at the broadest level. Many of these patients could absolutely flourish with psychoanalytic psychotherapy. These are the patients who have become stuck in their lives in a lacuna in a family or social setting which simply did not meet their needs. Before being offered psychoanalytic psychotherapy, they would have to have demonstrated a proclivity for hard work, delayed gratification, and a high level of general tolerance, determination, and patience, and have a core of benevolence for their fellow human beings. Careful patient selection would allow those schizophrenic patients who could benefit from psychoanalytic psychotherapy to flourish, with enough baseline support. No-one is suggesting pouring money into any bottomless pit. But to give these carefully identified patients their opportunity for co-operating with psychiatrists, to learn where they have been making their mistakes, to try out their own potential for themselves, and to fulfil their core desires to give to society when this has been impossible for them earlier in their lives, is part of Aneurin Bevan's intention for his NHS. Their clinical need is to be able to use their minds. The science underlying how they could use their minds, and how they could learn to use their minds, is documented (see Parts II, III, IV and V herein). Hope needs to be given to clinicians thinking about training in psychoanalytic psychotherapy, and then in applying this skill to working with schizophrenic patients. The more clinicians who train in this way, the better will be the opportunities for intelligent schizophrenic patients with all the attributes necessary for satisfactory completion of their treatment to progress onwards in their lives and flourish like their healthily developed contemporaries.

In March 2011, The Department of Health published "The NHS Constitution" (Department of Health, 2011). This describes seven principles and six core values by which the NHS serves the British people, and, in its more easily accessible form, "The Handbook to the NHS Constitution", is readily available to the public on the gov.uk website. The seven principles expand Aneurin Bevan's three central principles upon which he based his concept of the NHS in 1948:

Principle 1

The first principle, that "The NHS provides a comprehensive service available to all" summarises the first two of Aneurin Bevan's own three principles, and is generally intended for psychiatric patients as much as for medical and surgical patients. It declares the service is available to British people irrespective of gender, race, disability, age, sexual orientation, religion, belief, gender reassignment, pregnancy and maternity, or marital or civil partnership status. This outlook helps to unite British people as a nation in mutual self-care and social support, although unfortunately we too often tend to depend upon services at times when we could equally well help ourselves and each other as independent citizens. Elderly and frail people, and unsupported children, fall to health and social services for care when families are not forthcoming in taking responsibility for them. Mentally ill individuals are often too difficult for families to understand or take proper care of them without medical attention, and without the NHS's help these patients fall victim to destitution too often. This first principle states that the NHS has to help particularly those sections of society that fall below the national average in prosperity, and so refers particularly to schizophrenic patients in danger of destitution.

Principle 2

The second principle, that "Access to NHS services is based on clinical need, not an individual's ability to pay", emphasises, as it says, that mentally ill patients deserve to be treated and helped to the best psychological health they can achieve even though they may be impoverished. Accessing these individuals' goodwill can be key to helping them to recover their minds and set out on a future path that will allow them to flourish in their lives in a capacity acceptable to them, into which they will put their energy and application. It is a sad day when people who have been helped do not reciprocate this effort and waste all the help they have been given. Ward or health centre care needs to be strict in that lackadaisical attitudes will not be tolerated because there are so many other patients needing help that lack of co-operation wastes time and the resources of everyone. But where severe mental illness has afflicted a patient it is generally found that kindness and care brings about the best results, and that the grateful patient will be keen to give everything they can to co-operate with their carers and try their best to succeed at their own future life. These patients can get help with NHS charges, and information is available for overseas visitors wanting to use NHS facilities.

Principle 3

The third principle, that "The NHS aspires to the highest standards of excellence and professionalism" is adhered to by all NHS staff in their working lives. Today's stressful hospital environments and GPs' surgeries make it difficult to live up to, however. Junior doctors' strikes have been precipitated by fears for this principle if the doctors are squeezed too hard regarding their working hours and salaries. The use of agency staff, operating theatres and other hospital premises all have to be pared down to the bone to make the required savings for budgetary requirements, and maintaining clinical standards in face of these cuts is a very tall order. Clinical procedures have to be safe, effective, and focused on patient experience. Staff need to be fully trained, led by senior clinicians, and committed also to research that might improve patient care. Above every other concern is patient safety. In psychological treatments this is as true as in every other area of clinical care. Strong bonds between staff members on psychiatric wards and their patients is the best way of ensuring safety for the patients. Trust delivers much the best and surest results, above mere rules and statements and strictness in ward management. When psychiatric patients feel valued, and this in itself needs to be nurtured on the ward, they are much more likely to take proper care of themselves. This form of professionalism brings out the best in psychiatric patients, and also General Practice care of psychologically vulnerable patients. Respect, dignity, compassion, and care are how both patients and staff should be treated in the NHS, because this approach brings about patient safety, good experience, and good outcomes, as Aneurin Bevan would have wished.

Principle 4

The fourth principle, that "The NHS aspires to put patients at the heart of everything it does", prevents any deviation from the central business of treating patients' disorders among NHS staff or supporting agencies. The NHS should encourage patients' efforts to support themselves and their families, and fully respond to their carers. Psychiatric patients are particularly at risk here because often they do not know and cannot tell how best to look after themselves; they feel, and are, particularly helpless due to their condition, and if they do not have a specific carer or family member with their interests at heart, which is often the case, they are perilously in need of the NHS. This is often much more so for psychiatric patients than for general medical or surgical patients. Psychiatric services bear a great deal of responsibility on behalf of their patients on account of this set of circumstances, which is by no means uncommon. Arranging social care is challenging in today's NHS because of lack of residential accommodation, for example, community psychiatric care, and day hospital places. The services rely on the patients' goodwill to co-operate with what provision can be made, and to make the best of it. Those psychiatric patients who are provided with the opportunity of psychoanalytic psychotherapy may still be very vulnerable, but will be doing their best to stick to the arrangements made for them so that they can move on in their lives by learning to accommodate their illness and live with it. With "patient centred care" they will find their best outcome with the health services, which is the goal of the NHS. Psychiatric patients' needs are particularly acute because they are so unable to help themselves in a general way, not simply in relation to a particular operation or a specific episode of an illness, but in their relationship to their own life. Given their opportunity with skilled help, however, they may learn enough to become set on their way in a learning mode so that they can begin to help themselves, and thus relinquish to some extent their dependence on the NHS.

Principle 5

Principle 5 states that "The NHS works across organizational boundaries and in partnership with other organizations in the interest of patients, local communities and the wider population". This principle is enacted by psychiatric hospitals in their care for psychiatric patients who have received their treatment, when their hospital staff make arrangements for transfer of the patient from hospital or from their community setting towards sheltered employment, more satisfactory sheltered housing, or further education. The most alert patients may already be responding well to treatment and be keen to make their own arrangements. But even they may need some help to get started. All psychiatric patients' journeys are long ones compared with those who require a single operation or course of medication to recover. On this long journey the psychiatric patient may have to engage with a series of different organisations, in different places of accommodation, in different communities. But, by co-ordinating a patient's treatment and management, the patient may emerge as a good contributor to society, with strengths and unique insights that can be applied to help others. As ever, the humanitarian aspects of psychiatric patients' lives is important for its own sake, but often these patients really want to give back to society, inspired as they may be by other people, the media, or just in themselves as a solution to the frustrations they have lived with for so long, being unable to function properly. In today's world, 2018 and onwards, there is much more recognition of these tendencies, and much more is being done to help patients make their own contribution. In individual communities there is a wide range of charitable organisations working with psychiatric and other patients, and peer specialists and peer supporters who have recovered from their own illness and now help others towards integration and orientation forwards in life; they work with the NHS and can help patients where they are based, so that familiar surroundings help the patients' integration. This is particularly helpful for psychiatric patients who may be very anxious or frightened about their future.

Principle 6

The sixth principle states that "The NHS is committed to providing the best value for taxpayers' money and the most effective, fair and sustainable use of finite resources". Patients who are suitable for psychoanalytic psychotherapy are as entitled as any other to receive help from the NHS, even if the actual therapy requires payment not funded by it. If the patient's family can pay the therapist's fees, this will be required. Very occasionally individual therapy of this kind can be paid through other clinical sources, but this possibility should not be relied upon. Sometimes psychoanalysts will accept slightly lower fees if a patient has difficulty paying, or may rarely waive the fees, but they have to support themselves like everyone else so this also is seldom the financial basis of a therapy. Psychoanalytic psychotherapy is a very stressful, highly sensitive, extremely finely tuned treatment, and only a small proportion of patients could make use of it. The NHS usually provides the hospital care for such patients, together with arrangements for temporary accommodation out of hospital. Through this treatment patients even with extremely serious mental illnesses such as schizophrenia and schizoaffective disorder may be able to recover themselves successfully, when no other known treatment could achieve the same result. Medication is commonly prescribed for these patients, either on a temporary or more usually a long-term basis. Psychoanalytic psychotherapy is useful to society because if it releases patients who are bound and restricted by illness back to full functioning, then everyone gains. The hospital provision has been shown to be well worthwhile as far as taxpayers' money is concerned. Supportive therapies such as occupational therapy for those patients who require ongoing support while they learn about their illness are also good value to the taxpayer; these patients, too, may be liberated to their maximum extent from the limitations of their condition, and return to work and some fulfilment in life.

Principle 7

Principle 7 holds that "The NHS is accountable to the public, communities and patients that it serves". The British public do voice their complaints along with their wishes, hopes, and trust in connection with the NHS, although they are deeply attached to it and sometimes are pleased to think they can influence, if not run, it by vociferously making their views known, which is, indeed, generally welcomed. The NHS staff consist of entirely dedicated, honourable and selfless people who return to work every day aiming to uphold the NHS's principles with their skills. There are some instances where work related stress creates fraught environments as far as staff relations are concerned, and this is highly undesirable. The great majority of staff are very good people with a highly ethical approach to their work, and all the public should be deeply grateful to them. The staff are the first to be upset when standards in their department fall below what they should be. Between the Government, NHS Trusts, Hospital Management Boards, and heads of departments, everyone is trying to pull the NHS along effectively. Psychiatric patients are often not in a position to understand their management until many years after their treatment has been completed. But when they have recovered, they may retrospectively be profoundly grateful for the care they have received from the NHS as well as from other sources. In these instances, the NHS staff have done an excellent job in providing the facilities the patient has needed in order to work on themselves and become well.

Six core NHS values

The values that predominate within the NHS include 6 officially established aspirations that run through the whole of the NHS's work. "Working together for patients" means that everyone in the NHS organises themselves towards the best outcome for patients, including prioritising patients' interests and admitting mistakes, and attending to local communities' interests. "Maintaining respect and dignity" ensures that individual patients feel comfortable within the treatment environments, that their trust in the healthcare system will be respected through truthfulness and kindness, and that communications will be clear and open. "Commitment to quality of care" can be maintained only when the staff themselves are properly treated and cared for by their employers in the NHS. Feedback is sought from patients. This allows the highest quality of service to continue being implemented, and helps patients to feel their voice is being heard. "Compassion" is a basic aspect of healthcare that has existed within healing communities for thousands of years. Hippocrates wrote "I will keep my life and my art in purity and holiness" in approximately 400BC, and this is the fundamental attitude all doctors subscribe to. Nurses traditionally are moved by patients' pain and try to do everything they can to alleviate their suffering. "Improving lives" is connected to Principle 5, where the patient can best be helped in their life by resolving their problems through agencies working together. Through relating the different problems a patient may have to each other, the different agencies may together achieve an outcome that changes the patient's prospects and enables them to care for themselves more effectively. This is the ideal, but is nowhere more relevant than for psychologically disturbed patients who cannot handle several big issues at once when this would be needed for them to emerge into a brighter life. With the co-ordinated help of several different agencies, such as a community psychiatric nurse, a sheltered housing agency, medical staff in a hospital supervising a suitable medication regime, and a local day centre, the patient may be able to find some satisfaction in life again, making friends and perhaps finding work. Those who emerge completely out of their illness with psychoanalytic psychotherapy have even more reason to be grateful for the expertise of their healthcare staff. Their life may have been transformed by their treatment, allowing them to flourish as never before; or, perhaps, they have become able to re-engage with life as it was for them before a deeply traumatic event that profoundly affected them adversely. "Everyone counts" is the sixth value, providing the NHS with common ground for every person, everywhere in Britain, including destitute schizophrenia sufferers on the streets of large and small cities.

Funding is a very, very large obstacle to creating facilities in the NHS that everyone wants to see. There just is not the finance available to run the services that would lead everyone to feeling content. For example, currently £2.6 billion has been set aside as part of a Sustainability and Transformation Plan (STP) for the NHS, where NHS Hospital Trusts, community hospitals, the Nuffield Trust, local councils, care home agencies, and others are engaged in discussions about how best to manage the balance between social care provision and the financial and bed occupancy needs of hospitals. But last year the NHS hospitals acquired a deficit of some £1.8 billion, with at least the same sized deficit expected next year. So all of the STP provision is, in practice, already accounted for, with none left over for future creative management in social care. It is also asserted by some that even this welcome idea of the STP is being rushed through without addressing the problems with sufficiently deep consultative thought.

Some difficult principles would help, but are unlikely to be popular; prevention is better than cure (eg. persuade people to try harder not to become obese, with help and care in prescribing, to stop smoking, to eat well using scarce money wisely, and to take more exercise); to work with each other to derive plans that save money (eg. in hospitals, sharing facilities, working with flexitime to make working and restful hours more effective, and returning to hospitals for cleaning and re-use NHS equipment such as crutches and wheelchairs originally provided at discharge home from hospital); promoting people's self-care sensibly (but dissuading them from buying risky medications on the internet or self-treating in other ways, eg. with drastic purging); to check on local frail elderly and other needy neighbours in a community spirit, to prevent them becoming seriously debilitated from neglect. Trust, education, and calmness from those who are in positions to understand the issues most directly affecting the public are a good place to start in trying to help the population. Discussions and clear lines of communication, especially listening to the public, will identify some possible factors clearly, which then have to be ascertained more widely before any change is to be effected in practice. Some very good psychiatric care is being currently practised, such as much improved Early Intervention services for young people and particularly cases of first episode psychosis, such as in Cambridgeshire and Peterborough, although gaps are recognised such as in the transition from child to adult psychiatric care, and even here, initiatives are being enacted to bridge the gap; and the STAR Project, Support, Treatment And Recovery, in Southampton. Good provision with Early Intervention will save much stockpiled work for the future where young people pass years not being understood, and arrive in adulthood debilitated and confused; and a comprehensive, overall treatment and recovery service is likely to achieve high general efficacy.

Sustainability and Transformation Plans are today's efforts to continue to uphold Aneurin Bevan's 1948 vision embodied in the NHS's principles and values. They have been compiled in order to save £22bn over two years while doing so. Everyone wants the NHS to work both for patients and for its staff, and it seems that its valuable staff and the funds to run it are the two most pressing factors upon which it wholly depends. Clear thinking and good communication between the agencies involved in specific problems must be a good way to work through the arguments and arrive at the best available solutions. Educating the public about diet, exercise, and self-care despite society's hazardous and sometimes truly dangerous tendencies, not least regarding the upbringing of children, must be high on the list for curbing serious problems before they begin. Ill-afforded extravagances relating to social one-upmanship, throwing caution to the winds, and self-neglect could all be addressed by society if we cared more in a basic way about each other so that we each learned good ways to feel better about ourselves; addressing these would save the NHS billions. Community spirit, self-help, moderation, tolerance and initiative where appropriate, and taking the longer view would all help people get the most out of life together in a much safer and healthier way. Government policies regarding housing and pensions could also support the population if politicians responded capably to the evident need. Recognition of patients' dignity, hope, and their own capacity for initiative, including that of psychiatric patients, are good ways to help them best to help themselves. The NHS staff need just the same recognition, respect and dignity to carry out and to carry on their essential work. If attitudes became more finely tuned to what is important regarding culture then people's health would likely improve greatly. At present there is so much good and vital work being done that it needs protecting and cherishing, together with recognition and understanding of its good foundation of knowledge, determination, and application of good, sound sense. Some of this is being done. Psychiatric patients' needs are being addressed by brave, determined, and thoughtful clinicians within the psychiatric, psychological, and psychoanalytic specialties, but to serve patients optimally, research work needs to be discussed and its arguments worked through so that knowledge can be agreed upon and enacted by the clinicians. Very many people know a lot about different things, so consensus is difficult to arrive at. Knowledge, arrived at in different ways but discussed openly, should be at the scientific core of the Medicine practised in the NHS. Patients in such a system are indeed truly blessed by all the good staff who put into practice not only this knowledge but also all Aneurin Bevan's original, and the later derived, principles, and the NHS Constitution's values. Psychiatric patients are today beginning to benefit as they should, like other patient groups. And once psychiatric illness has been optimally treated, individuals with resolved psychiatric illness should be encouraged like everybody else to think for themselves in a kindly and tolerant society, and to contribute to it as best they are able.

CHAPTER 26

THE HUMAN MIND'S STRUCTURAL AND CONSTITUTIONAL BEAUTY

The human mind manifests beauty both structurally, in its elemental form during psychoanalytic therapy of schizophrenic illness, and constitutionally, in its compassionate and generous relations to others, especially when these others are ill, vulnerable, or in some otherwise needy or compromised state such as being at a very young or very great age.

The PPCC model in its pentapointed state structurally illustrates in several ways the Golden Ratio. This Golden Ratio is a mathematical ratio widely to be found within art and architecture, and in nature due to its remarkable properties involving harmony, regeneration and balance, and other patterns. It holds that in a line divided in this ratio, the ratio of the shorter length to the larger of the two resulting lengths is the same as the ratio of the larger length to the whole length; it illustrates how every entity in the universe reflects unity in its relationship with the whole, fitting into the universe in perfect harmony. All tiny realities matter, thereby, because individually they incrementally reflect each larger aspect of the greater whole. Through the PPCC model's Golden Ratios it becomes philosophically mandatory to emphasise the justice of trying to restore every patient to their individual integrated state, reflecting the naturally integrated whole of their community; and this is quite apart from the humanitarian and social imperative to alleviate their human suffering.

Numerically, the Golden Ratio states that

$$\text{Phi} = \frac{(1 + \text{square root of } 5)}{2} = 1.618033 : 1$$

and that

$$\text{Phi} = \frac{2.618033}{1.618033} = \frac{1}{0.618033} = 1.618033 : 1$$

THE HUMAN MIND'S STRUCTURAL AND CONSTITUTIONAL BEAUTY

This ratio exists within the PPCC's pentapointed, paranoid-schizoid model of the schizoaffective mind in its neutral, accessible state, in which its psychotic part (its Determining Orientation) is separated from its communicable, non-psychotic part (its Observations). Thus the patient's great difficulties with her original representational world receive balance and beauty through the PPCC model, with its potential for future development in therapy. Several different instances of the Golden Ratio are to be found within the PPCC model (see Figure 16). And it may be of philosophical interest that the prehensile extremities of the anthropoid apes' limbs with their five digits, ie. four digits and an opposable thumb, demonstrate the same (4 + 1) pattern as human minds illustrated by the PPCC model with its 4 analysand variables + 1 analyst variable. No-one can fathom or explain the philosophical beauty of this phenomenon of the human mind corresponding in nature to the human body. But this interest is philosophical, only. No theological, sacred or divine properties are discussed here.

The PPCC construct's shape is that of the Golden Ratio pentagram (see Figures 2a and 16). These figures illustrate how at every larger or smaller scale, the Golden Ratio applies to the lengths sectioned off along the PPCC construct's sides and interior boundaries. Over the centuries, this shape has had many meanings, from magical to anarchical to spiritual connotations. The Golden Pentagram with its patterns around the number five may also be found in cross-sections of apples (Hemenway, 2008, p. 15). The pentapointed PPCC construct was initially derived principally through distributing five groups of ideas evenly in a visual form. Henceforward, this diagram was observed to display relational properties of the human mind; usefully, albeit also beautifully.

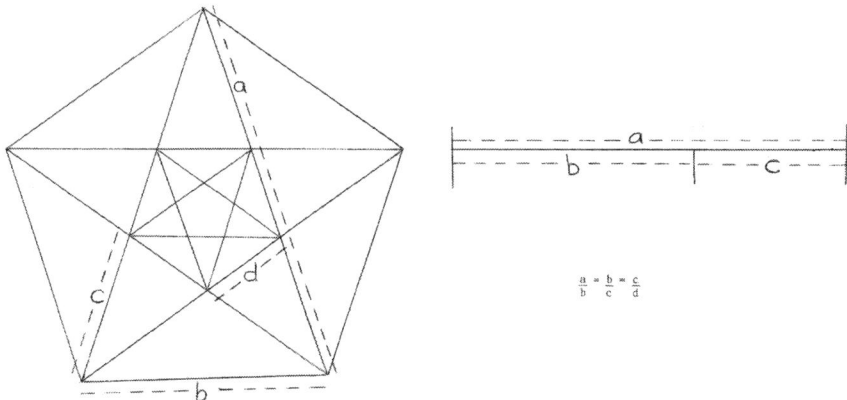

Figure 16 Illustration of the PPCC construct and the Golden Ratio pentagram

The Golden Ratio is also described as the Golden Proportion, the Golden Section, the Golden Mean, the Golden Rectangle, the Golden Spiral, the Golden Triangle, and the Golden Angle. All of these forms interrelate mathematically, and also bear a relationship to the Fibonacci series of numbers: 0, 1, 1, 2, 3, 5, 8, 13, 21, 34, 55, 89, 144, 233, 377, 610, 987, 1597, 2584, 4181, where each number is the sum of the previous two numbers. The ratios between successive Fibonacci numbers approach Phi, or 1.618033. The Fibonacci series possesses many mathematical properties, and the ubiquity and growth potential inherent in these mathematical properties as well as their perfection and consistency are among the reasons for their indefinable value:

> *"The power of the Golden Section to create harmony arises from its unique capacity to unite the different parts of a whole so that each preserves its own identity, and yet blends into the greater pattern of a single whole."*
> Gyorgy Doczi (1981) The Power of Limits (p.13)
> (quoted in Priya Hemenway, The Secret Code, p.12)

Phi, the Greek symbol for the Divine Proportion that was first put into words by the Greek mathematician Euclid, is also expressed as (1+ square root 5) ÷ 2, as mentioned above (Hemenway, 2008). The numerical value of Phi permeates each of the Golden forms described, and provides the link between their interrelationships that is to be found in the physical world, as widely instantiated, and in the psychological world, as has recently been described in this volume. It has been pointed out (Ulmer et al, 2009) that "evidence exists that Phi is also present in the design of the human body. For example, in the 'perfect' body, Phi can be found by splitting certain distances (such as head to pelvis, or fingertip to wrist) into numerous segments – for example, mouth and nose are found at Phi proportions of the distance between the eyes and the chin."

The Golden Rectangle, based on Phi, is found widely in architecture, for example in the Parthenon on the Acropolis, Athens, and in many Gothic cathedrals. This proportion, the Golden Proportion in an oblong, is pleasing to the eye and structurally sound when built upon.

Many sea shells such as Nautilus illustrate the Golden Spiral (Hemenway, 2008). The Golden or Fibonacci or logarithmic Spiral (not an Archimedes spiral, where the distance from the centre point grows at a fixed rate) can be initiated utilising the first numbers of the Fibonacci series: 0, 1, 1, 2, 3, 5, 8, 13, 21. The cochlea in the human ear, which establishes balance and hearing, comprises

2.75 spiral turns and allows us to hear up to ten octaves of sound. Pythagoras' discovery that musical notes can be expressed as mathematical ratios extends to the relationship that is formed when these notes are graphed. The graph forms the shape of the Golden Spiral. When it is stretched into three dimensions it becomes the shape of the cochlea (Hemenway, 2008, p. 132).

Golden Triangles are isosceles triangles that form a continuous succession of ever-diminishing or ever-increasing triangles; thus a freshly drawn internal line, drawn from one of a Golden Triangle's baseline angles to construct an isosceles triangle, bisects, at its base, a baseline in the relative lengths of the Golden Ratio, thus creating a new Golden Triangle. Golden Spirals may be created using either Golden Rectangles or Golden Triangles (Hemenway, 2008, p. 128) (see Figure 17).

If we measure the angles between successive petals on a developing rose bloom, appearing in a generative spiral, we find that the angles between them are about 137.5 degrees. This angle is called the Golden Angle, and is found by multiplying 360 degrees by Phi, the ratio formed by successive Fibonacci numbers. The Fibonacci numbers also appear in the genealogy of honeybees, and in the numbers of petals of many flowers,

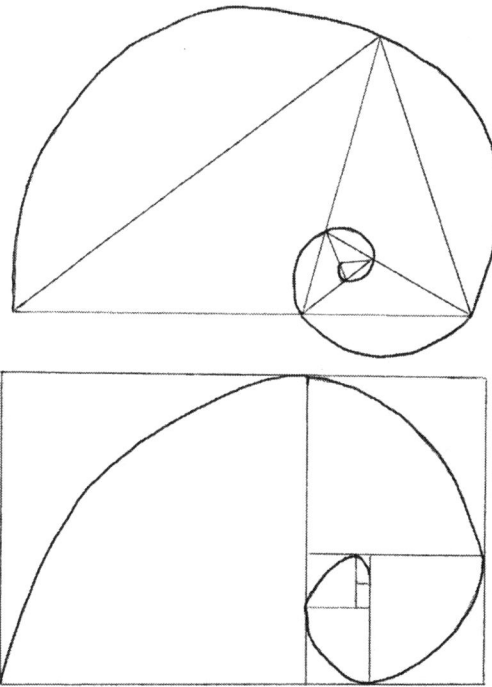

Figure 17 Golden Spirals created from Golden Triangles and Golden Rectangles

particularly for example daisies. Daisy flowers with 13, 21, 34, 55 or 89 petals are all quite common (Hemenway, 2008).

The Fibonacci series is found within the structures of pineapples and sunflowers. These forms are not actually symmetrical; the numbers of clockwise and counterclockwise spirals are not, in fact, equal. They reveal a pattern of successive Fibonacci numbers (Hemenway, 2008, p. 138). Thus the number of spirals in two directions may be 21 and 34, or they may be 8 and 13. There is a biological explanation for this (Hemenway, 2008), a revelation that Alan Turing of Bletchley Park was creatively seeking in his mathematical explorations of biological phenomena. The reason offered by Priya Hemenway for the spiral patterns is that each bud in its sequential formation at the plant's growing-tip cone seeks the maximum space available to it. Numbering the buds 1, 2, 3, 4, 5... in order of appearance illustrates the process. Buds 1 and 2 separate the three-dimensional growing-tip cone into a larger and a smaller section. The next bud 3 then finds it easiest to move into the larger section, forcing bud 4 into the smaller section. As the plant grows in this fashion the buds continue to grow into the largest space they can find, developing into the spirals that we see. This author believes Alan Turing would have been delighted to learn of this three-dimensional botanical explanation of the structure of sunflower seed-heads provided by Priya Hemenway.

Following on from Priya Hemenway's work in "The Secret Code" (Hemenway, 2008, p. 138), describing how successive sunflower buds emerge in the sunflower's growth-cone into the larger of the spaces available to them, this author has developed a simple worked example showing the directions that, on this occasion, successive buds have taken (see Figure 18a). Spirals have then been demonstrated within these ever-expanding consecutive numbers as they take their place in concentric rings that accommodate successive buds. The spirals result from the fact that the buds occupy the largest space available to them in a consecutive process. The worked example shows how spirals develop in both directions (see Figure 18b), even if not replicating precisely logarithmic spirals as found in sunflower seed-heads themselves. Spirals have been coloured in one direction, representing spirals of sunflower seeds, while linear spirals in the opposite direction represent equivalent but not self-coloured spirals (see Figure 18c).

In this example there are five spirals (coloured) in one direction, and three spirals (linear) in the opposite direction. In the diagrams of this worked example, potential further spaces may be observed for seeds of the pale green spiral to locate into, and similarly, to a lesser extent, potential spaces

THE HUMAN MIND'S STRUCTURAL AND CONSTITUTIONAL BEAUTY

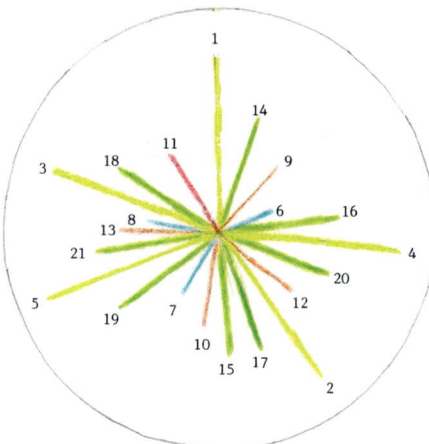

Figure 18a Diagram showing the relative positioning of each bud where there is most space for it in the developing sunflower's growth cone

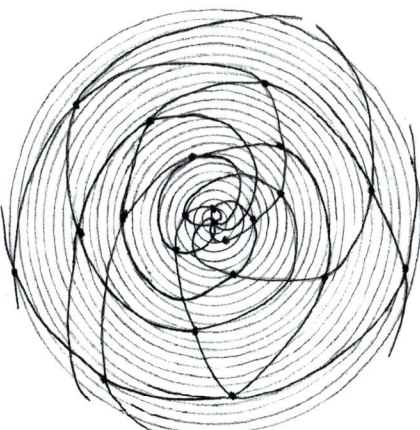

Figure 18b Projected developing spirals in both directions, a Fibonacci number of spirals in each direction, in a sunflower seed-head, in accordance with Figure 18a

for seeds in the yellow spiral to develop into. The darker green spiral may yet find spaces in the outer reaches of the sunflower seed-head as it enlarges.

The sunflower seed organisation is illustrated in detail because it demonstrates how biological processes in nature conform to the Golden Ratio's characteristics in practice. The schizoaffective patient studied in this volume made a small study of her own mind: her ideas fell into five naturally-occurring groups which she displayed on a pentapointed diagram while

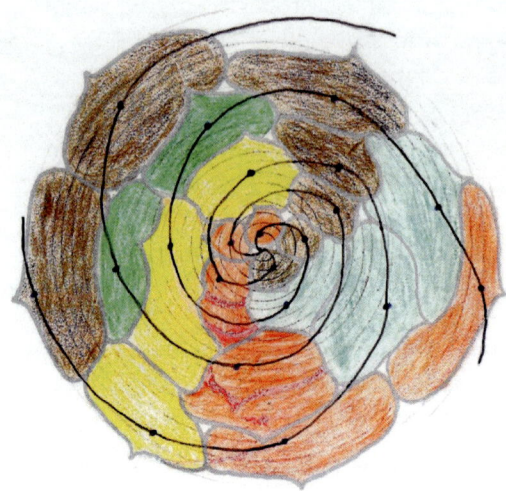

Figure 18c Projected developing spirals of seeds in a sunflower seed-head anticipated by the theoretical botanical process described by Priya Hemenway, as depicted in Figures 18a and 18b; thus mental life as illustrated by the PPCC is connected to life on earth exemplified in sunflower seed-heads by the Golden Ratio

knowing nothing about Golden Ratios or the Golden Pentagram or about psychoanalysis. Her simple diagram provided her with intense satisfaction, pleasure, and relief while engulfed by her distress at her illness. It was, perhaps, nature's own way of helping her find her own harmony, just as, equally, nature bestows life to sunflower seed-heads according to the properties of Fibonacci numbers and of the Golden Ratio. Figure 18 illustrates, as an example via Fibonacci numbers, the ubiquitous relevance to life on earth of the Golden Ratio. The sunflower seed-head, as a botanical phenomenon, demonstrates spirals enumerated by Fibonacci numbers, and is thus connected by the Golden Ratio with the phenomenon of the human mind represented by the PPCC construct: a patient's Representational World with its constituent variables, confirmed by a psychiatry textbook.

Every psychological health worker has their own inspirations and ideals that they work towards, through helping their patients; and commonly their patients' responses to the daily help that they give is their motivation in itself. Most like nothing better than to see the results of their work as a team: patients who have calmed and then understand and forgive seemingly impossible obstacles. This rarely happens overnight, and sometimes not at all. But sometimes very hard therapeutic work over a number of weeks can create a catharsis, to be witnessed by many people present at the time it happens, for example in a group meeting, where a member of the group may, all of a sudden, articulate cathartically everything about their life that they have so far found impossible to express or admit to themselves, for a deep psychological reason which perhaps has manifested as anxiety with depression. Here the beauty of the human mind comes to the fore in both the giver and in the receiver of the beauty of psychological, verbal treatment as compassionate therapy, acting towards this excellent result through the human spirit. Balance, whether or not of the Golden Ratio, is restored. Nature has been helped, and can be described in terms similar to the human hand's four fingers working with one thumb, ie. the human mind's four analysand (patient) variables working with the fifth, analyst, variable in the patient's individual therapy that she may have been attending and working hard at, in addition to her group work.

No-one can say how much or little there is a philosophical analogy here; but the Shorter Oxford Textbook of Psychiatry (Gelder et al, 2006, p. 89) specifies the four analysand core variables ("Dreams" are a form of representation; "Observations" are applied thought; fantasies are one mode of the "Determining Orientation"; and "Experiences" include childhood experiences and those up to and including the present time), and the PPCC includes the fifth, analyst, variable, as a result of data scientifically obtained in the original schizoaffective patient's valid, objective study. The human prehensile thumb and four digits form a beautiful, practical instrument for enabling human development and creativity, the human hand; and the PPCC's structural beauty as a form rich in the Golden Ratio represents the potential for constitutional growth from the mind's strongly balanced core structural variables, albeit describing a patient's unpleasant representational world, into the richness and constitutional beauty of human mental health.

Gyorgy Doczi illuminates further:

"When we share our own limitations with the limitations of others, as we do in the golden relations of neighbors, we complement our own and others' shortcomings, creating thereby living harmony in the art of life, comparable to the harmonies created in music, dance, marble, wood and clay. It is possible to live in this way because the proportions of reciprocal sharing, nature's own golden proportions, are built into our own nature, into our bodies and minds which are, after all, part of nature. The basic pattern-forming processes of nature, which have shaped the human hand and mind,

can continue to guide whatever the hand and mind are shaping, when the hand and mind are true to nature."

Gyorgi Doczi (1981)
The Power of Limits (p.141)

Here Gyorgy Doczi indicates that "nature's own golden proportions" are built into our minds as well as into our physical attributes. The human mind is prevented by schizophrenic psychosis from achieving its productive shaping activities that are enjoyed in health. But the PPCC model's shapes continue to illustrate the mind's own shapes during its process of recovery from illness. The problematic mind depicted by the golden proportion-rich PPCC construct is that of a schizoaffective patient, nonetheless quiescent despite her problems, in her neutral state between psychotic episodes. The Golden Ratios of the PPCC's pentagram, or pentapointed mode, denote the schizoaffective patient's strength and psychological beauty in counteracting her illness which, because of the natural history of the diagnosis, usually resolves, with treatment, in early adult life. And the constitutional beauty of the shaping relationship between psychoanalyst and patient is also included as part of the structural beauty of the PPCC pentagram.

The charitable, loving and giving nature of healthy human minds is to be found ubiquitously in the world. Everywhere, in families and communities, love for babies, spouses, parents, and people of all kinds and characteristics is to be seen, flourishing and lively. These communities are rendered resilient by their outlook and effects on the world around them. Tyranny, hatred, death, and destruction tend to self-destruct in the face of sufficient goodness, properly applied. What survives in the world, in almost every instance, is the result of loving feeling and actions. Everyone in the world knows very well what is good, and also what is bad even if they persist with the most outrageously inhuman behaviour; and in between exist, if they only could identify them, the majority of the remaining issues that must be discussed rather than being acted upon aggressively before being given adequate thought. Generosity, altruism, and bravery can lead to a priceless self-sacrificial tendency to promote humanitarian freedom and safety, as in the armed services and police defending life and liberty, and the protection of human life as in fire crews and lifeboat sailors. Patience, tolerance, long-suffering, and benevolence towards others are well developed in most mental health patients, as they recover, because their experiences have been so painful to them. The sense that each one makes of their own predicaments and their own endeavours, leading to their own emergence into health, is very beautiful to those who love them. Creativity often blossoms at such times. And the human spirit is absolutely inextinguishable. It just depends on its energetic and optimal application of applied clear forward thinking and active vigilance, when this is really needed, to secure its own future growth and potential.

Psychiatry's medical responsibility for the mental health of the population could enact success in fulfilling this objective in some instances by adopting these goals. Some reactive, paranoid schizophrenic and schizoaffective patients who have endured thoroughly disadvantageous circumstances during their development could, if they adhere to their own lofty aspirations that meet their therapists' therapeutic objectives, be lifted out of their condition by their own supported efforts. In this way, the mental health of some of the population could be improved.

The patients' disadvantageous circumstances if replaced by expert therapy and supportive circumstances could offer them new life, like a heart transplant match. Implant the heart, instigate the therapy, and work with the patient to adopt this new thinking. This way, the patient's new thinking could substitute effectively their schizophrenic illness.

CHAPTER 27

MOTIVATION: THE PATIENT EXPERIENCE AND THE HUMAN SPIRIT IN ALL ITS GUISES

The experience of having a schizophrenic illness is surely one of the most frightening, bewildering, and miserable states of awareness known to humankind. The patient can see no end to it. The daily onslaught of confusion, loneliness, and sadness must be endured, for no very obvious reason, and towards no very clear purpose. Day after day is suffered with no logical or evident outcome for all the pain lived through. Life really seems to have no point to it at all.

So if the patient is fortunate enough to have helpful possible connections to psychological therapy, or if they are approached through the care agencies from which they have so far received care, with a view to tackling their mental illness, the chances are that an intelligent patient will leap at the opportunity offered to them. A great deal rides on their own personal characteristics; whether or not they are capable of personal recovery through psychoanalytic psychotherapy is dependent solely upon their own response to it, given sufficient support over the treatment period regarding hospital care, accommodation, finance, and a therapist who is skilled and capable of guiding them through their stages of recovery. This treatment is fraught with challenges, at every one of which it could fail, and the final outcome depends ultimately on the patient themselves. Mutual trust, open warmth, vigilance, consistency, and a firm line held by staff are all good guidelines for the hospital care as well as for the individual psychotherapeutic care, and good liaison between these is also essential.

It is the human spirit that sustains schizophrenic patients through their suffering, for there is little else that could explain their fortitude. The loving awareness of loved ones in a caring role accounts for much of what keeps many schizophrenia sufferers together, in their lives. Gratitude, even cheerfulness when the patient has received help to stabilise themselves in terms of medication, affect regulation skills, social skills, and financial management, may emerge and help the patient to tolerate a steady state in their condition. Their human spirit connects with the goodness of their carers and hospital staff, and allows them to survive the specific unpleasantness that they personally experience.

The human spirit is the remarkable ingredient in human nature that has been with us since we emerged out of the forest, living through hunting among nature's provision, and began to cultivate and farm the land around our settlements. For as long as we have experienced challenges in our lives and risen to meet them, our human spirit has helped us to withstand the difficulties we have encountered, and to overcome them.

Right up to the present day, the resilience of the human spirit has been a hallmark of our social, cultural, technological, artistic and, in every sense, developmental directions of evolution. Where we have met obstruction, we have found our way round it; where difficulties threatened, methods of overcoming these have been developed. We have never doubted that we can succeed in our enterprises if these were really needed by our societies, or even if simply to fulfil a need to stretch ourselves, like landing on the moon, or indeed on Mars, from curiosity; and so good results have generally been forthcoming.

The spirit of schizophrenic patients lies at the other end of the spectrum of human achievement from that which builds monuments and bridges, entire cities, and scientific fields of expertise and civilisations. Schizophrenic patients survive from day to day, knowing only what they already know, with closed minds, and finding it difficult to learn. Chronic schizophrenic patients are not, on their own, likely to achieve much change in their role in life, although with enough help their experience of life may be considerably improved. Nonetheless, Dr Michael Robbins chose to treat chronically paranoid schizophrenic patients, one of whom, who recovered completely from her schizophrenic illness, developed a very successful career in education, got married, and successfully adopted and raised a young man from a deprived early background. Of particular note in this case was the fact observed by Dr Robbins that this young woman was particularly intelligent, with a large vocabulary; he was able to sustain his relationship with her over a period of eleven years or so, through all the difficulties that both she and he encountered during her treatment.

Newly-ill, acutely disturbed young patients have the world before them. Their spirits are fully alive and very upset indeed at the turn their lives are taking. They object vociferously at what is wrong, for them, and heed no-one in their expressions of distaste, fear, and anger. This manifestation of their human spirit is like the young infant's who is objecting heartily at being left alone for too long, or who is hungry, or whose bath is too hot or too cold. The human spirit is our own protector to begin with, and then it finds its outlets in helping society through other people; everyone has their own human spirit, first to help ourselves, and then to help others collectively.

Schizophrenic patients' human spirit does become damaged if, as patients, they have to make too many depressing compromises to their illness in order to manage their lives. This happens particularly if the duration of untreated psychosis is too long. If they lose touch with who they are during the process of adjustment to their illness then, unhappily, depression is likely to set in as a very unwelcome concomitant to their schizophrenic illness for the long term unless the patient is actively related to, intensely and personally. Some cope remarkably well with this blunting effect on their perception of themselves and their world. But group therapy as soon as they are stabilised, and plenty of human contact may keep open their spiritual connections to the world as they have come to know it. Catching their self-expressiveness while this is still fresh, for example in art therapy or active music therapy, can be most effective in preserving the schizophrenic patient's natural, innate potential until this can be utilised to its own maximal and optimal extent in daily work and congress with others. If the patient's human spirit can be engaged early in psychoanalytic psychotherapy then it seems almost possible that nothing is lost and the patient may eventually contribute productively as themselves to the life around them. This treatment is likely to remove blocks in their psychology and free their spirit ever more effectively, so that the patient begins to flourish as never before. This is so, even though very hard and painful, difficult early work must be done in therapy while the patient works through the worst of their psychological blocks and obstructions, that is their faulty perceptions, terrible experiences, incorrect assumptions, undesirable self-realisations, sometimes atrocious memories, and all the other contributory factors of their illness.

When the schizophrenic patient has addressed all these unpleasant aspects of their early life, and of themselves, and then has found strength to address a possible future for themselves, their life becomes more like normal, healthy people's experiences of life. When psychological blocks have been removed and the patient begins to experience some returns on their efforts, the whole world opens up to them. Some schizophrenic patients, for example Sara, as described in Part V herein, early on can feel extremely angry at the extent to which blocks and restrictions and false limits and assumptions have been inflicted upon them in their early environments. But, if their human spirit is sufficiently forgiving, these limits may be dismissed quietly, to let their spirit flourish.

The human spirit is principally creative and has, in addition, elements of love, compassion, spirituality, endeavour, and self-awareness. It is indomitable. It has allowed humankind to explore every habitat on earth, including the depths of the oceans, the heights of mountains, the coldest Poles, isolated islands, and the hottest deserts, jungles, and wildernesses, and to inhabit some of these for long intervals of time, sometimes permanently. Thus humankind's spirit has allowed people to explore the earth widely as well as to explore our own internal nature and all of our creative potential. It seems that all of this endeavour is enacted for its own rewards. Men and women are curious, and venture forth individually in life as well as in cultural and societal groups. The rewards they seek are many and various, and presumably are considered to validate the effort put into achieving them; for human striving continues.

Schizophrenic patients have usually begun to flounder before they reach their first symptoms. They cease to be attracted to the possibility of rewards. Their curiosity has been dampened by then because of the unpleasantness of the confused and saddened experiences they have been living through in their environments up to this point. Failure to be sufficiently assertive has allowed their awareness to implode; when their illness breaks out into symptoms their mind has given up the effort of being curious and engaging with the whole world around themselves. One main structural feature of schizophrenic psychology is that the patient has found their collective experience to be so unpleasant that they unconsciously withdraw completely from this world that they find so unbearable. Effective treatment therefore aims to detect any tenuous possible connection that can be made with the surviving human spirit that has become so withdrawn, to draw it out, learn about it, and then strengthen it. If it is there it will have similarities to the human spirit that climbed Mount Everest. The lively schizophrenic patient was just not as fortunate as the mountaineer in being able to make strong and good connections with their early environments and the people in them as they tried to develop, eg. as Wilfred Bion's "Links" of love, hate, and knowledge (Bion, 1962, pp. 42-44). There are also genetic factors at work; and no-one knows for certain whether a particular schizophrenic patient will be strong enough to pull through the treatment even after a very careful history and assessment. But schizophrenic patients have rarely felt entirely at ease or comfortable with other people, this probably being connected with their discomfort with one or more persons in their immediate early environments. If they are given a good chance to reverse this developmental psychological awkwardness and relate constructively with, instead, a personable, kind, intelligent psychoanalyst, they may be enabled to "find themselves" within the analyst's company. This is the beginning of their psychological recovery, or even their own discovery of themselves for the first time. If no progress is made, they can still be helped to adjust to their life, and their session times with the analyst allocated to another schizophrenic patient who has shown promise. £60,000 per year is spent on each untreated schizophrenic patient's maintenance in Britain, when for the same money they might equally well be treated and helped back to work and a fruitful life; this time in their life might just as well be spent working as meandering through it, idling quietly.

The human spirit identifies beauty and tries to enhance it. Clinicians recognise health and healthy signs in their patients and try to build on these as they help their patients to progress. This is a motivating process for clinicians. Patients' motivation, especially in young adults, is to rectify what they see as being very wrong in their lives. Together, and mutually reinforcing each other, the two participants in treatment, clinician and patient, seek to strengthen the health that is already there within the patient. This germ of life and growth, like the growth-cone in a sunflower seed-head, or a tiny Golden Ratio pentagram within successively larger, growing pentagrams, needs to be detected and identified, and then nourished and nurtured into a chance of life that is as richly deserved as a patient receiving a transplanted heart. As noted, doing nothing costs the country £60,000 a year for each schizophrenic patient. This money could be so much better spent if it supported a treatment. Even if a particular patient's treatment was not successful, the money would still otherwise have been spent on maintaining an untreated patient.

Careful patient selection on the basis of the qualities required for a successful treatment, secure funding arrangements, good or excellent hospital ward accommodation when required, with groups, and a skilled psychiatrically-trained psychoanalyst are the main practical requirements for enabling the clinician's and his or her patients' human spirits to flourish. Life might just as well be spent enacting aspiration as condoning destitution. Early intervention and its sustained application are both desirable aspects of optimally preserving the patient's spirit. Preserving the germinal growth-cones of these young schizophrenic patients who show potential like a beautiful sunflower seed-head could harvest worthwhile and even valuable contributors to society who will subsequently possess an unusually rich understanding of aspects of life that society greatly needs. Simply giving these young people the opportunity to learn about themselves, most effectively in psychoanalytic psychotherapy but, alternatively, also in other ways, is the humane and ethical answer that enables them to take their place and make their best contribution to society. Achieving this would ensure that both they and their clinicians feel their work has been done well. The patients' self-helping psychological skills engendered in therapy by an active, skilled, and faithful psychoanalyst render, as accessible, unparalleled potential life-skills, from which the responding patients and all their subsequent endeavours will benefit. But to reach efficacy, this possibility does require consultant psychiatrists to be able to recognise it, and refer likely prospective candidates among their patients to a psychoanalyst for psychoanalytic psychotherapy, so that their hopes for mental health can become a reality.

REFERENCES

Abraham, K (1924). Selected Papers of Karl Abraham. Translators D Bryan and A Strachey. London: Hogarth Press Ltd and the Institute of Psychoanalysis (1949).

Andrews, A; Knapp, M; McCrone, P; Parsonage, M; Trachtenberg, M (2012). Effective interventions in schizophrenia, the economic case: a report prepared for the Schizophrenia Commission. Personal Social Services Research Unit (PSSRU), London School of Economics and Political Science, London, UK. London: Rethink Mental Illness.

Baethge, C (2007). Biological treatment of schizoaffective disorders. In The Overlap of Affective and Schizophrenic Spectra, Eds. A. Marneros and H Akiskal. Cambridge, New York: Cambridge University Press.

Beauchamp, T; Childress, J (1989). Principles of biomedical ethics. 3rd Ed. New York, Oxford: Oxford University Press.

Bion, W (1962). Learning from Experience. London: Karnac.

Bion, W (1963). Elements of Psychoanalysis. London: Karnac.

Bion, W (1967). Second Thoughts. London and New York: Karnac.

Bollas, C (2013). Catch them before they fall: the psychoanalysis of breakdown. East Sussex, New York: Routledge.

Bouvet, C; Petot, J-M; Diot, E; Ettaher, N; Hasan, O (2018). From medical insight to narrative insight: insight as a support for the therapeutic relationship. Psychosis, **10**(4): 275-285.

Britton, R (1998). Before and after the depressive position; Ps(n)➔D(n)➔Ps(n+1). In Belief and Imagination: Explorations in Psychoanalysis. R Britton. East Sussex: Routledge.

Cannon, M; Jones, P; Murray, R (2002). Obstetric complications and schizophrenia: historical and meta-analytic review. American Journal of Psychiatry, **159**: 1080-1092.

Cardno, A; Gottesman, I (2000). Twin studies of schizophrenia: from bow-and-arrow concordances to Star Wars Mx and functional genomics. American Journal of Medical Genetics, **97**: 12-17.

Cullberg, J (1991). Recovered versus non-recovered schizophrenic patients among those who have had intensive psychotherapy. Acta Psychiatrica Scandinavica, **64**: 242-245.

REFERENCES

Cullberg, J; Levander, S (1991). Fully recovered patients who received intensive psychotherapy: a Swedish case-finding study. Nordisk Psykiatrisk Tidsskrift, **45**: 253-262.

Curtis, L (2011). Unit costs of health and social care 2011. Kent, UK: PSSRU at University of Kent.

Daniels, N (1985). Just health care. Boston, Massachusetts: Cambridge University Press.

Daniels, N (2008). Just health: meeting health needs fairly. New York: Cambridge University Press.

Davidson, L; Chinman, M; Sells, D; Rowe, M (2006). Peer support among persons with serious mental illness: a report from field. Schizophrenia Bulletin, **32**(3): 443-450.

Deegan, P (1996). Recovery as a journey of the heart. Psychiatric Rehabilitation Journal, **19**(3): 91-98.

Department of Health (2011). The NHS Constitution. In The Handbook to the NHS Constitution. www.gov.uk

Department of Health (2015). Reference Costs 2014-2015. November 2015. Referencecosts@dh.gsi.gov.uk

Department of Health (2017). Reference Costs. Referencecosts@dh.gsi.gov.uk. Cost Collection Team, Room 2S07, Quarry House, Quarry Hill, Leeds LS2 7UE.

Doczi, G (1981). The Power of Limits: proportional harmonies in nature, art and architecture. Colorado 80301: Shambhala Publications, Inc.

Evans, M (2016). Making Room for Madness in Mental Health. London: Karnac.

Fazel, S; Langstrom, N; Hjern, A; Grann, M; Lichtenstein, P (2009a). Schizophrenia, substance abuse, and violent crime. Journal of the American Medical Association, **309**(19), 2016-2023.

Fazel, S; Gulati, G; Linsell, L; Geddes, J; Grann, M (2009b). Schizophrenia and violence: systematic review and meta-analysis. PLOS Medicine. **6**(8), p.e1000120.

Fonagy, P; Lemma, A (2012). Does psychoanalysis have a valuable place in modern mental health services? Yes. BMJ 2012; 344:e1211 doi:10.1136/bmj.e1211 (Published 20 February 2012).

Fonagy, P; Target, M (2003). Psychoanalytic Theories: perspectives from developmental psychopathology. London and Philadelphia: Whurr Publishers Ltd.

Freedman, R; Adler, L; Gerhardt, G; Waldo, M; Baker, N; Rose, G; Drebing, C; Nagamoto, H; Bickford-Wimer, P; Franks, R (1987). Neurobiological studies of sensory gating in schizophrenia. Schizophrenia Bulletin, **13**: 667-678.

Freud, S (1917). Mourning and Melancholia. In The Standard Edition of the Complete Psychological Works of Sigmund Freud. Ed. J Strachey. Vol. XIV. London: Vintage, (2001).

Freud, S (1933). Figure: Freud's latest model of a healthy mind. New Introductory Lectures on Psycho-Analysis. In The Standard Edition of the Complete Psychological Works of Sigmund Freud. Ed. J Strachey. Vol XXII. London: Vintage, (2001). 78.

REFERENCES

Freud, S (1940). Splitting of the ego in the process of defence. In The Standard Edition of the Complete Psychological Works of Sigmund Freud. Ed. J Strachey. Vol. XXIII, pp. 271-278. London: Vintage, (2001).

Friedman, D; Squires-Wheeler, E (1994). Event-related potentials (ERPs) as indicators of risk for schizophrenia. Schizophrenia Bulletin, **20**: 63-74.

Friedman, S; Smith, L; Fogel, D; Paradis, C; Viswanathan, R; Ackerman, R; Trappler, B (2002). The incidence and influence of early traumatic life events in patients with panic disorder: a comparison with other psychiatric outpatients. Journal of Anxiety Disorders, **16**(3): 259-72.

Fulford, K; Thornton, T; Graham, G (2006). Oxford Textbook of Philosophy and Psychiatry. New York: Oxford University Press: 676.

Gelder, M; Harrison, P; Cowen, P (2006). Shorter Oxford Textbook of Psychiatry. 5th Edition. Oxford: Oxford University Press: 89.

Gillon, R (1994). Medical ethics: four principles plus attention to scope. BMJ 1994; 309:184. (Published 16 July 1994).

Guntrip, H (1968). Schizoid Phenomena, Object Relations and the Self. Hogarth.

Hartmann, H (1939). Ego Psychology and the Problem of Adaptation. New York: International University Press, 1958.

Hemenway, P (2008). The Secret Code. Koln: Evergreen.

Henderson, C; Flood, C; Leese, M; Thornicroft, G; Sutherby, K; Szmukler, G (2004). Effect of joint crisis plans on use of compulsory treatment in psychiatry: single blind randomised controlled trial. British Medical Journal, 329: 136. (Published 15 July 2004). doi: https://doi.org/10.1136/bmj.38155.585046.63

Herman, D; Conover, S; Felix, A; Nakagawa, A; Mills, D (2007). Critical Time Intervention: an empirically supported model for preventing homelessness in high risk groups. The Journal of Primary Prevention, **28**(3-4), 295-312.

Herman, D; Conover, S; Gorroochurn, P; Hinterland, K; Hoepner, L; Susser, E (2011). A randomized trial of critical time intervention to prevent homelessness in persons with severe mental illness following institutional discharge. Psychiatric Services, **62**(7), 713-719.

Hingley, S (2006). Finding meaning within psychosis: the contribution of psychodynamic theory and practice. In: Evolving psychosis: Different stages, different treatments. Eds. Johannessen, J-O; Martindale, B and Cullberg, J. 200-214. London and New York: Routledge.

Hinshelwood, R (1989). A Dictionary of Kleinian Thought. London: Free Association Books.

Hinshelwood, R (1994). Clinical Klein. London: Free Association Books.

Hippisley-Cox, J; Pringle, M (2005). Report to the Disability Rights Commission. Health Inequalities experienced by people with Schizophrenia and Manic Depression: Analysis of general practice data in England and Wales. http://leeds.ac.uk/disability-studies/archiveuk/pringle/Qresearch_%20initial_analysis_gen_practice_data.pdf

Holowka, D; King, S; Saheb, D; Pukall, M; Brunet, A (2003). Childhood abuse and dissociative symptoms in adult schizophrenia. Schizophrenia Research, **60**: 87-90.

REFERENCES

Ingraham, L; Kety, S (2000). Adoption studies of schizophrenia. American Journal of Medical Genetics, **97**: 18-22.

Jackson, M (2001). Weathering the storms: psychotherapy for psychosis. London and New York: Karnac, 334.

Jackson, M (2015). Creativity and psychotic states in exceptional people. New York and East Sussex: Routledge.

Jackson, M; Williams, P (1994). Unimaginable storms: a search for meaning in psychosis. London: Karnac.

Joseph, B (1981). Defence mechanisms and phantasy in the psychological process. Bulletin of the European Psycho-Analytical Federation, **17**: 11-24.

Kandel, E (1999). Biology and the future of psychoanalysis: a new intellectual framework for psychiatry revisited. American Journal of Psychiatry, **156**(4), 505-524.

Kelly, G (1955). The psychology of personal constructs. New York: Norton.

Kendler, K; McGuire, M; Gruenberg, A; O'Hare, A; Spellman, M; Walsh, D (1993). The Roscommon Family Study. I. Methods, diagnosis of probands and risk of schizophrenia in relatives. Archives of General Psychiatry, **50**: 527-540.

Khanom, H; Samele, C; Rutherford, M (2009). A missed opportunity? Community sentences and the mental health treatment requirement. London, UK: Sainsbury Centre for Mental Health.

Klein, M (1935). A contribution to the psychogenesis of manic-depressive states, 1935. In: Love, Guilt and Reparation and other works 1921-1945. London: Vintage, (1998): 276.

Klein, M (1946). Notes on some schizoid mechanisms, 1946. In: Envy and Gratitude and other works 1946-1963. London: the Hogarth Press, (1984):14.

Klein, M (1952). The origins of transference. In: Envy and Gratitude and other works 1946-1963. London: the Hogarth Press, (1984): 53.

Larkin, W; Morrison, A (2006). Trauma and psychosis. London and New York: Routledge: 37.

Leff, J; Williams, G; Huckvale, M; Arbuthnot, M; Leff, A (2013). Computer-assisted therapy for medication-resistant auditory hallucinations: proof-of-concept study. British Journal of Psychiatry. (Published June 2013). **202**(6): 428-433; doi: 10.1192/bjp.bp.112.124883.

Leonard, S; Gault, J; Hopkins, J; Logel, J; Vianzon, R; Short, M; Drebing, C; Berger, R; Venn, D; Sirota, P; Zerbe, G; Olincy, A; Ross, R; Adler, L; Freedman, R (2002). Association of promoter variants in the a7 nicotinic acetylcholine receptor subunit gene with inhibitory deficit found in schizophrenia. Archives of General Psychiatry, **59**: 1085-1096.

Liddle, P (1987). The symptoms of chronic schizophrenia. A re-examination of the positive-negative dichotomy. British Journal of Psychiatry, **151**: 145-151. doi: 10.1192/bjp.151.2.145.

Lucas, R (2009). The Psychotic wavelength. London and New York: Routledge.

Mahler, M (1971). A study of separation-individuation process and its possible application to borderline phenomena in the psychoanalytic situation. The Psychoanalytic Study of the Child, **26**: 403-24.

REFERENCES

Mangalore, R; Knapp, M (2007). Cost of schizophrenia in England. Journal of Mental Health Policy and Economics, **10**(1): 23-41.

Marneros, A; Akiskal, H (2007). The overlap of affective and schizophrenic spectra. Cambridge and New York: Cambridge University Press.

Marshall, M; Lewis, S; Lockwood, A; Drake, R; Jones, P; Croudace, T (2005). Association between duration of untreated psychosis and outcome in cohorts of first-episode patients: a systematic review. Archives of General Psychiatry, **62**(9): 975-83.

Martindale, B; Summers, A (2013a). The psychodynamics of psychosis. Advances in Psychiatric Treatment, **19**: 124-131. doi: 10.1192/apt.bp.111.009126.

Martindale, B; Summers, A (2013b). Using psychodynamic principles in formulation in everyday practice. Advances in Psychiatric Treatment, **19**: 203-211. doi:10.1192/apt.bp.112.010181.

Ministry of Justice (2011). Costs per place and costs per prisoner by individual prison. http://www.justice.gov.uk/downloads/statistics/prison-probation/prison-probation-performance-stats/prison-costs-summary-10-11.pdf

NHS Blood and Transplant (2009). Taking organ transplantation to 2020: A UK Strategy. The Economic case for organ transplantation. www.nhsbt.nhs.uk

NICE (2009). National Institute for Health and Clinical Excellence (2009). Schizophrenia: Core Interventions in the Treatment and Management of Schizophrenia in Adults in Primary and Secondary Care (updated edn). British Psychological Society/Royal College of Psychiatrists.

Panksepp, J (1998). Affective neuroscience: the foundations of human and animal emotions. New York: Oxford University Press.

Platt, S; Halliday, E; Maxwell, M et al. (2006). Evaluation of the first phase of Choose Life. Final Report. Edinburgh: Scottish Executive.

Rang, H; Dale, M; Ritter, J; Flower, R; Henderson, G (2012). Rang and Dale's Pharmacology. 7th Edition. Edinburgh: Elsevier Churchill Livingstone.

Read, J; Perry, B; Moskowitz, A; Connolly, J (2001). The contribution of early traumatic events to schizophrenia in some patients: a traumagenic neurodevelopmental model. Psychiatry: Interpersonal and Biological Processes, **64**: 319-345.

Repper, J; Carter, T (2011). A review of the literature on peer support in mental health services. Journal of Mental Health, **20**(4): 392-411.

Rey, H (1994). Universals of psychoanalysis in the treatment of psychotic and borderline states. Factors of space-time and language. London: Free Association Books.

Rid, A; Biller-Andorno, N (2009). Justice in action? Introduction to the mini-symposium on Norman Daniels' "Just health: meeting health needs fairly". Journal of Medical Ethics, 2009; **35**: 1-2. doi: 10.1136/jme.2008.025783.

Robbins, M (1993). Experiences of schizophrenia: an integration of the personal, scientific and therapeutic. New York: The Guilford Press.

Robbins, M (2011). The primordial mind in health and illness: a cross-cultural perspective. London and New York: Routledge.

REFERENCES

Robbins, M (2012). The successful psychoanalytic therapy of a schizophrenic woman. Psychodynamic Psychiatry, **40**(4): 575-608.

Rosenbaum, B (2009). Early and sustained dynamic intervention in schizophrenia. Psychiatria Danubina, **21**(1): 132-134.

Rosenbaum, B; Valbak, K; Harder, S; Knudsen, P; Koster, A; Lajer, M; Lindhardt; Winther, G; Petersen, L; Jorgensen, P; Nordentoft, M; Andreasen, A (2005). The Danish National Schizophrenia Project: prospective, comparative longitudinal treatment study of first-episode psychosis. British Journal of Psychiatry, **186**: 394-399.

Rosenbaum, B; Harder, S (2007). Psychosis and the dynamics of the psychotherapy process. International Review of Psychiatry, **19**(1): 13-23.

Saha, S; Chant, D; Welham, J; McGrath, J (2005). A systematic review of the prevalence of schizophrenia. PLOS Medicine, **2**(5): p.e141. http://www.plosmedicine.org/article/info%3Adoi%F10.1371%2Fjournal.pmed.0020141

Saha, S; Chant, D; McGrath, J (2007). A systematic review of mortality in schizophrenia. Archives of General Psychiatry, **64**(10): 1123-1131.

Sandler, J (1972). The role of affects in psychoanalytic theory. In J Sandler (Ed), From Safety to the Superego: Selected Papers of Joseph Sandler (1987). 285-300. New York: Guilford Press.

Sandler, J (1987). From Safety to the Superego: Selected Papers of Joseph Sandler. New York: Guilford Press.

Sandler, J (1989). Toward a reconsideration of the psychoanalytic theory of motivation. In A Cooper; O Kernberg; E Person (Eds), Psychoanalysis: Toward the Second Century. 91-110. New Haven, CT: Yale University Press.

Sandler, J; Rosenblatt, B (1962). The concept of the representational world. Psychoanal St Child, **17**: 128-45.

Segal, H (1981). The work of Hanna Segal: Delusion and Artistic Creativity and other psychoanalytic essays. London: Free Association Books, Maresfield Library (1986).

Seymour, L; Rutherford, M (2008). The Community Order and the Mental Health Treatment Requirement. London, UK: Sainsbury Centre for Mental Health.

Shedler, J (2010). The efficacy of psychodynamic psychotherapy. American Psychologist, **65** (2): 98-109. doi: 10.1037/a0018378.

Singleton, N; Bumpstead, R; O'Brien, M; Lee A; Meltzer, H (2000). Psychiatric morbidity among adults living in private households. International Review of Psychiatry, **15**(1-2): 65-73.

Slade, E; McCarthy, J; Valenstein, M; Visnic, S; Dixon, L (2012). Cost savings from assertive community treatment services in an era of declining psychiatric inpatient use. Health Services Research, 1-23.

Sohn, L (1999). Psychosis and violence. In P Williams (Ed), Psychosis (madness). London: Institute of Psycho-Analysis (1999).

Sokol, D (2013). "First do no harm" revisited. BMJ 2013; 347: f6426.

Solms, M and Turnbull, O (2002). The Brain and the inner world. London: Karnac.

Steggles, G (2012). The process of recovery of a schizoaffectively disordered mind: a psychoanalytic theory of the functional psychoses, the psychodynamic

REFERENCES

pentapointed cognitive construct theory. BMJ Case Reports; doi: 10.1136/bcr-2012-006683.

Steggles, G (2014). PhD Thesis. University of Essex, Albert Sloman Library.

Steggles, G (2015a). Stages in the psychological resolution of schizophrenia. Frontiers in Psychology. Vol. 6 (86), March 2015.

Steggles, G (2015b). Psychoanalytic psychotherapy for schizophrenia and schizoaffective disorder. In Schizophrenia Treatment, SM Group Publishers, www.smgebooks.com December 2015.

Steggles, G (2016). Psychological progress in schizophrenic patients undergoing psychoanalytic psychotherapy. International Journal of Psychology and Psychoanalysis 2:012. Vol 2(1).

Steggles, G (2018). Visually conceptualizing psychoanalytic resolution of schizophrenia and schizoaffective disorder. International Journal of Psychiatric Research, 2018; 1(1): 1-4.

Steiner, J (1979). The border between the paranoid-schizoid and the depressive positions in the borderline patient. British Journal of Medical Psychology, **52**: 385-91.

Steiner, J (1987). The interplay between pathological organizations and the paranoid-schizoid and depressive positions. International Journal of Psycho-Analysis, **68**: 69-80.

Steiner, J (2009). Rosenfeld in Retrospect. Essays on his clinical influence. London and New York: Routledge.

Susser, E; Lin, S (1992). Schizophrenia after prenatal exposure to the Dutch hunger winter of 1944-1945. Archives of General Psychiatry, **49**: 983-988.

Susser, E; Neugebauer, R; Hoek, H; Brown, A; Lin, S; Labovitz, D; Gorman, J (1996). Schizophrenia after prenatal famine: further evidence. Archives of General Psychiatry, **53**: 25-31.

The Schizophrenia Commission (2012). The abandoned illness: a report from the Schizophrenia Commission. London: Rethink Mental Illness.

Ulmer, H; Kelleher, C; Dunser, M (2009). George Clooney, the cauliflower, the cardiologist, and phi, the golden ratio. BMJ2009; 339:64745.

UNOS (2011). UNOS Transplant Living. United Network for Organ Sharing in the USA. Average costs in 2011.

Verdoux, H; Geddes, J; Takei, N; Lawrie, S; Bovet, P; Eagles, J; Heun, R; McCreadie, R; McNeil, T; O'Callaghan, E; Stober, G; Willinger, M; Wright, P and Murray, R (1997). Obstetric complications and age at onset in schizophrenia: an international collaborative meta-analysis of individual patient data. American Journal of Psychiatry, **154**: 1220-1227.

Wasserman, D; Wasserman, C (2009). Suicidology and suicide prevention. Oxford: Oxford University Press.

Williams, P (1999). Psychosis (madness). London: Institute of Psycho-Analysis.

Williamson, P (2006). Mind, brain and schizophrenia. New York: Oxford University Press.

REFERENCES

Winnicott, D (1953). Transitional objects and transitional phenomena. International Journal of Psycho-Analysis, **34**: 1-9.

Winnicott, D (1965). The Maturational Process and the Facilitating Environment, 140-52. New York: International Universities Press.

Zetzel, E (1970). The Capacity for emotional growth. The International Psycho-Analytical Library No. 86. Toronto: The Hogarth Press Ltd.

TABLE OF FIGURES

Figures that are annotated in their legend by © BMJ 2017 are reproduced with permission by Copyright 2012 BMJ Publication Group from the following reference:

Steggles, G (2012). The process of recovery of a schizoaffectively disordered mind: a psychoanalytic theory of the functional psychoses, the psychodynamic pentapointed cognitive construct theory. BMJ Case Reports 2012: doi:10.1136/bcr-2012-006683.

Figure 6 is reproduced with permission by the editors of the "Standard Edition of the Complete Psychological Works of Sigmund Freud" (Freud, 1933).

Dr Michael Robbins' Seven Stages of the resolution of schizophrenia by psychoanalytic psychotherapy are reproduced with permission, in Figures 14 and 15, from his book "Experiences of Schizophrenia: An Integration of the Personal, Scientific and Therapeutic" (Robbins, 1993).

Figure 1: A schizoaffective patient's original representational world. (colour plate)
Figure 2a: The PPCC model in the paranoid-schizoid position.
Figure 2b: The PPCC model illustrating affect regulation. (colour plate)
Figure 3: The PPCC model in the depressive position.
Figure 4: Closure of the PPCC's vertex.
Figure 5: The endpoint of the recovery process: the patient's mind maturing "with all its corners rubbed off".
Figure 6: Freud's latest model of a healthy mind.
Figure 7: The overall PPCC sequence of recovery from schizophrenia.
Figure 8a: The development of the PPCC adaptation for depression.
Figure 8b: Adaptation of the PPCC construct for depression.
Figure 9a: The development of the PPCC adaptation for mania.
Figure 9b: Adaptation of the PPCC construct for mania.

TABLE OF FIGURES

Figure 10a: The development of the PPCC adaptation for schizophrenia.

Figure 10b: Adaptation of the PPCC construct for schizophrenia.

Figure 11: The PPCC illustrating the processes towards illness and towards resolution in schizophrenia.

Figure 12: A combination of internal and external factors of the mind leading to a mental outcome.

Figure 13: Comparison of the mental processes of Bion's and Fodor's theories of thinking with Freud's theory of depression.

Figure 14: Dr Michael Robbins' Seven Stages of the resolution of schizophrenia by psychoanalytic psychotherapy, illustrating the coinciding of Dr Robbins' therapeutic perspective, Dr Gillian Steggles' PPCC model, and the patient's perspective.

Figure 15: Summary of Dr Robbins' Seven Stages of the resolution of schizophrenia by psychoanalytic psychotherapy, paralleled by changes in the PPCC model: Robbins (and PPCC).

Figure 16: Illustration of the PPCC construct and the Golden Ratio pentagram.

Figure 17: Golden Spirals created from Golden Triangles and Golden Rectangles.

Figure 18 illustrates a worked example of the derivation of spirals in a sunflower seed head according to the process described by Priya Hemenway in "The Secret Code" (2008) (p.138) where each successive bud occupies the largest space available to it in the developing sunflower's growth cone. Figure 18 illustrates as an example the ubiquitous relevance to life on earth of the Golden Ratio, via Fibonacci numbers in the case of the sunflower seed head, thus connecting the human mind's PPCC construct phenomenon with a botanical phenomenon.

Figure 18a: Diagram showing the relative positioning of each bud where there is most space for it in the developing sunflower's growth-cone. (colour plate)

Figure 18b: Projected developing spirals in both directions, a Fibonacci number of spirals in each direction, in a sunflower seed head, in accordance with Figure 18a.

Figure 18c: Projected developing spirals of seeds in a sunflower seed head anticipated by the theoretical botanical process described by Priya Hemenway, as depicted in Figures 18a and 18b; thus mental life as illustrated by the PPCC is connected to life on earth exemplified in sunflower seed heads by the Golden Ratio. (colour plate)

ACKNOWLEDGEMENTS

My principal, and most wholeheartedly grateful, acknowledgements are to my esteemed and tremendously admired colleague in Massachusetts, USA, Dr Michael Robbins MD. Dr Robbins' lifetime's work has been the psychoanalytic psychotherapeutic alleviation of their symptoms in his paranoid schizophrenic patients.

To allow me to include verbatim two of his most excellent case reports as clinical studies in this volume has been an act of unparalleled generosity, and I thank him again for this tremendous permission. All references to my work in this context should cite his name and his expertise, which is no less than his very due desserts.

Although declining on a number of occasions joint authorship of this volume or any other volume incorporating my PPCC Theory, Dr Robbins has continued to develop his own views of The Primordial Mind in his many other publications which are not cited here. His ideas are useful in contemplating the nature of the germinal schizophrenic mind as it encounters its successive and often adverse environments. My work with my PPCC Theory is quite separate from Dr Robbins' work and should not be linked to it except in this volume, where the complete and absolute correspondence between our two sets of results, from the therapeutic, and from my patients', perspectives may be appreciated.

I am indebted to the staff of University College London for their undiminishing support and encouragement over the past forty-six years, for inviting me to use their libraries and to enjoy countless seminars, lectures, and conferences, and to meet themselves, especially in the Psychoanalysis Unit; Professor Peter Fonagy allowed me to become attached to it while I studied independently, which I greatly appreciated. Likewise, I am very grateful to the staff and students at the Institute for Psychiatry, Psychology and Neuroscience in Camberwell, and to the staff and patients at the Maudsley Hospital in London, similarly, for their advice and friendship and

ACKNOWLEDGEMENTS

my introduction to the rigours of psychiatry. And, equally, I am deeply indebted to the staff at Essex University in the Department of Psychosocial and Psychoanalytic Studies for their patience and generosity to me while I was learning to encompass my academic identity.

I am immensely grateful to both Professor R D Hinshelwood and Dr Miomir Milovanovic for their generosity and hard work in producing an enlightening Foreword and Introduction, which set out for psychiatrists who may doubt the veracity of the theory and efficacy of psychological treatments the thinking behind the success of these approaches.

I owe an unbounded debt to British psychiatry and its exponents, particularly to Professor Julian Leff, Professor R D Hinshelwood, the late Dr Leslie Sohn, and the late Dr Murray Jackson. Britain's adopted medical ethics as practised in its National Health Service are unparalleled anywhere in the world. When mentally ill patients, like physically ill people, ask for help from British psychiatrists, they can be sure that the best possible of the treatments and management available will be given them, in a humane and considered way. This leads to a very heavy workload for British psychiatrists in terms of their own strength and goodwill. This book's premise is an acknowledgement of that workload, its intention being to relinquish a growing number of those very ill patients who suffer from schizophrenic illness from their patient lists and NHS care, once they are able to shoulder much of their own condition's management for themselves, with a grateful and cheerful mindset; thus with greatly improved mental health, and saving the NHS an estimated £1.8 million, less the costs of treatment, per schizophrenic patient life.

My other main acknowledgement is to Mr Trevitt Steggles, who has funded my latter academic work unstintingly and with utmost generosity. Over many years he has allowed me to persevere in developing my study, taking part in contemporary academic thinking, and pursuing my profession sufficiently to write up this volume. My thanks, again wholeheartedly, are to him for his generosity, patience and consistent support.

INDEX

A10 nucleus   92-93
"abandoned illness"   259
Abraham, Karl   6, 98
accountability to public of NHS   278
acute psychosis (see acute schizophrenia)
Advanced Treatment Directives (ATDs)   242
adversity   39
affect regulation   95, Figure 2b
Alanen, Yrjo   6
alienation   4
alignment of Freud's, Bion's and Fodor's theories   76, 77, Figure 13
Alzheimer   2
Analysand PPCC variables   50, Figure 2a
Analyst PPCC variable   50, Figure 2a
analyst's boundaries   96
analyst's incorporation   98
anger   95
anhedonia   244
Anticipatory Pleasure Skills training   23, 31, 34, 244
Assertive Community Treatment (ACT)   240
autonomous conflict-free ego functions   97
autonomy of patient   42, 264, 266, Figure 14
Avatar Therapy   23, 115, 243, 254

baby, neglected   293-294
Baethge, Christopher   29, 30
Barnard, Christiaan   255
Beauchamp and Childress, ethicists   263
beauty of the human mind   282-291
Bell, David   127
Benedetti, Gaetano   125
beneficence for patient   265-267
Bevan, Aneurin   269-281
Bion, Wilfred R   6, 17, 43, 55, 60, 76, 94, 95, 99, 120, 135
blocks, psychological   294
Bollas, Christopher   35
boundaries in therapy   96, 110
brain diseases   2-3
brainstem reticulum   92
British Medical Journal (BMJ)   126, 263
Britton, Ronald   99

Cambridgeshire and Peterborough EIS   280
CARE   91
chlorpromazine 3, 197
closure of the vertex   (see vertex)
cochlea   284
cochlear implant
   cost   255
   value   255
Cognitive Analytic Therapy (CAT)   254
Cognitive Behavioural Therapy (CBT)   23, 43, 84, 85, 242, 254

INDEX

cognitive functioning, damage to 255-256
cognitive resolution   95
comfort blanket   59
communication difficulties   17-18, 251
communication skills   251, 264
compassion   34, 270
conflict   120
constructive thinking   37
construing
   looser   61, 79, Figure 3
   tight   61, Figure 2a
containment   95, Figure 4
"corners rubbed off"   82, 138, Figure 5
cost of therapy (see schizophrenia)
cost of treatment (see schizophrenia)
cost to society (see schizophrenia)
countertransference   93, 94, 104, 113, 116
criminal justice system   21
Criminal Justice System Diversion (CJSD)   239
Crisis Resolution Home Treatment (CRHT)   241
Critical Time Interventions (CTI)   240
Cullberg, Johan   128-129
curiosity of psychoanalyst   116

Daniels, Norman   267
de Chavez, Manuel Gonzalez   129
defence mechanisms   97
delusional system   105
delusions 15, 40, 105, 106
   "patches"   41
dental care   244-245
dependence of patient   34
depression   16, 67, 68, 76, 93, 95, 100, Figures 8a, 8b
   psychotic   16
depressive position   52, 61, 79, 81, 99, Figure 3
   alternation with paranoid-schizoid position   61, 99
determination of the patient   22-23, 34

Determining Orientation PPCC variable   50, Figure 2a
diagnosis of "schizophrenia"   34
Diagnostic and Statistical Manual (DSM)   188, 217, 259
differentiation   100, Figures 14 and 15
disappointment in the patient   23
Disorganization Syndrome (Liddle)   73, 93, 173-175, 224-225, 231
Doczi, Gyorgy   284, 289-290
dopamine hypothesis 3, 92-93
dorsal tegmentum   91, 92
dreams   106-107
   recurring   107
Dreams/Representations PPCC variable   50, Figure 2a
drives   97
DSM-III-R   39, 259
dynamic movements of PPCC model   54

Early Intervention Services (EIS)   31, 33, 36, 237, 256
Edward   121, 122
ego
   affect regulation   95-96
   boundaries   94-100
   conflict-free functions   97
   foundational   91
   localization in PPCC model   91-92
eidetic imagery   52, 58
Electroconvulsive Therapy (ECT)   238
Emily   130, 132, 141-183
   psychoanalytic psychotherapy   141-170
   visualization of therapy   171-178
   commentary on visualization   179-183
emotional abuse   40
emotional drives   91
emotional neglect   39
emotional outbursts   109
emotions   62, 106
empowerment   265

INDEX

encouragement 114
enlightenment 101
environmental factors 5, 267
ERTAS 91, 92
ethics 34, 117
Evans, Marcus 18, 41, 43
evenly suspended positive regard 116
executive functions 91-92
experience, clinical 139
Experiences PPCC variable 50, Figure 2a
Extended Reticular and Thalamic Activating System (ERTAS) 91-92
External Reality 50-51, 62, 79, 89-91, 97, 98, 111, 133, Figure 2a

Fairbairn, Ronald 99, 120
families 25
Family Therapy 23, 84, 238-239
fear 14
FEAR 91
feeling states 61, 97
Fibonacci numbers 284-288
fixed abode 14
Flechsig 2
floundering patient 295
Fodor, Jerry 43, 55, 68, 76, Figure 13
Freud, Sigmund 6, 43, 55, 68, 69, 76, 89, 93, 118, 254, Figure 13
    latest model of a healthy mind Figure 6
Fromm-Reichmann, Frieda 123

GABA-ergic interneurones 92-93
germ of life and growth 296
Gillon, Raanan 263-266
glutamatergic stimulation 92-93
Golden Ratio 282-291, Figures 16, 17
Golden Ratio pentagram 283, Figure 16
"good enough containment" 95
gratitude 292
group psychodynamic psychotherapy 243

hallucinations 106
    auditory 15, 23, 106
    second person 15
    visual 40
harm 249
healthy human minds 290
heart transplant operation 255, 257, 266, 268, 270, 291
Hingley, Susan 39, 43, 259
Hippocrates 263
Hippocratic oath 263
homelessness 21, 35, 240
hopes, the patient's 23, 24, 31, 82, 84, 85, 90, 115, 268, 290-297
hopelessness 23, 24, 31, 292, 294
HPA axis 83
human spirit 292-297
5-hydroxytryptamine (5HT) 93
hypothalamus 91, 92

id 89, 94, 97
identity of baby 100
ill feeling 114
independence 13, 42, Figure 14
indignation of patient 95
Individual Placement and Support (IPS) schemes 238
initiative of the patient 34
insight of the patient 42
inspirations and ideals 44, 288
integration 100, 138, Figures 14 and 15
Internal Space 50-51, 61-62, 79, 80, 89, 90, 94-98, Figure 2a
internal good object 61, 83, 98, 99, 136
interpretations 107
    accuracy 108
introversion 31
isolation 18-19
International Society for the Psychological and Social Treatment of Schizophrenia and other Psychoses (ISPS) 260

INDEX

Jackson, Murray   17, 60, 120, 125-126
Jung, Carl Gustav   119
justice for patients   265-268

Kandel, Eric   42, 44, 93
Kendler, Kenneth   3-4
kidney transplants   257-258
Klein, Melanie   52, 79, 94, 98, 99, 103, 119, 120, 122, 176, 226

"large man"   15, 41
Leff, Julian   243
Liddle, Peter   73, 91, 93, 173-175, 224-225, 231
"links" of Bion   295
lithium carbonate 29
locus coeruleus   91, 92
Lotterman, Andrew   127
loving awareness   292
Lucas, Richard   17, 18, 42, 60, 120, 125
LUST   91

Mahler, Margaret   100
mania   16-17, 67, 69-70, 95, 100, Figures 9a, 9b
Mars   293
Martindale, Brian   40-44, 128
maturing patient   Figures 5, 14, 15
Maudsley Hospital   243
"me" and "not-me"   59, 89, 94
medications
    antipsychotic   28-30, 38, 101, 106, 135, 238, 259
    side-effects   28-29
    stabilizing   29-30, 254
mental effort   24-25
Mental Health Act   242
Mental Health Treatment Requirement (MHTR)   239
mental representations   99
Mildred   122
mind and brain   3, 4
"mirroring"   95
monitoring   110

moon   293
morale, good   38
motivation   31, 115, 137, 292-297
motivational interviewing   244, 254
Mount Everest   295

narcissism   94, 100
narcissistic organization   99
narrative, patient's   107
National Health Schedule for Schizophrenia (NHSS)   xix, 30, 32, 37, 84, 85, 183, 235-260
National Health Service (NHS)   8, 39, 84, 269, 273
    best value in   277
    clinical need in   274
    comprehensive service of   274
    funding   279
    highest standards in   275
    organisational boundaries in   276
    patients at heart of   275
    principles and values   269-281
National Institute for Health and Care Excellence (NICE)   20, 42
National Institute of Mental Health (NIMH)   4
Nautilus   284
Need Adapted approach   6
negative symptoms   13, 103
neuroleptics, atypical   39
neuropsychoanalysis   7, 93
neuropsychoanalytic aspects of the PPCC model 91-93
"New Intellectual Framework for Psychiatry Revisited" (Kandel) 93
n-methyl-D-aspartate (NMDA) receptors   32, 92-93
non-maleficence for patients   265, 266
non-psychotic part of mind   17-18, 60-61, 73, 79, 81, 101, Figure 2a
non-psychologically-orientated readers   80
nucleus accumbens   93

INDEX

olanzapine   21
Observations PPCC variable   50, Figure 2a
Open Dialogue approach   6, 8
optimism of patient   34, 35
orientation in time, place and person   54, 95
outrage of patient   95
Outreach Services   31, 42, 241
overall PPCC sequence of resolution   56-58, 65-66, 83, Figure 7

PANIC 91
Panksepp, Jaak   89, 91, 92
parabrachial nuclei   91, 92
paranoia   14
paranoid delusions   15
paranoid-schizoid position   52, 61, 67, 74, 79, 81, 99, Figure 2a
   alternation with depressive position   61, 99
"parasitism" in a patient   102, 133, Figure 14
Parthenon   284
pathological organization   99
"pathosymbiosis"   103, 112, Figures 14 and 15
patience, the analyst's   112-113
patient safety   246-253
patient selection   37, 73, 101, 266, 296
peace of mind   19
peer-support workers   241
pentagram of PPCC   283, Figure 16
pentapointed PPCC   Figure 2a
pentasided pyramid   53, 54, 56, 59, 62-63, 82, 95, 137, Figures 4, 5 and 7
periaqueductal grey (PAG)   91, 92
personality loss by patient   34
PhD Thesis   99
phenothiazines   39
Phi   282
physical health maintenance   240
physical neglect   39

PLAY   91
police cells   36
positive symptoms   103
PPCC construct's source   48
PPCC construct's original interest   48
PPCC model   43, 47 et seq, 81, 95
   and psychoanalytic concepts   52
   and psychotic and non-psychotic parts of the mind   60-61
   dynamic movements between its stages   54
   for affect regulation   Figure 2b
   for depression   68, 93, 95, Figures 8a, 8b
   for mania   69, 93, 95, Figures 9a, 9b
   for schizophrenia   67, 70-75, 79-85, 92-93, 95, Figures 10a, 10b, 11
   original role   58
   overview   55, 80, 83
   spatial correlations   62
   useful projections   54
   use of geometric shapes   59
PPCC model's concepts
   inclusion/rejection   57, 79, 98, Figures 1, 2
   solidity/containment   57, Figure 4
   process of evolution   49, 57, Figure 7
PPCC Theory   xviii, 56, 63, 75, 89, 99-101, 133, 135
predictability   248
prefrontal cortex   91-93
pre-pulse inhibition   28
presentations, common patient   102
prima facie moral principles   263, 266
prison place cost   22
prisons   36
"process" schizophrenia   39
projective identification   73, 100, 119-121, 135
"protopathosymbiosis"   133, Figures 14 and 15
Provisions for patients, society's   36
Psychiatry

INDEX

concepts 101
Kaplan and Sadock's Comprehensive Textbook 1-2
history of "modern psychiatry" 2-3
psychoanalysis 254
    results of psychoanalytic work 259
psychoanalytic psychotherapy 30, 31, 36, 37, 38, 39, 43, 47-66, 71-75, 82-84, 91, 94-101, 122-123, 132-139, 183, 237, 242, 245, 255-257, 259, 266-268, 272, 273, 297
psychoanalytic concepts 52, 100, 101
psychoanalytic understanding 44, 101, 259-260
psychodynamic principles 40-44, 260
Psychomotor Poverty Syndrome (Liddle) 73, 93, 173-175, 224-225, 231
psychosis
    acute 18-19, 37, 40-41, 81
    chronic 18-19
    episode of 96, 98, 100, 103, 256
    illness 39, 101, 105-106, 137
psychotic part of the mind 17-18, 60-61, 79, Figure 2a
psychotic wavelength 18, 71
public regard for patients 34

Quality Adjusted Life Years (QALYs) 266

rage 95
RAGE 91
raphe nuclei 91, 92
"reactive" schizophrenia 39
Reality Distortion Syndrome (Liddle) 73, 173-175, 224-225, 231
recovery 241
regard for the patient 116-117
relatives 111
relationships, good staff 247
reliability
    of patients 248
    of psychotherapy unit's clinical systems 248
representational world 50 et seq, 67, 79, 80, 83, 90-92, 96, 98-100, 113, 133, 137, 138, 172-173, 180, 223-224, 230, Figure 2a
Representational Theory of Mind (Fodor's) 76, Figure 13
research project 48-49
resilience
    of staff 251
    of the human spirit 293
resolution of illness 44, 54, 59-60, 82, 85
restrictions affecting staff 249
revolving door policy 35, 39
"rewrite her history" 81-82
Rey, Henri 124
risks 252-253
Robbins, Michael 4-7, 30, 42, 43, 67, 73, 85, 94, 102-104, 129-131, 132-139, 293
robustness of patients 248
Rosenbaum, Bent 47, 127-128
Rosenblatt, Bernard 51, 90, 91
Rosenfeld, Herbert 6, 94, 120-121

safety
    of a child 97
    of patients 246-253
sanctuary, lack of 19, 33-38
Sandler, Joseph 51, 90, 91, 97
Sara 94, 130, 132, 185-234, 294
    psychoanalytic psychotherapy 185-221
    visualization of therapy 222-228
    commentary on visualization 229-234
schizoaffective disorder 15, 79, 89-101, Figure 2a
    compared with schizophrenia 15, 79-85, 237
    pharmacotherapy 29-30
    research case study patient 48-49

INDEX

schizophrenia
    acute   14-15, 18, 33-37, 79-85, 267, Figures 7, 10a, 10b, 11
    affect regulation in   95
    alcohol misuse   21, 30
    birth vulnerabilities   27-28
    chronic   14-15, 18, 31, 33, 35-36, 267, 293, 294, Figures 10b, 11a
    co-morbidity with substance abuse   21, 30-31
    costs
        cost drivers   20
        cost to families   22, 24-26
        cost to public sector   20
        cost to society   20-26
        cost to patients themselves   22-24, 272
        cost of therapy   20, 44, 255
        cost of treatment   256-259
        direct costs   20
        hospital costs   21
        premature mortality   26
        suicide   13, 16, 26
        tax revenue lost   21
        unpaid care   20
    criminal justice system   21
    distinguishing features   100
    drug abuse   30
    economic output   22
    EEG changes   28
    employment rate   21
    environmental factors   5-6
    foetal growth abnormalities   27
    genetic factors   28
    guilt feeling in families   25
    homelessness   21
    hypertelorism   27
    inpatient time   21
    maternal starvation   27-28
    mortality rate   21
    motivation   31, 296
    narcissism   94
    new classification of symptoms (Liddle)   73, 173-175, 224-225, 231
    obesity   21
    physical concomitants   27, 31, 83
    physical management   29
    PPCC model in   67, 70-75, 80-83, Figures 2a, 2b, 4, 5, 7, 10a, 10b, 11
    presentations   102, 295
    smoking in   21, 30-31
    survival value   24
    symptoms   104
    tax revenue lost due to   21
    theories of:
        dopamine hypothesis   3, 92-93
        neurodevelopmental hypothesis   6
        sociodevelopmental-cognitive model   6
        developmental risk factor model   6
Schizophrenia Commission Report   20, 33, 237, 256, 259
Schizophrenic Global Perspectives   64, 72-73, 90-91, 172-173, 180, 223-224, 231-233
scope, of ethical principles   263, 266
Searles, Harold   6, 123
security, lack of   14
SEEKING   91
Segal, Hanna   6, 94, 103, 120, 121
SELF (Jaak Panksepp's) see Simple Ego-type Life Form
self-awareness   42
self-belief   24
self-care   17
self-compassion   34
self-confidence   82
self-damaging habits   21
self-defence   97
self-discipline   31
self-doubt   31
self-efficacy   34
self-esteem   22, 31
self-harm   13
self-help   14, 23, 24, 33

INDEX

self-identity 37
self-preservation 97
self-regard 82
self-scrutiny 37
self-sufficiency 138
self-understanding 82
Semrad, Elvin 125, 230
sexual abuse 39
sexuality 112
siblings 25-26
side-effects of medications (see medications)
Simple Ego-type Life Form (SELF) 89, 91, 92, 98
small study of schizoaffective patient 48, Figure 1
Social Services 23
Social Skills Therapy 23, 84, 239
Sohn, Leslie 17, 60, 120, 126-127
Solms, Mark 7, 93
sourness in the patient 114-115
sphere, final stage 55, 64-65, Figures 5, 7
spirit, emerging human 293
Stages of the resolution of schizophrenia by psychoanalytic psychotherapy (Dr Robbins) 73, 100, 132-139, Figures 14 and 15
staff
    role of 31, 101, 246-247, 256, 266, 268, 270-273, 291
    needs of 249-251
Steiner, John 99
stigmatising 4
substance misuse treatment 239-240
suicide 13, 16
Sullivan, Harry Stack 6, 124
Summers, Alison 40-44
sunflowers 286-288, Figures 18a, 18b, 18c
superego 89, 94, 97
supervision, clinical, of staff 250
Support, Treatment and Recovery (STAR) project, Southampton 280

suppressing the patient 4
Sustainability and Transformation Plan (STP) 279-281
symptom control 104

Tamminga, Carol 2
"talking therapies" 254
tectum, mesopontine 91, 92
thalamus 91, 92
"The NHS Constitution" 273
The Shorter Oxford Textbook of Psychiatry 43, 51, 79, 90, 289
therapeutic alliance 52, 81
therapeutic termination 138
third person voices 15
training of staff 256
transference 73, 93, 94, 96, 103, 122
    healing 97
    psychotic 120
transitional object 58-59
transplant programme in UK 259
trust 47, 292
Turing, Alan 286

unconscious fantasies 97

variables of PPCC model 47 et seq, 51, 73, 79, 81, 90-93, 98, 100, 289, Figure 2a
ventral tegmental area (VTA) 93
ventromesial cortex 92
versatility of PPCC model 76-78
vertex, closure of 53, 59, 62-63, 74, 81-82, 97, Figure 4
vigilance 246
violence 109
violent crime 21-22
vulnerability of patients 282

ward staff 42, 81
ward visit 106
Williams, Paul 127
Winnicott, Donald 58, 95
withdrawal from the world 100